Obstetrics and Gynaecology

First edition authors:

Nick Panay
Ruma Dutta
Audrey Ryan
J A Mark Broadbent

Second edition authors:

Maryam Parisaei
Archana Shailendra
Ruma Dutta
J A Mark Broadbent

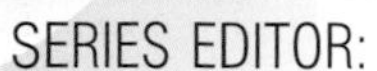

3rd Edition

CRASH COURSE

SERIES EDITOR:

Dan Horton-Szar

BSc(Hons) MBBS(Hons) MRCGP

Northgate Medical Practice

Canterbury

Kent, UK

FACULTY ADVISORS:

Shreelata T Datta

LLM, MBBS, BSc (Hons), MRCOG

Consultant in Obstetrics and Gynaecology,

King's College Hospital, London UK

Ruma Dutta

BSc, MBBS, MRCOG

Consultant in Obstetrics and Gynaecology,

Hillingdon Hospital NHS Trust, Middlesex, UK

Obstetrics and Gynaecology

Chidimma Onwere

MBBS BSc MRCOG

Specialist Registrar in Obstetrics and Gynaecology, St. Mary's Hospital, Imperial College Healthcare NHS Trust, London, UK

Hemant N Vakharia

MBBS BSc(Hons) MRCOG

Specialty Registrar in Obstetrics and Gynaecology, Barnet and Chase Farm NHS Hospitals Trust, London, UK

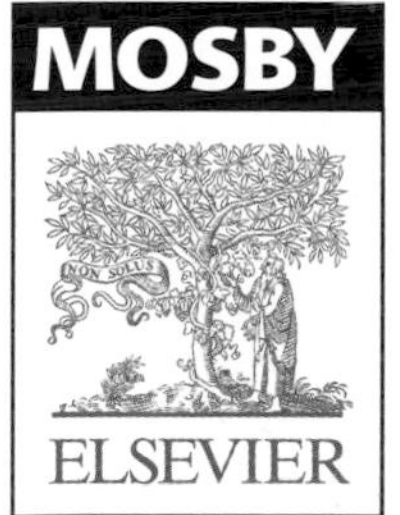

Edinburgh London New York Oxford Philadelphia St Louis Sydney Toronto 2015

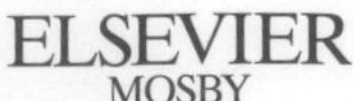

Commissioning Editor: Jeremy Bowes
Development Editor: Fiona Conn
Project Manager: Andrew Riley
Designer: Christian Bilbow
Icon Illustrations: Geo Parkin
Illustration Manager: Jennifer Rose

First edition 2004

Second edition 2008

Third edition 2014

Updated Third edition 2015

Reprinted 2015

ISBN: 978-0-7234-3870-0

British Library Cataloguing in Publication Data
A catalogue record for this book is available from the British Library

Library of Congress Cataloging in Publication Data
A catalog record for this book is available from the Library of Congress

Notices
Knowledge and best practice in this field are constantly changing. As new research and experience broaden our understanding, changes in research methods, professional practices, or medical treatment may become necessary.

Practitioners and researchers must always rely on their own experience and knowledge in evaluating and using any information, methods, compounds, or experiments described herein. In using such information or methods they should be mindful of their own safety and the safety of others, including parties for whom they have a professional responsibility.

With respect to any drug or pharmaceutical products identified, readers are advised to check the most current information provided (i) on procedures featured or (ii) by the manufacturer of each product to be administered, to verify the recommended dose or formula, the method and duration of administration, and contraindications. It is the responsibility of practitioners, relying on their own experience and knowledge of their patients, to make diagnoses, to determine dosages and the best treatment for each individual patient, and to take all appropriate safety precautions.

To the fullest extent of the law, neither the Publisher nor the authors, contributors, or editors, assume any liability for any injury and/or damage to persons or property as a matter of products liability, negligence or otherwise, or from any use or operation of any methods, products, instructions, or ideas contained in the material herein.

Printed in China

Last digit is the print line: 10 9 8 7 6 5 4 3 2

Series editor foreword

The *Crash Course* series first published in 1997 and now, 17 years on, we are still going strong. Medicine never stands still, and the work of keeping this series relevant for today's students is an ongoing process. These new editions build on the success of the previous titles and incorporate new and revised material, to keep the series up to date with current guidelines for best practice, and recent developments in medical research and pharmacology.

We always listen to feedback from our readers, through focus groups and student reviews of the *Crash Course* titles. For the new editions we have completely re-written our self-assessment material to keep up with today's 'single-best answer' and 'extended matching question' formats. The artwork and layout of the titles has also been largely re-worked to make it easier on the eye during long sessions of revision.

Despite fully revising the books with each edition, we hold fast to the principles on which we first developed the series. *Crash Course* will always bring you all the information you need to revise in compact, manageable volumes that integrate basic medical science and clinical practice. The books still maintain the balance between clarity and conciseness, and provide sufficient depth for those aiming at distinction. The authors are medical students and junior doctors who have recent experience of the exams you are now facing, and the accuracy of the material is checked by a team of faculty advisors from across the UK.

Dr Dan Horton-Szar

Preface

As medicine progresses in the 21st century, the specialty of obstetrics and gynaecology continually evolves, combining medical, surgical and practical components which must be grasped by the contemporary medical student. Often in the space of only eight weeks, this must seem like an overwhelming task.

As part of the Crash Course series, this third edition continues to give the essential information in a clear concise manner, combining up-to-date text with tables, figures and algorithms. It gives vital information as well as hints and tips that focus on how important it is to take a good history. Obviously this is necessary in any branch of medicine, but the personal nature of this specialty makes it even more crucial. Similarly, examination of the patient is described in a sensitive manner. After covering management for each topic, the popular self-assessment section has been updated in line with current examination techniques.

In addition to imparting the factual knowledge needed to pass examinations, we hope that this book will give today's students the encouragement to find out more for themselves; to gain clinical experience and not to just learn lists. With a similar basis for both sides of the specialty, actual practice on the shopfloor is so diverse that there is something that every student can find to engage them. We hope this textbook is an essential guide to introduce students to a unique and very rewarding specialty, capturing its diversity and its challenges.

Chidimma Onwere

Hemant Vakharia

Shreelata Datta

Ruma Dutta

Dedication

To my excellent parents for all their encouragement and my dear husband Tochi for all his love and support.

Chidimma Onwere

To my father, mother and brothers for all their amazing support, to my wife for her endless love and patience and to my gorgeous daughter for making it all worthwhile!

Hemant Vakharia

To my grandfathers, who continually inspire me, to my parents who kept me going as a student and to my patients, who keep me going as a doctor.

Shreelata Datta

To my dad, who would have been proud to see my name in print, and to my mum, who is. Also to Paul, Jack and Sadie for all their patience and love.

Ruma Dutta

Contents

Taking a history

Objectives

By the end of this chapter, you should be able to:

- Understand how to take a history for obstetrics and gynaecology.

The history plays a vital role in obstetrics and gynaecology, often giving pointers to a diagnosis that is not always evident from examination and investigation of the patient alone. Many women are embarrassed by having to discuss their personal problems, especially to someone who is often younger than they are, so it is important to overcome this by developing a confident, but sensitive manner. Always introduce and present yourself in an acceptable manner, be courteous and friendly without being overfamiliar, and always pay attention. Remember to ask who has accompanied the patient – do not assume it is her partner – and consider whether she may want to answer personal questions in front of a family member.

THE PATIENT'S DETAILS

It is surprising how often the patient's details are omitted from a history. Always record the following:

1. Name, date of birth, age and address (sticky labels with this information are usually available)
2. Marital status, ethnic group and occupation
3. The date, time and place of the consultation
4. Source of referral, e.g. GP referral, self-admitted to A&E, labour ward.

HINTS AND TIPS

It is useful to get into the habit of writing certain details in the top right hand corner of the clerking sheet so they are not omitted, for example:

- Age
- Parity
- Date of last menstrual period (LMP)
- Date of last smear.

PRESENTING COMPLAINT

The presenting complaint may be documented in the referral letter or the casualty card, but this does not always correlate with what the patient perceives as the main problem. It is therefore vital to ask the patient what she sees as her primary complaint and document this — preferably in her own words. If there are multiple symptoms, document each one in order of severity.

During the examination, investigations and treatment never lose track of the presenting complaint, otherwise management plans may not always be appropriate. For example, it would not be helpful to suggest a MIRENA coil for treatment of menorrhagia to a woman whose main concern is trying for a pregnancy. Conversely, the presenting complaint might be a cover for a different problem that the patient has difficulty discussing. For example, the patient may complain about vaginal discharge, although her main concern is pain during intercourse. Always ask if there is anything else bothering the patient that she wishes to discuss.

HISTORY OF PRESENTING COMPLAINT

Details of the history of the presenting complaint should be ascertained:

- **How long has the complaint been present?** For example, a woman might complain that she has always had heavy periods but they have only been a problem for the last 2 years.
- **Was the onset of symptoms sudden or gradual?** For example severe hirsutism of rapid onset is more likely to be due to an androgen-producing tumour.

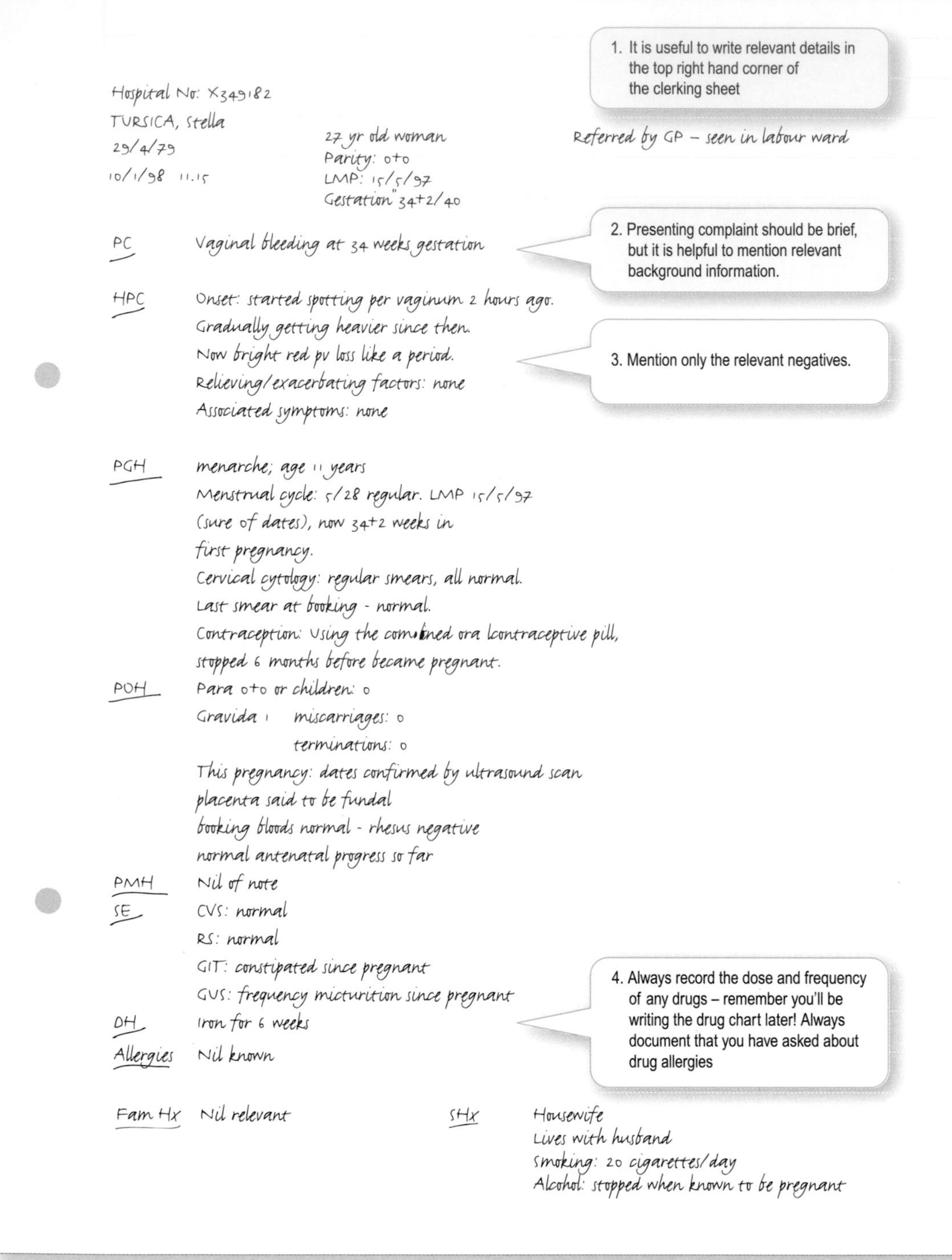

Fig. 1.1 Obstetric clerking.

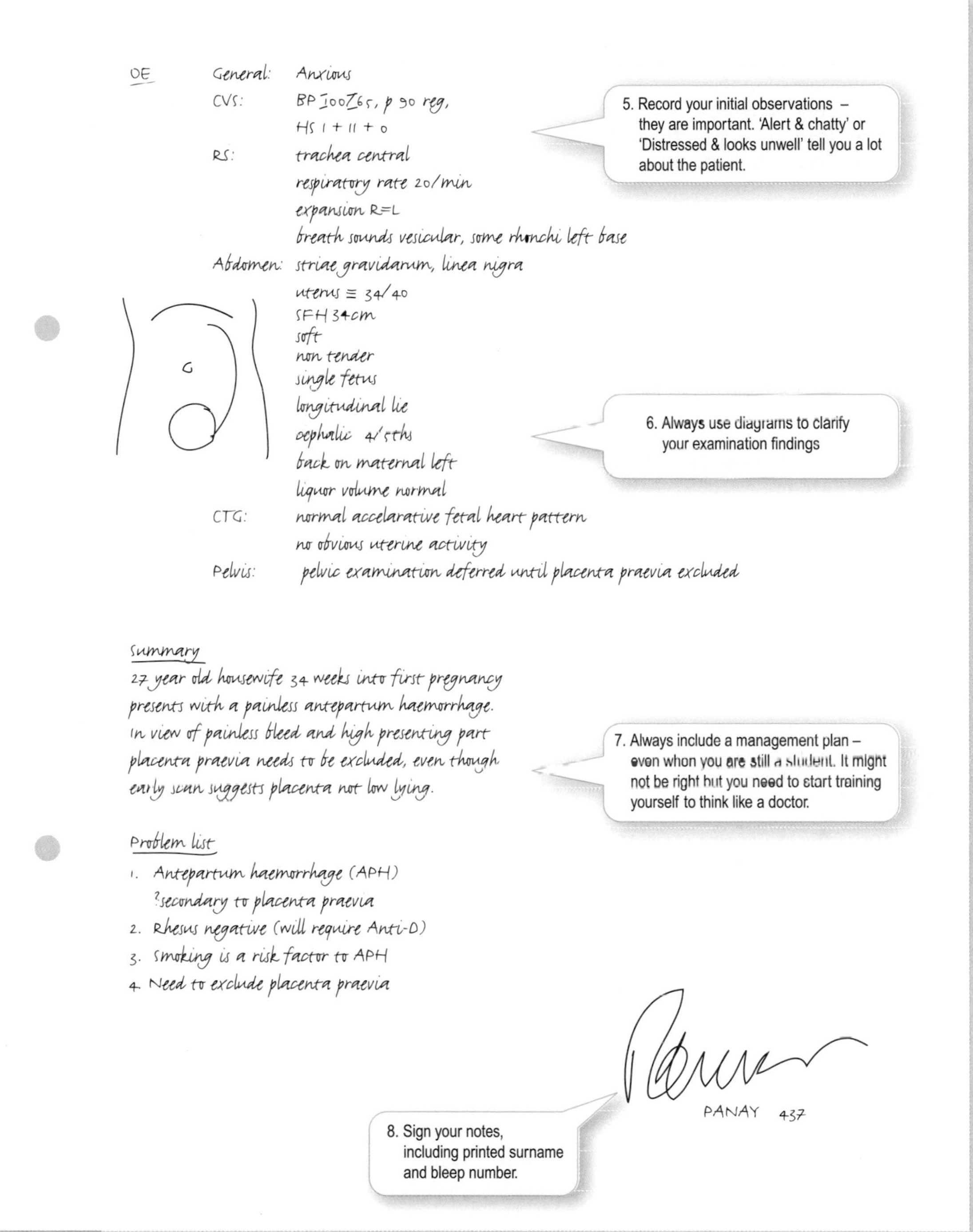

Fig. 1.1 Obstetric clerking —cont'd

- **Was the onset associated with a previous obstetric or gynaecological event?** For example, stress incontinence and childbirth.
- **Are there any relieving or exacerbating factors?** For example symptoms of prolapse are often worse on standing and better on lying down.
- **Are there any associated symptoms?** For example the painful periods of endometriosis are sometimes associated with deep dyspareunia (deep pelvic pain with intercourse).

If pain is the presenting complaint, then the following characteristics should be noted:

- **Site**: is the pain pelvic or abdominal? For example ovarian pain can be felt quite high in the abdomen.
- **Severity**: how severe is the pain and to what extent does it disrupt everyday life? For example the cyclical pain of endometriosis might necessitate regular time off work.
- **Onset**: sudden or gradual? For example the pain from a torted ovarian cyst is usually of very sudden onset.
- **Character**: is the pain sharp/knife-like, dull, heavy/dragging, colicky, stretching or twisting? Many adjectives have been used to describe pain or discomfort of gynaecological origin. For example women with uterine prolapse might describe a pulling or a dragging pain/sensation, dysmenorrhoea might be likened to labour pain.
- **Duration**: is the pain constant, intermittent, what is the frequency if intermittent? The pain of a degenerating fibroid in pregnancy will be constant whereas the pain of threatened premature labour will be intermittent and frequent.
- **Radiation**: does the pain radiate? For example endometriosis pain might radiate to the back or into the upper thighs.
- **Relieving/exacerbating features**: does anything make the pain better or worse and this should include self-prescribed analgesia? For example endometriosis symptoms are usually cyclical and associated with menstruation.
- **Associated symptoms:** for example symptoms of peritonitis or advanced malignancy.

PAST GYNAECOLOGICAL HISTORY

Menstrual history

The following characteristics of menstruation and the menstrual cycle should be noted:

- Age at menarche
- Last menstrual period (LMP) = 1st day of last period
- Menstrual cycle: usually denoted as 5/28, where the numerator is the length of the period in days and the denominator is the length of the cycle in days from 1st day to 1st day. If period and cycle length are variable the shortest and longest are noted, e.g. 3–10/14–56
- Menstrual flow: whether light, normal or heavy. This is often very subjective, therefore if heavy, the presence of clots, flooding, night time soiling and the number of sanitary pads/towels used should be noted
- Menstrual pain or dysmenorrhoea: is the pain mild, moderate or severe? Has it been present since menarche or is it of recent onset. Is the pain worse before (primary dysmenorrhoea) or during the period (secondary dysmenorrhoea)?
- Associated symptoms: for example bowel or bladder dysfunction, nausea
- Other bleeding: intermenstrual bleeding (IMB), postcoital bleeding (PCB), pre- or postmenstrual spotting
- Age at menopause.

HINTS AND TIPS

A useful way to ask sensitive questions may be to consider a logical order: after menstrual cycle, ask about bleeding between periods (IMB), then bleeding after intercourse (PCB) and then pain with intercourse (dyspareunia) either superficial (around the opening of the vagina) or deep.

COMMUNICATION

Particularly for women who come from countries in the Horn of Africa (e.g. Somalia, Eritrea, Ethiopia), either themselves or their families, a history should be elicited regarding female circumcision or female genital mutilation (FGM). This procedure usually occurs as a child in their country of origin, being illegal in the UK since 2003. It is defined as all procedures involving partial or total removal of the external female genitalia or other injury to the female genital organs, whether for cultural or other non-therapeutic reasons. As an adult, it can cause significant problems including dyspareunia, recurrent urinary tract infections, trauma and haemorrhage during childbirth, as well as psychological issues. Such a history must therefore be approached in a sensitive manner.

Sexual activity and contraception

Has the patient ever been sexually active? Is the patient currently sexually active or in a relationship? Does the patient suffer from dyspareunia and if so is it superficial or deep? Is she or her partner using contraception and if so what? If she is on the pill or has a MIRENA coil was it prescribed for contraceptive purposes or menstrual disorder?

Cervical screening

Has the patient undergone regular cervical screening? When was the last smear taken? Have there ever been abnormal smears? Has she had the vaccination for human papilloma virus (HPV)?

Vaginal discharge

Is vaginal discharge present and if so is it normal for the patient or abnormal? If abnormal, what is the colour and consistency and is it irritant? Was the onset associated with a change in sexual partner? Is there a history of sexually transmitted infection?

PAST OBSTETRIC HISTORY

The parity and gravidity should be noted. Parity denotes the number of livebirths or stillbirths after 24 weeks gestation and gravidity the total number of pregnancies including the current one if pregnant (see Chapter 2). Use of the terms 'parity' and 'gravidity' can become very complicated, especially with a history of multiple pregnancies. An alternative way of documenting previous pregnancies is to document the number of:

- C = Children
- M = Miscarriages
- T = Terminations.

Document the details of each pregnancy:

- The number of children with age and birth weight. Note any complications of pregnancy, labour and the puerperium.
- The number of miscarriages, their gestation and complications if any.
- The number of terminations of pregnancy, their gestation, method and indication and complications if any.

PAST MEDICAL HISTORY

This should include previous surgery, for example sterilization. Medical disorders such as hypertension or diabetes may be relevant to suitability for surgery or because they are risk factors for complications in pregnancy. Psychiatric history is particularly important in obstetrics, for planning both antenatal and postnatal care.

SYSTEMS ENQUIRY

A brief systems enquiry should be made with particular reference to:

- general symptoms: weight gain or loss, loss of appetite
- gastrointestinal tract: change in bowel habit, especially with menstruation
- genitourinary system: urinary frequency, nocturia, dysuria, incontinence.

DRUG HISTORY

A careful drug history should be taken and should include hormonal contraception and HRT, which are often overlooked by the patient. Drugs are important for pregnancy, e.g. anti-epileptics can be associated with fetal neural tube defects, or β blockers with intra-uterine growth restriction.

ALLERGIES

Document all known or suspected allergies.

FAMILY HISTORY

For gynaecology, enquire as to a family history of ovarian, uterine and breast disease. In obstetrics, diabetes, hypertension and pre-eclampsia may all have relevance to the current pregnancy.

SOCIAL HISTORY

Occupation, smoking habits and alcohol consumption should be noted. If gynaecological surgery is contemplated, what is the support network at home? Should social services be involved in planning the appropriate care for the newborn baby?

Further reading

RCOG, 2009. Female Genital Mutilation Management RCOG green top guideline 53 May 2009. Royal College of Obstetricians and Gynaecologists, London.

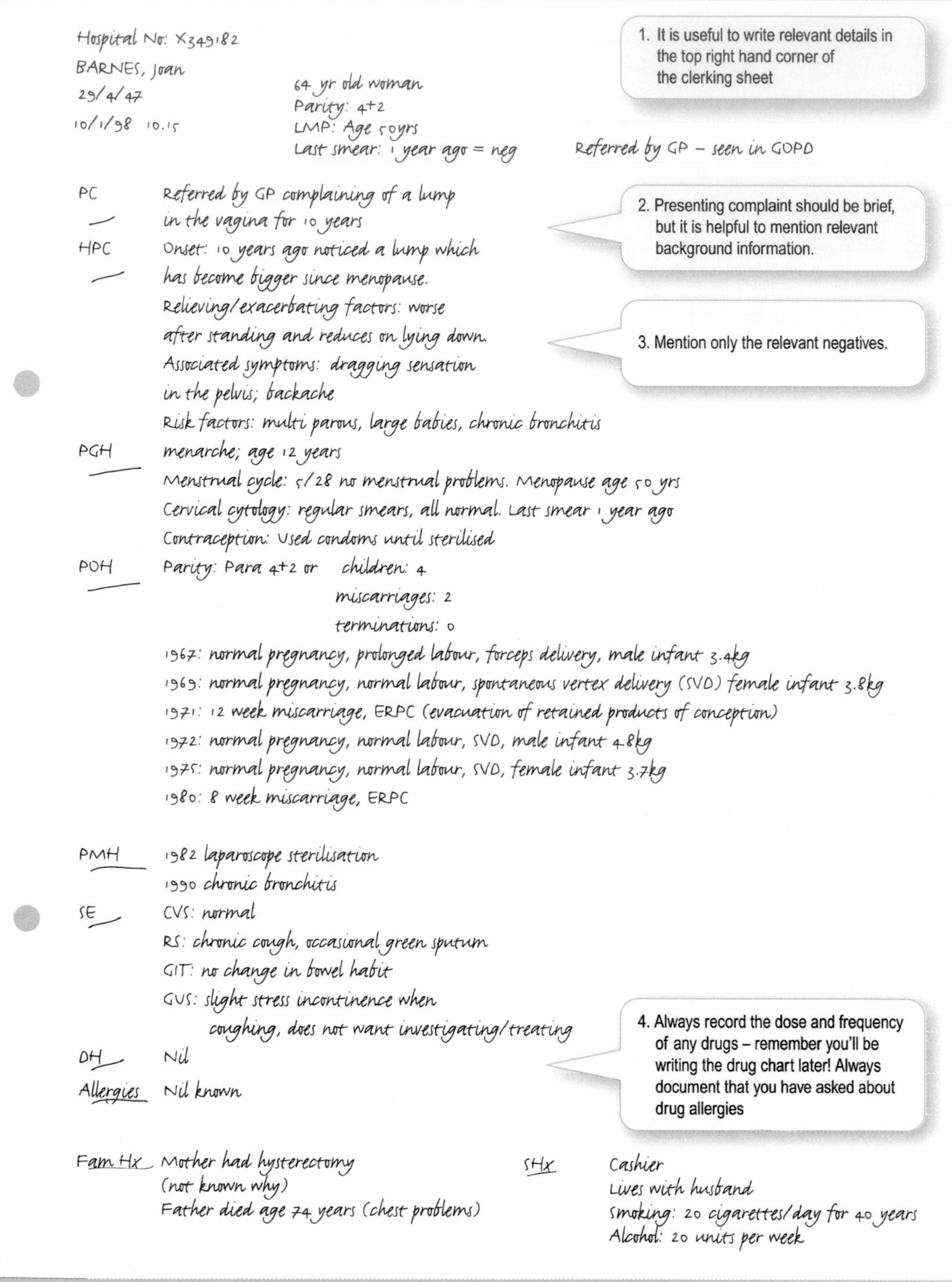

Hospital No: X349182
BARNES, Joan
29/4/47
10/1/98 10.15

64 yr old woman
Parity: 4+2
LMP: Age 50yrs
Last smear: 1 year ago = neg

Referred by GP – seen in GOPD

1. It is useful to write relevant details in the top right hand corner of the clerking sheet

PC — Referred by GP complaining of a lump in the vagina for 10 years

2. Presenting complaint should be brief, but it is helpful to mention relevant background information.

HPC — Onset: 10 years ago noticed a lump which has become bigger since menopause.
Relieving/exacerbating factors: worse after standing and reduces on lying down.
Associated symptoms: dragging sensation in the pelvis; backache
Risk factors: multi parous, large babies, chronic bronchitis

3. Mention only the relevant negatives.

PGH — menarche; age 12 years
Menstrual cycle: 5/28 no menstrual problems. Menopause age 50 yrs
Cervical cytology: regular smears, all normal. Last smear 1 year ago
Contraception: Used condoms until sterilised

POH — Parity: Para 4+2 or children: 4
miscarriages: 2
terminations: 0
1967: normal pregnancy, prolonged labour, forceps delivery, male infant 3.4kg
1969: normal pregnancy, normal labour, spontaneous vertex delivery (SVD) female infant 3.8kg
1971: 12 week miscarriage, ERPC (evacuation of retained products of conception)
1972: normal pregnancy, normal labour, SVD, male infant 4.8kg
1975: normal pregnancy, normal labour, SVD, female infant 3.7kg
1980: 8 week miscarriage, ERPC

PMH — 1982 laparoscope sterilisation
1990 chronic bronchitis

SE — CVS: normal
RS: chronic cough, occasional green sputum
GIT: no change in bowel habit
GUS: slight stress incontinence when coughing, does not want investigating/treating

DH — Nil

Allergies — Nil known

4. Always record the dose and frequency of any drugs – remember you'll be writing the drug chart later! Always document that you have asked about drug allergies

Fam Hx — Mother had hysterectomy (not known why)
Father died age 74 years (chest problems)

SHx — Cashier
Lives with husband
Smoking: 20 cigarettes/day for 40 years
Alcohol: 20 units per week

Fig. 1.2 Gynaecology clerking.

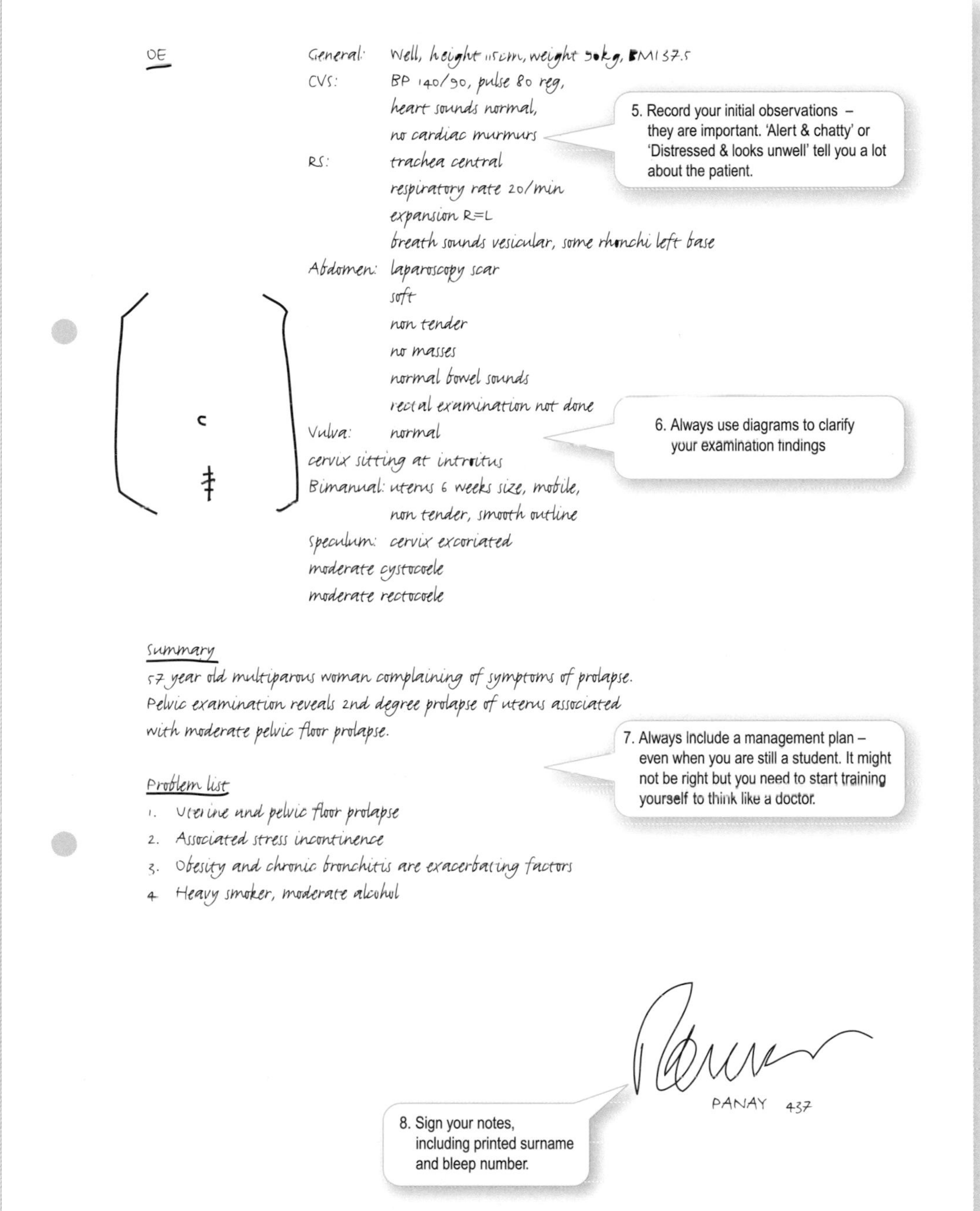

Fig. 1.2 Gynaecology clerking—cont'd

Antenatal booking and prenatal diagnosis

Objectives

By the end of this chapter, you should be able to:
- Understand what happens at an antenatal booking why it is important
- Understand how to take a booking history and what screening investigations are done
- Understand what prenatal diagnosis is and to whom it is offered.

ANTENATAL BOOKING

The antenatal booking appointment is arguably the most important visit a patient will make during their pregnancy. Ideally it will occur before the tenth week of pregnancy and is almost universally conducted by trained midwives. During this visit it is paramount to:

- take a thorough history to identify risk factors for the pregnancy
- educate the patient about key 'do's and don'ts' in pregnancy.

Identifying a patient's risk factors allows their care to be tailored and any additional medications or investigations to be arranged. It is worth noting that during a booking visit, sensitive information may be disclosed. Therefore, it is important to take the history in a sensitive and confidential manner.

History taking

Current pregnancy

An essential step in any booking visit is an accurate estimation of the gestational age. Most commonly this is calculated using the first day of the patient's last menstrual period (LMP) and an obstetric wheel. The obstetric wheel will give both the current gestational age as well as an estimated date of delivery (EDD). Naegele's rule can also be used as an estimate (Fig. 2.1). However, national screening guidelines advise that all patients are offered an ultrasound scan between 11 and 14 weeks for the most accurate EDD, by measuring the fetal crown-rump length (CRL), as well as offering Down's syndrome screening.

HINTS AND TIPS

An ultrasound scan between 11+4 and 14+0 weeks' gestation will:
- measure the CRL to calculate the EDD
- confirm a viable pregnancy
- diagnose multiple pregnancy and check chorionicity
- examine for fetal anomalies
- perform screening test for Down's syndrome.

The history includes whether or not it is a planned pregnancy and whether any fertility treatment was required in order to become pregnant. Patients who have undergone fertility treatment are at risk of multiple pregnancy (see Chapter 18) and/or may have had complications thus far such as ovarian hyperstimulation syndrome (OHSS).

Past obstetric history

A thorough enquiry about previous pregnancies and outcomes is essential as this may allow interventions in this pregnancy to reduce the risk of a further adverse outcome, e.g. prescribing low-dose aspirin 75 mg daily for patients with a previous pregnancy complicated by pre-eclampsia.

When documenting previous pregnancies there is a widely accepted method of doing so using the letters G and P. G stands for 'GRAVIDITY' and refers to the number of pregnancies the patient has had including the current one. P denotes 'PARITY' and states the number of children the patient has delivered **above 24 weeks of gestation**. As an adjunct to this method, add the number of miscarriages or terminations a patient has had by documenting this after the parity.

Fig. 2.1 Naegele's rule.
In situations where one does not have access to an obstetric wheel, using Naegele's rule is an easy way of estimating the due date. The rule assumes the patient has a 28 day cycle and the EDD is calculated by adding 7 to the first day of the LMP and deducting 3 from the month of the LMP. eg. if a patient's LMP was 5/4/2012 then the EDD would be:

05	04	2012
+7	−3	
12	01	2013

HINTS AND TIPS

Catherine is 31 weeks in her third pregnancy; her 1st child was born at 38 weeks. Between these pregnancies, she had a miscarriage at 9 weeks. So her obstetric history is documented as G3 (this is her third pregnancy) P1 + 1 (she has had one child born after 24 weeks of gestation and one pregnancy before 24 weeks).

Past medical history

Identification of co-existing medical problems is essential in pregnancy. For some disorders, early management plans may be appropriate to reduce the risk of adverse fetal and maternal outcomes (see Chapter 23). In some instances, it is better to initiate changes even before pregnancy and therefore some hospitals run preconception clinics. Optimizing conditions such as pre-existing diabetes and epilepsy will improve outcomes. For example, many of the epilepsy medications are teratogenic and modification of the drug regimen may reduce this risk.

Drug history and allergies

Enquiry should be made about what medications the patient may be taking including over-the-counter supplements. Folic acid should be recommended in the first trimester and specialist advice may be needed if the patient has been taking any potentially teratogenic medications.

Family history

Some diseases are relevant with regards to a family history, such as hypertension or diabetes. For example, a family history of Type II diabetes in a first degree relative confers an increased risk of developing gestational diabetes. These patients should be screened by way of a glucose tolerance test (GTT). Any genetic conditions which run through the family may prompt referral to a geneticist +/- invasive testing.

Social history

Consideration should be given to the patient's occupation in order to minimise any risk she may be exposed to. For example a nursery teacher who has not had chicken pox should be advised on how to minimize the risk and how to seek help should she come into contact with a child who has chicken pox. Other occupations to make note of are healthcare workers (infectious diseases), vets (toxoplasmosis) and chefs/butchers (food-borne infections such as listeria, salmonella and toxoplasmosis).

Smokers should be offered referral to a specialist smoking cessation clinic and educated about the risks to their pregnancy. In addition alcohol abuse and illicit drug use should be identified with referral to the appropriate drug and alcohol service and education about the risks to pregnancy made as a priority. Social services may need to be informed so that appropriate postnatal care plans can be made for mother and baby. This may include those with a mental health history or teenage patients. Support is vital with a history of domestic violence.

Examination

At a booking visit the examination of a patient will generally be limited to measurement of the patient's blood pressure and recording their height and weight to allow calculations of their body mass index (BMI).

Investigations

There is a nationally agreed set of investigations which should be offered to patients to allow screening for certain conditions in order to minimize their risk if present. A booklet has been produced by the UK national screening committee for patients to understand when they will be offered certain screening tests during their pregnancy and what the baby will be offered in the first few weeks after birth (see references).

Full blood count

A full blood count (FBC) is an important investigation as it allows for the detection of anaemia and assessment of the platelet count. Anaemic patients can then be further investigated by measurement of their ferritin, folate and vitamin B12 levels if indicated.

With a lower normal range for haemoglobin in pregnancy, due to the normal physiological changes that occur, the most common reason for anaemia is iron deficiency which can be managed with iron supplements. Low platelets (thrombocytopenia) may indicate an underlying issue such as idiopathic thrombocytopenia which is an autoimmune condition that can affect the fetus. Severe cases may need specialist haematologist advice.

Haemoglobin electrophoresis

Haemoglobinopathies are disorders of haemoglobin structure and are more common in certain ethnic groups. Thalassaemia and sickle cell disease are screened for to allow identification of fetuses at risk of having the condition. Both conditions are autosomal recessive so in order for the individual to be affected they need to have two defective copies of the gene. Patients can be asymptomatic carriers of the condition without knowing. For example, in the UK there are estimated to be around 240 000 carriers of sickle cell.

Thalassaemia

The thalassaemias are denoted either α- or β- depending upon the affected haemoglobin chain. α-thalassaemia is common in people of South East Asian descent and β-thalassaemia is common in people of Cypriot and Asian descent. During pregnancy, if the mother is found to be a carrier her partner should also be screened. Based on his results, invasive testing may need to be considered.

Sickle cell disease

Sickle cell disease is also an autosomal recessive condition. People with one defective copy of the gene are referred to as sickle cell trait. Around 1:10 people of African-Caribbean descent have sickle cell trait and therefore screening can identify at-risk fetuses.

Both conditions can render the patient anaemic and supplementation with iron and folate may be required. It is, however, important not to iron overload these patients. Pregnant patients with sickle cell disease (i.e. two defective genes) should be managed in a specialist centre under a multi-disciplinary team.

Blood group and antibody screen

Knowledge of a patient's blood group and antibody status is very important in pregnancy. Certain antibodies can cause haemolytic disease of the newborn (HDN) and, therefore, blood is screened at booking and again at 28 weeks to ensure antibodies have not developed. Those who have the particular antibodies will need regular blood tests to quantify the levels and may require close surveillance in a fetal medicine unit if the levels rise.

The most common antibodies causing HDN are the rhesus antibodies. Those that are rhesus negative will be offered anti-D prophylaxis.

HINTS AND TIPS

Rhesus blood group system and anti-D

The rhesus (Rh) blood group system is one of a number of systems and within it are many known antigens.

In pregnancy the most important antigen is the D antigen. Those patients who have one or two copies of the Rh-D antigen gene will be Rh positive. Those patients who do not have copy of the gene will be Rh negative.

In pregnancy, if a Rh negative patient has a partner who is Rh positive their offspring may be Rh positive. During the pregnancy fetal blood may enter maternal circulation and cause antibodies to develop to the D-antigen. In subsequent pregnancies these antibodies may then cross the placenta and attack fetal red cells causing anaemia and subsequent fetal hydrops +/- stillbirth.

To prevent this, a patient should be offered anti-D immunoglobulin. This can be given:

- in one dose at 28 weeks or in divided doses at 28 and 34 weeks
- postnatally
- if a potentially sensitizing event has occurred, i.e. any event which may cause the passage of fetal cells into maternal circulation such as abdominal trauma, bleeding in pregnancy after 12 weeks, amniocentesis and others.

Screening for infection

In pregnancy a number of infections can have a detrimental effect on the health of both the mother and fetus. Therefore screening will allow modification of their management to minimize the risk, not only in this pregnancy but also future pregnancies.

Rubella

Rubella in pregnancy can have severe consequences for the fetus such as microcephaly. The risk of transmission is greatest in the first trimester and fetuses can develop congenital rubella syndrome.

The purpose of identifying those patients not immune to rubella is to offer these patients postnatal vaccination (usually in the form of the MMR vaccine, a live vaccine) and advise contraception for 3 months.

Education of those at risk of catching rubella (nursery nurses, school teachers, healthcare professionals) includes advice to avoid contact with people known to have the infection.

Syphilis (Treponema pallidum)

Syphilis is a sexually transmitted infection which can be easily treated. Fetal infection can lead to non-immune hydrops and stillbirth. The risk of transmission to the fetus can be dramatically reduced by treating the mother. Patients identified with syphilis should be referred to a genito-urinary medicine (GUM) clinic for:

- treatment
- screening of other sexually transmitted infections
- contact tracing including partner.

Hepatitis B

Hepatitis B is a viral infection transmitted:

- sexually
- vertically (mother to fetus)
- via blood.

The patient should be referred to a liver physician if she has not been seen previously and her liver function tests monitored. Again, partner testing is recommended as well as any existing children she may have.

Post-natal vaccination of the fetus has been shown to reduce the risk of transmission. Patients who have the hepatitis E-antigen (HBeAg) carry the highest risk of transmitting the infection to the fetus.

Hepatitis C is also a viral illness which is transmitted sexually, vertically (mother to fetus) or via blood. Current guidelines, however, do not recommend routine screening.

Human immunodeficiency virus

Human immunodeficiency virus (HIV) is a blood-borne virus also transmitted sexually, vertically and by blood. Although incurable, modern advances in management have increased the life-expectancy of affected individuals and significantly reduced the rate of vertical transmission (see Chapter 23).

Screening for HIV allows patients to commence on treatment if required and to assess how the patient should deliver. All cases should be managed by a multi-disciplinary team involving obstetricians, HIV specialists and specialist midwives.

Urinary tract infections

Urinary tract infections (UTIs) may be symptomatic or asymptomatic. In untreated asymptomatic cases, there is a significant risk of pyelonephritis and preterm birth. Current guidelines recommend screening for asymptomatic bacteriuria in all pregnant women by means of a midstream urine (MSU) culture.

Antenatal education

For some patients pregnancy can be a daunting time; especially those who are embarking on their first pregnancy or those who are very young. Therefore, education at booking is a vital step and the provision of clear (often written) information can be an invaluable tool to put patients at ease.

Topics that should be covered include:

- common symptoms in pregnancy (see Fig. 2.2)
- maternity benefits
- working during pregnancy
- dietary information:
  - Advice on a mixed diet with fruit, vegetables, fibre, lean meat, fish, lentils, starchy foods (bread/pasta, etc.) and dairy
  - Foods to avoid and why are shown in Figure 2.3
- smoking and alcohol:
  - Discussion about smoking cessation is essential plus referral to specialist services if accepted
  - Alcohol consumption should be avoided completely in the first trimester and, ideally, throughout pregnancy. Those who choose to drink should be advised to drink no more than 1–2 units a week and to avoid binge drinking.

Fig. 2.2 Common symptoms in pregnancy.

Nausea and vomiting
Usually resolves by 16 -20 weeks Eating little and often and regular antiemetics can help
Heartburn
Avoid large meals and lying supine soon after food Reduce caffeine and foods with high fat content Antacid preparations
Constipation
Increase fibre in diet, avoid dehydration
Haemorrhoids
Haemorrhoid creams, avoidance of constipation
Varicose veins
Compression stockings can be helpful Elevation of legs Avoid prolonged periods of standing
Backache
Advice on posture, massage and water exercising can help
Symphysis Pubis Dysfunction (SPD)
Physiotherapy referral for advice and consideration of pelvic support devices

Fig. 2.3 Dietary precautions in pregnancy.

Soft cheeses, unpasteurised milk/cheese, Raw fish (sushi)	Risk of infection with listeria which can lead to miscarriage and stillbirth
Unwashed salad, fruit, vegetables Raw meats	Risk of Toxoplasmosis infection which can lead to miscarriage, stillbirth or disability
Shellfish (oysters) Raw eggs	Risk of food poisoning
Caffeine	Limit intake to 300mg per day

- medications, vitamins and supplements:
  - It is important to emphasize that most medications have insufficient data to be deemed 100% safe in pregnancy and therefore their use should be limited to occasions when they are absolutely necessary. Complementary medicines again have little or no safety data.
  - Advise on the importance of taking folic acid (400 μg od) during the first 12 weeks to reduce the risk of neural tube defects.
- driving/air travel:
  - Appropriate positioning of the seatbelt, i.e. wearing it above and below the bump NOT over.
  - Long-haul flights are independently associated with an increased risk of venous thromboembolism. Therefore, unless travel is essential it may be advisable to avoid it especially when there are other risk factors such as raised BMI. Compression stockings have been shown to reduce this risk.
- exercise:
  - Moderate exercise is safe in pregnancy, although patients should be informed of the risks with contact sports and other forms of vigorous exercise.
- pets:
  - Toxoplasmosis risk from cat faeces and contaminated soil, therefore avoidance of handling cat litter and wearing gloves when gardening as well as hand washing should be advised.

Further antenatal care

Depending upon the classification of risk, ongoing antenatal care in pregnancy may be delivered by general practitioners, midwives, obstetricians or a combination of all three. Generally low-risk patients in their first pregnancy will have around 10 visits spread throughout their pregnancy and those who have had a baby before and are low risk will have seven visits. In patients for whom issues have been identified, the schedule of care will need to be modified according to their individual needs.

Screening for chromosomal abnormalities

National guidelines recommend offering all patients a screening test for Down's syndrome (trisomy 21). In this disorder, the fetus has three copies of chromosome 21. Future problems include severe learning difficulties and cardiac and gastrointestinal tract abnormalities.

Combined screening test

Depending on the gestation, ultrasound combined with certain blood tests is used as part of the screening programme. Between 11 and 14+0 weeks gestation, patients who opt to have the test will undergo an ultrasound assessment (Fig. 2.4), which measures the nuchal translucency (NT). They will also have a blood test to measure serum levels of β-human chorionic gonadotrophin (βHCG) and pregnancy-associated plasma protein A (PAPP-A).

NT is an ultrasound observation and refers to the black space seen on ultrasound within the back of the fetus' neck. The width of this space is measured – on average, fetuses affected with Down's syndrome have an increased NT. It should be remembered that not all fetuses with an increased NT will have Down's syndrome.

Once the patient has undergone these tests, the results are combined to calculate a risk score which denotes the risk of the fetus of having Down's syndrome, for example 1 in 2000, i.e. this is only a **screening test**. In the UK

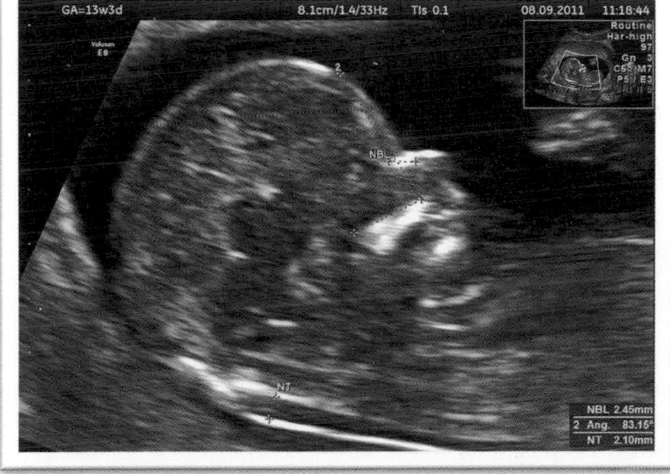

Fig. 2.4 Measurement of nuchal translucency.

guidance has recommended a cut off of 1 in 150 for consideration as 'high risk' and these individuals are counselled about the option of invasive testing, i.e. do they wish to proceed with a **diagnostic test**.

Triple or quadruple test

For those patients who book late or have missed the cut off for combined screening, they can be offered second trimester screening in the form of the triple or quadruple test. These are blood tests following which a risk score is also generated.

Ultrasound at 18–20 weeks

Patients will also be offered another scan ideally between 18 weeks and 20 weeks+6 days, which is known as the routine anomaly scan and looks for any problems of development in the fetus. Again, if abnormalities are detected, then it may be appropriate to offer invasive testing and prenatal diagnosis.

PRENATAL DIAGNOSIS

The introduction of screening programmes and increased awareness of certain genetic conditions has led to the option of prenatal diagnosis becoming a common diagnostic tool. It is estimated that around 5% of pregnant patients are offered invasive prenatal diagnostic tests (30 000 patients in the UK).

As mentioned above, patients are offered screening for chromosomal abnormalities such as Down's syndrome. These tests are NOT diagnostic and only offer a risk score. In individuals who are deemed high risk, prenatal diagnosis offers a way of establishing a diagnosis as to whether the fetus does indeed have the condition suspected by the screening. Also, parents who are carriers for certain conditions may wish to know whether or not their child is affected by the condition. Undergoing prenatal diagnosis allows the couple to be prepared for the needs of the child if they choose to continue with the pregnancy or indeed opt for a termination of pregnancy. Furthermore, it allows medical teams to modify antenatal care and to prepare for the delivery and needs of the baby once born.

Techniques

Ultrasound

As mentioned above, ultrasound is used at a number of stages in pregnancy. The early scan allows for the measurement of nuchal translucency (NT) and later, the anomaly USS (18–20 weeks) allows for a more detailed assessment of any structural anomaly. Although often not realized by patients, this indeed is a form of prenatal diagnosis. Any anomaly identified may prompt further diagnostic interventions such as amniocentesis or fetal blood sampling.

Amniocentesis

The term amniocentesis is derived from the Greek words *amnion* (referring to the amnion of the fetal membranes) and centesis, from *kentēsis* a puncture, i.e. a puncture of the amnion. The aim of the procedure is to obtain a sample of amniotic fluid from which fetal cells can be harvested. The fetal cells are then cultured and undergo testing to establish the fetal karyotype (the number and visual appearance of the chromosomes in the cell). Results take:

- 2–3 days using the polymerase chain reaction (PCR) technique
- up to 2 weeks from a culture.

Another use of amniocentesis is for diagnosis of suspected fetal infection where the amniotic fluid can be sampled and tested, e.g. cytomegalovirus infection.

The procedure is carried out after 15 weeks of pregnancy; those done prior to this are associated with a higher risk of fetal loss and limb abnormalities. Under ultrasound guidance, a needle is passed through the anterior abdominal wall into the amniotic cavity. Amniotic fluid is then aspirated and the needle withdrawn. Figure 2.5 shows the technique.

As with any medical procedure there are associated risks, therefore before undergoing the procedure it is essential that patients understand the risks and weigh up whether the benefits outweigh the risks. An amniocentesis carries a 1% risk of miscarriage and 0.1% risk of serious infection.

> **HINTS AND TIPS**
>
> Both an amniocentesis and chorionic villous sampling are considered a potentially sensitizing event and therefore the administration of anti-D immunoglobulin to RH negative mothers is recommended.

Chorionic villous sampling

Chorionic villous sampling (CVS) is a technique used to obtain a sample of chorionic villi from the fetal placenta. It can be carried by the transabdominal route or less commonly, the transcervical route, and again is done under continuous ultrasound guidance (Fig. 2.6). CVS is usually performed between 11 weeks

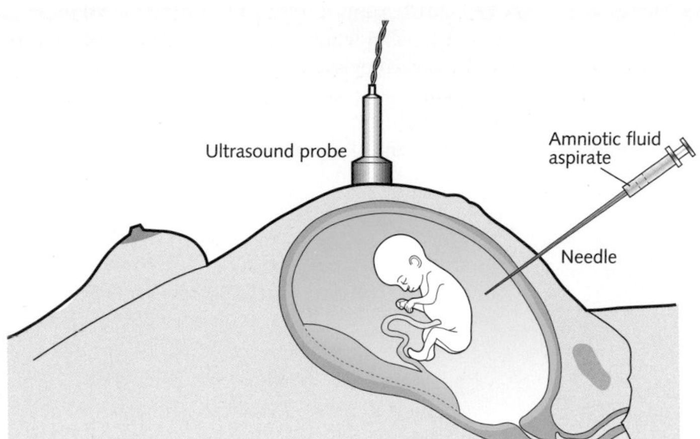

Fig. 2.5 Amniocentesis. Both an amniocentesis and chorionic villous sampling are considered a potentially sensitizing event and therefore the administration of anti-D immunoglobulin to RH negative mothers is recommended.

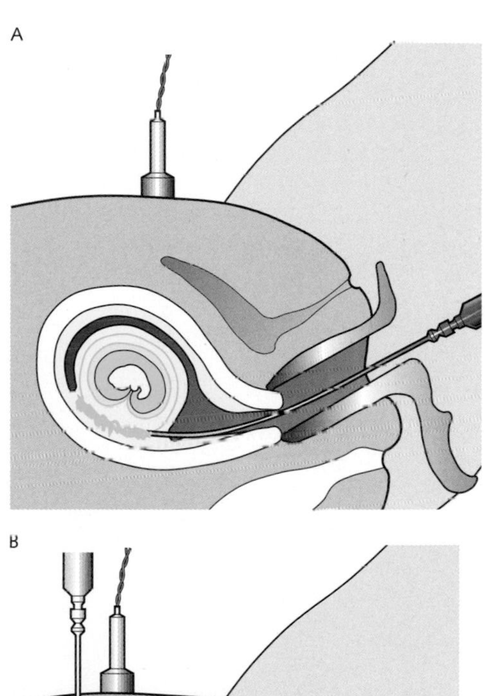

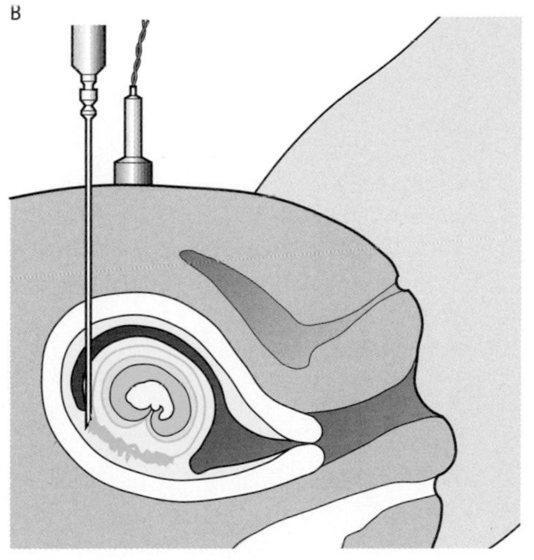

Fig. 2.6 Chorionic villous sampling (CVS) (A) Transcervical. (B) Transabdominal.

and 13 weeks + 6 days and should not be performed before 10 weeks due to concerns about increased loss rates and limb abnormalities.

The rate of miscarriage following a CVS is generally thought to be greater than that of an amniocentesis, however data from specialist units where a large number of procedures are carried out have shown that the loss rates may actually be very similar. As with an amniocentesis there is a 0.1% chance of serious infection.

As CVS is performed earlier than amniocentesis, the patient has the choice of an earlier surgical termination which patients may find more acceptable. However, there is the risk of placental mosaicism that can yield an inconclusive result requiring further testing.

Fetal blood sampling

Fetal blood sampling (FBS) in prenatal diagnosis involves the aspiration of fetal blood using a transabdominal approach under ultrasound guidance. It is important to recognize that this is very different to the fetal blood sampling performed in labour when a sample of blood is obtained from the fetal scalp. The technique can be used to detect fetal anaemia or fetal thrombocytopenia. However, the use of middle cerebral artery Doppler assessment has largely replaced FBS for diagnosis of anaemia. FBS also allows the transfusion of blood or platelets if required.

Further reading

Leslie, K., Papageorghiou, A., 2011. Invasive Procedures in Oxford Desk Reference Obstetrics & Gynaecology. Oxford University Press, London.

Nelson-Piercy, C., 2010. Handbook of Obstetric Medicine, fourth ed. Informa Healthcare, London.

NICE, 2010. NICE Guidelines – Antenatal Care. National Institute for Health and Care Excellence, London. Available online at: guidance.nice.org.uk.

NHS Fetal Anomaly Screening Programme. Available online at: http://fetalanomaly.screening.nhs.uk.

RCOG, 2010. Amniocentesis and Chorionic Villus Sampling, Green-top Guideline No. 8. Royal College of Obstetricians and Gynaecologists, London.

UK National Screening Committee, 2013. Screening Tests for You and Your Baby Booklet. Available online at: www.screening.nhs.uk/annbpublications.

Examination 3

Objective

By the end of this chapter, you should be able to:

- Understand the basic techniques of antenatal and gynaecological clinical examination.

GENERAL EXAMINATION

General examination of the patient is extremely important and is often overlooked. Ensure that the patient is comfortable and not unduly exposed. Obstetric patients should not be examined flat on their backs because of the risk of postural supine hypotensive syndrome: when lying flat, the pregnant uterus compresses the aorta and reduces blood flow back to the maternal heart. As a result, the patient feels faint. The following general assessment should be made quickly:

- General well-being
- Body mass index (BMI)
- Cardiovascular system, including pulse, blood pressure, cardiac murmurs and clinical signs of anaemia; oedema can affect the hands, the periorbital region, the legs and the sacral region
- Respiratory system.

The urine should be tested for the presence of sugar, protein and blood.

> **HINTS AND TIPS**
>
> A chaperone should always be used when performing an examination in obstetrics and gynaecology, regardless of whether the doctor is male or female.

ABDOMINAL EXAMINATION

Inspection

Inspection of the abdomen is an important part of the abdominal examination.

Surgical scars

Surgical scars are often overlooked because of successful attempts to produce cosmetically pleasing scars, e.g. transverse suprapubic and laparoscopy scars. Always check the umbilicus and pubic hairline. Multiple small scars might be present following minimal access surgical procedures.

Abdominal masses

Inspection for abdominal masses is important, although they might not be evident on inspection alone if the patient has an increased BMI. The size and shape of the abdomen should be noted.

Stigmata of pregnancy

Striae gravidarum (stretch marks) are caused by pregnancy hormones that stimulate the splitting of the dermis and can occur relatively early in pregnancy. New striae appear red and sometimes inflamed and can be sore and itchy, old striae from previous pregnancies are pale and silvery. They usually appear on the lower abdomen, upper thighs, buttocks and breasts.

Increased skin pigmentation can occur in pregnancy and results in the linea nigra – midline pigmentation from the xiphisternum to the symphysis pubis. Other areas that can undergo pigmentation in pregnancy include the nipples, the vulva, the umbilicus and recent abdominal scars.

Palpation

Before palpating the abdomen always enquire about areas of tenderness and palpate these areas last. Using the palm of the hand, gently palpate the four quadrants of the abdomen to elicit tenderness, guarding and rebound.

On discovering an abdominal mass, assess:

- size
- shape
- position
- mobility
- consistency.

You should ascertain whether the mass is arising from the pelvis. If you cannot palpate the lower aspect of the mass it is probably arising from the pelvis. Percussion can help outline the borders of a mass in an obese patient.

Auscultation

Auscultation of the abdomen is important to assess bowel sounds and in an obstetric patient the fetal heart should be auscultated using a pinard or a sonicaid.

Obstetric palpation

Uterine size

Uterine size is assessed by palpation and is a skill that is acquired through experience. A rough guide to the uterine size can be made from assessment of the fundal height in relation to the following anatomical landmarks: the symphysis pubis, umbilicus and xiphisternum, equivalent to 12, 20 and 36 weeks' gestation (Fig. 3.1). The fundus of the uterus should not be palpable abdominally until 12 weeks' gestation. By 36 weeks the fundus should be approximately at the level of the xiphisternum, following which it drops down as the fetal head engages into the maternal pelvis.

When palpating the uterine fundus, always start at the xiphisternum and work towards the umbilicus using the medial border of the left hand or the fingertips. This technique should ensure that you always palpate the upper extent of a pelvic mass. Measuring the distance from the fundus to the symphysis pubis in centimetres (the symphysis-fundal height SFH) is a more objective method of assessing fundal height than using topography alone. The SFH measurement ± 3 cm should equal the number of weeks amenorrhoea after 24 weeks' gestation, e.g. at 34 weeks' gestation the SFH should be between 31 and 37 cm.

Number of fetuses

The number of fetuses present can be calculated by assessing the number of fetal poles present. 'Fetal pole' is the term used to denote the head or the breech. In a singleton pregnancy, two poles should be palpable unless the presenting part is deeply engaged in the pelvis. In multiple pregnancies, the number of poles present *minus one* should be palpable. For example, four poles are present in a twin pregnancy and only three should be palpable as one is usually tucked away out of reach. More commonly, the patient has already had an ultrasound scan detailing the number of fetuses.

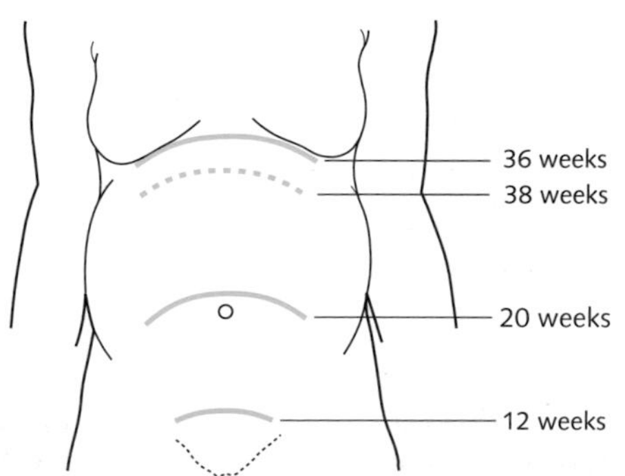

Fig. 3.1 Fundal height in relation to abdominal landmarks.

Fetal lie

This is the relationship between the long axis of the fetus and the long axis of the uterus. This can be longitudinal, transverse or oblique (Fig. 3.2).

Fetal presentation

This is the part of the fetus that presents to the maternal pelvis. If the head (also known as the vertex) is situated over the pelvis this is termed a 'cephalic presentation'. Three different types of cephalic presentation can occur, depending on the degree of flexion of the head on the fetal spine:

- A well flexed head will present by the vertex (the area bordered by the parietal bones and the anterior and posterior fontanelles).

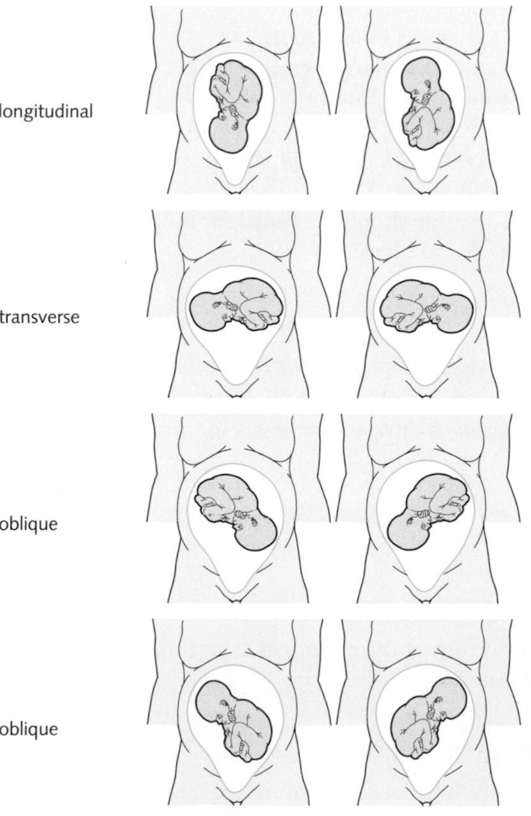

Fig. 3.2 The fetal lie. The relationship of the long axis of the fetus to the long axis of the uterus.

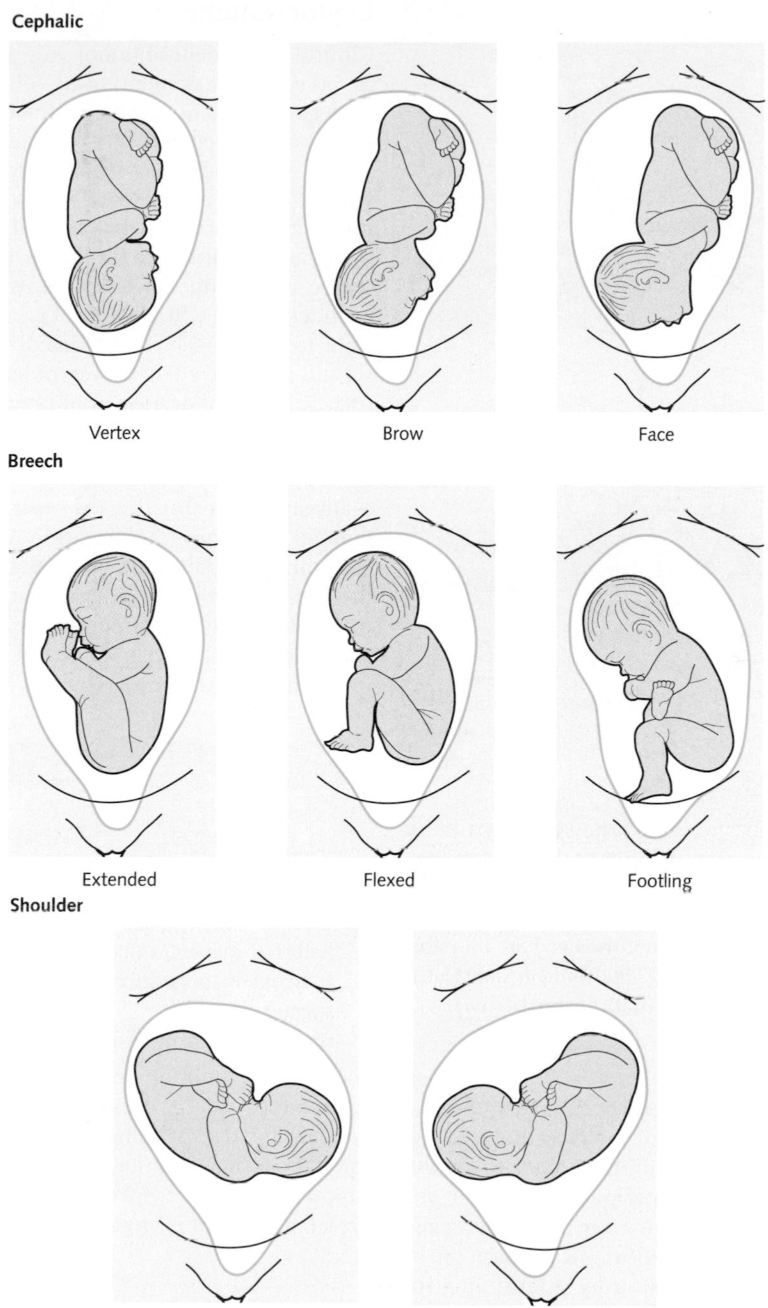

Fig. 3.3 The fetal presentation. The relationship of the presenting part of the fetus to the maternal pelvis.

- A partly extended head will present by the brow.
- A fully extended head will present by the face.

In a breech presentation the buttocks occupy the lower segment, and in an oblique lie the shoulder generally presents (Fig. 3.3). Any presentation other than a vertex presentation is called a malpresentation.

Engagement

The fetal head is said to be engaged when the widest diameter of the head (the biparietal diameter) has passed through the pelvic brim. Abdominal palpation of the head is assessed in fifths and is measured by palpating

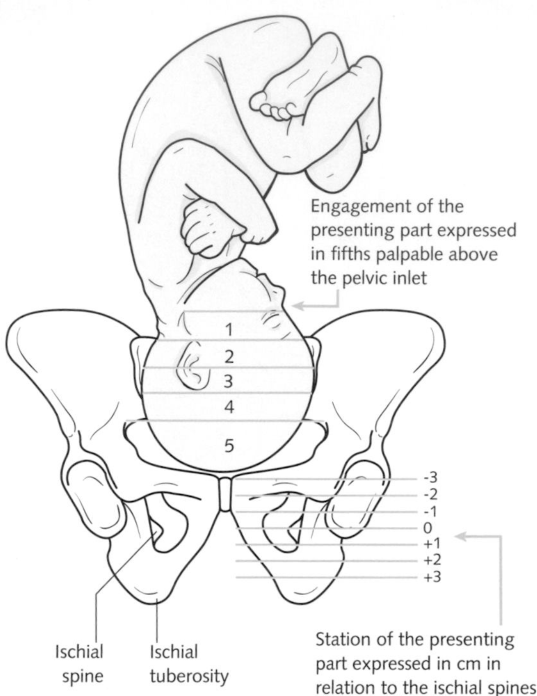

Fig. 3.4 Engagement of the fetal head.

the angle between the head and the symphysis pubis (Fig. 3.4). When three or more fifths of the head are palpable abdominally the head is not engaged because the widest diameter of the head has not entered the pelvic brim. When two or fewer fifths of the head are palpable the head is clinically engaged. This should equate to the station found on vaginal examination (see below).

Position

The position of the presenting part is defined as the relationship of the denominator of the presenting part to the maternal pelvis. The denominator changes according to the presenting part: the occiput in a cephalic presentation, the mentum (chin) in a face presentation and the sacrum in a breech presentation. The position can be assessed on abdominal palpation by determining the position of the fetal back. If the back lies:

- on the maternal left, the position is likely to be left occipitotransverse
- on the maternal right, the position is likely to be right occipitotransverse
- more posteriorly (i.e. towards the mother's spine), the position is likely to be left or right occipitoposterior
- anteriorly, the position is likely to be left or right occipitoanterior (Fig. 3.5).

The position of the presenting part can be assessed more accurately by vaginal examination.

Liquor volume

Clinical assessment of liquor volume is not as accurate as objective assessment using ultrasound. However, subjective assessment can alert the examiner to the possibility of reduced or increased liquor volume and instigation of the necessary investigations. Reduced liquor volume might be suggested when the uterus is small for dates with easily palpable fetal parts producing an irregular firm outline to the uterus. Increased liquor volume causes a large-for-dates uterus that is smooth and rounded and in which the fetal parts are almost impossible to distinguish. If suspected, an ultrasound scan should be ordered to assess objective measurements such as depth of deepest pool or amniotic fluid index.

Difficulty palpating fetal parts

Many students worry that they will not be able to ascertain all the above information during an obstetric abdominal palpation. It is not always possible even in the most experienced hands, but it is important to understand why this might be so. Figure 3.6 shows some situations when palpation of the fetal parts might prove difficult.

PELVIC EXAMINATION

Gynaecological pelvic examination

There are three important steps when performing a pelvic examination:

1. External inspection of the vulva
2. Internal inspection of the vagina and cervix via a speculum
3. Bimanual examination of the pelvis.

The most common position for carrying out a pelvic examination is the dorsal position with the woman lying on her back with her knees flexed. Make sure that the patient is as comfortable as possible and not too exposed. External inspection only can be performed on a patient who is virgo intacta.

HINTS AND TIPS

During a gynaecological examination the pelvic examination should always be preceded by inspection of the external genitals and vaginal walls.

External examination of the vulva

The presence of abnormal discharge on the vulva should be noted, as should the anatomy of the external genitalia (Fig. 3.7). Parting the labia with the left hand, the entire area should be carefully inspected for

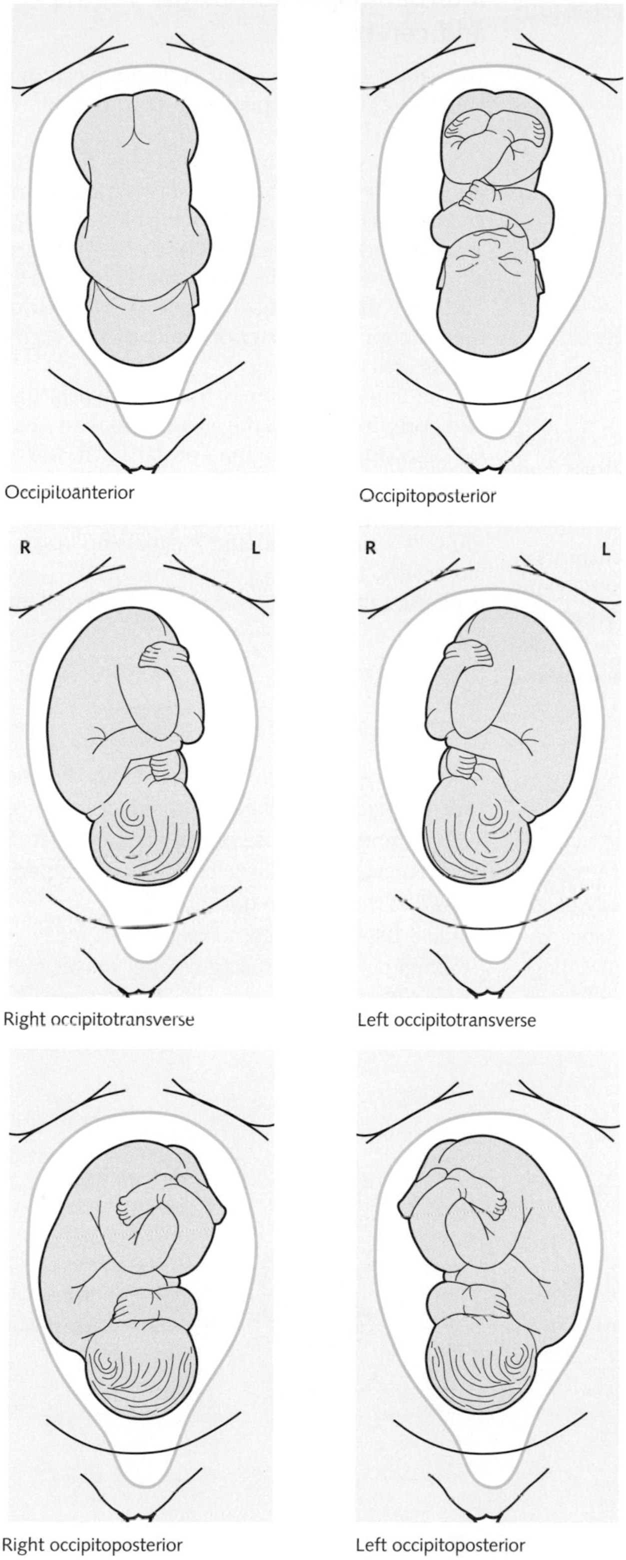

Fig. 3.5 The fetal position.

Occipitoanterior

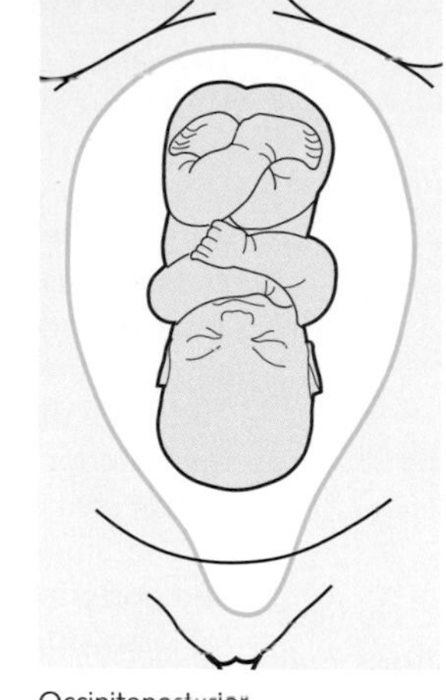

Occipitoposterior

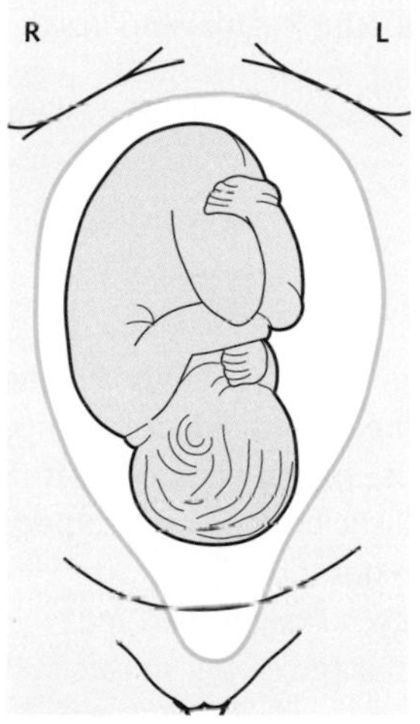

Right occipitotransverse

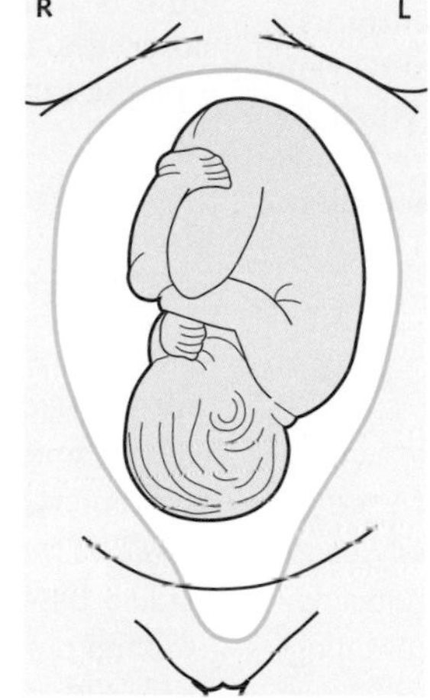

Left occipitotransverse

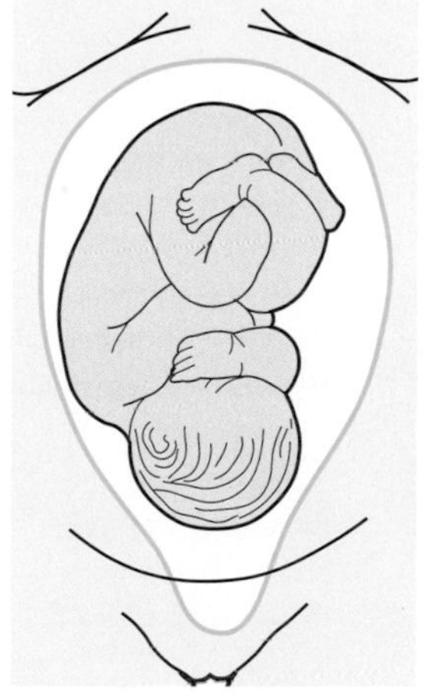

Right occipitoposterior

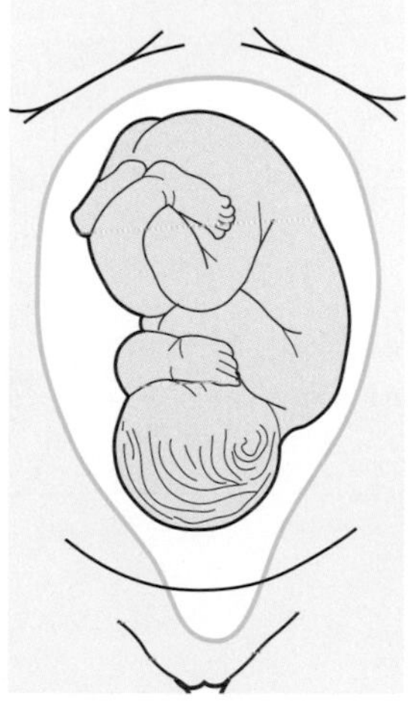

Left occipitoposterior

Fig. 3.6 Situations where fetal parts might be difficult to palpate.

Types of reason	Description
Maternal reasons	Maternal obesity Muscular anterior abdominal wall
Uterine reasons	Anterior uterine wall fibroids Uterine contraction/Braxton Hicks contraction
Fetoplacental reasons	Anterior placenta Increased liquor volume

inflammation, ulceration, swellings, atrophic changes and leucoplakia (white plaques) and the clitoris and urethral orifice inspected. A deficient or scarred perineum is a clue to previous trauma due to vaginal delivery. Vaginal or uterine prolapse through the introitus is assessed with and without the patient bearing down and stress incontinence might be demonstrated when the patient coughs. Assessment of prolapse can only be adequately made with the patient in the left lateral position using a Sims' speculum (see Chapter 15).

HINTS AND TIPS

Examination of the vulva includes assessment of female circumcision or female genital mutilation (FGM see Chapter 1), whether or not a history has already been elicited. The grading is shown in the RCOG guideline. All grades may be relevant to the patient's presenting complaint.

Internal inspection of the vagina and cervix

To inspect the vagina and cervix a speculum is used; either the Cuscos speculum (bivalve) or the Sims' speculum (Fig. 3.8).

The Cuscos speculum is used with the patient in the dorsal position and consists of two blades hinged open at the vaginal introitus. When the blades are opened, the anterior and posterior walls of the vagina are separated allowing the vaginal fornices and cervix to be visualized. The main disadvantage of the Cuscos speculum is that the anterior and posterior walls of the vagina cannot be assessed adequately.

The Sims speculum is used to inspect the anterior and posterior walls of the vagina and is an excellent tool for assessing uterovaginal prolapse. It was originally developed to examine vaginal fistulae. With the patient in the left lateral, or Sims, position the blade of the speculum is inserted into the vagina and used to retract either the anterior or posterior walls. Uterovaginal prolapse can then be assessed with the patient bearing down.

HINTS AND TIPS

Liquid-based cytology is the current technique for taking cervical smears and reduces the need to repeat smears because of inadequate/unsatisfactory specimens. A soft plastic brush is used to perform this and the cells are transported in fluid. Liquid-based cytology is likely to become routine practice for taking cervical smears in the near future.

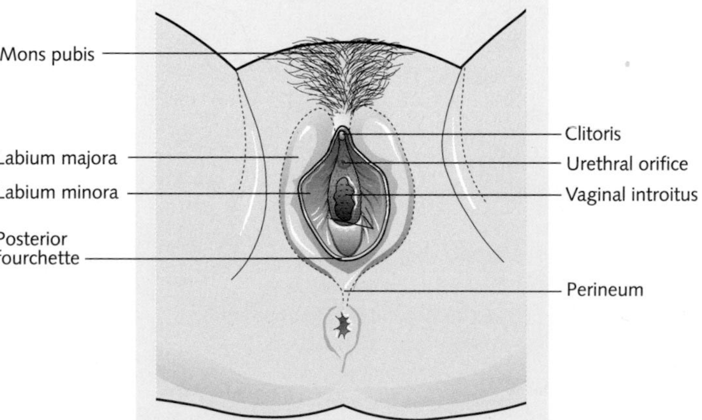

Fig. 3.7 The female external genitalia.

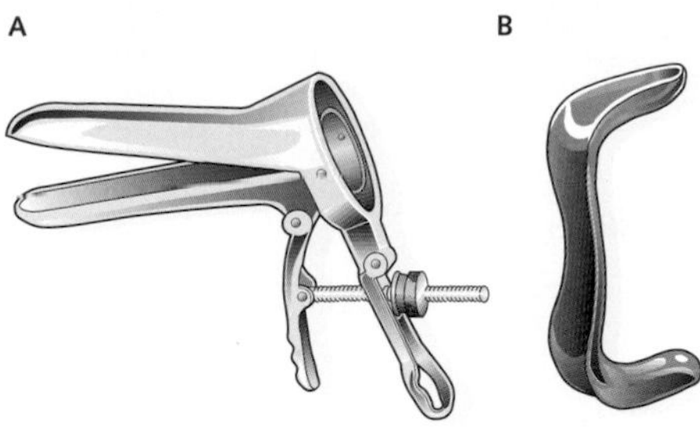

Fig. 3.8 (A) Cuscos. (B) Sims vaginal specula.

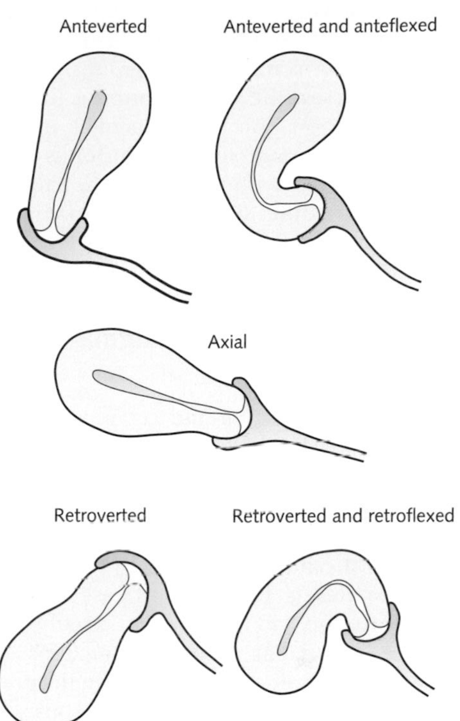

Fig. 3.9 Positions of the uterus.

Bimanual examination

It is usual to perform an internal examination using the lubricated index and middle fingers of the right hand. In nulligravid and postmenopausal women it might be necessary to use only the index finger. Palpation of the vaginal walls is important to exclude scarring, cysts and tumours that can easily be missed on inspection. The vaginal fornices should be examined for scarring, thickening and swellings that will suggest pelvic pathology. The size, shape, position, consistency, angle and mobility of the cervix should be assessed. Moving the cervix from side to side might elicit cervical motion tenderness and elevating the cervix anteriorly, thereby stretching the uterosacral ligaments, might cause pain in the presence of endometriosis.

The fingers of the right hand are then used to elevate or steady the uterus while the left hand palpates abdominally. An anteverted uterus is usually palpable between the two hands. A retroverted uterus is usually felt as a swelling in the posterior fornix and is not bimanually palpable unless it is flipped forward into an anteverted position and elevated into the anterior part of the pelvis. The different combinations of version and flexion of the uterus are shown in Figure 3.9. The size, position, consistency, outline and mobility of the uterus should all be noted. A pregnant uterus should feel soft and globular and roughly the size of an apple, large orange and grapefruit at 6, 8 and 12 weeks' gestation, respectively.

To examine the adnexa, the fingers of the right hand should be positioned in one of the lateral fornices and the adnexal region palpated between the two hands. Normal premenopausal ovaries are not always palpable depending on the size of the patient. Fallopian tubes and postmenopausal ovaries should not be palpable. If an adnexal mass is discovered, then its size, shape, consistency, mobility and whether it is fixed to the uterus or not should all be noted. The presence and degree of tenderness should be noted.

Obstetric pelvic examination

There are three components to the obstetric pelvic examination:

1. External inspection of the vulva
2. Internal inspection of the vagina and cervix
3. Vaginal examination.

> **HINTS AND TIPS**
>
> An obstetric examination is incomplete without a blood pressure check, urinalysis and auscultation of the fetus.

External examination of the vulva

The blood flow through the vulva and vagina increases dramatically in pregnancy. The vulva might look swollen and oedematous secondary to engorgement.

The presence of vulval varicosities should be noted. Note the presence of vaginal discharge or leaking amniotic fluid. In certain ethnic groups, it may be appropriate to assess the vaginal introitus for signs of female circumcision (or female genital mutilation FGM). This is important since the introitus may not allow vaginal delivery without offering the patient revision – this procedure should ideally occur before 20 weeks gestation.

Internal inspection of the vagina and cervix

Examination of the vagina and cervix with a sterile Cusco's speculum should be performed using an aseptic technique. Increased vaginal and cervical secretions are normal in pregnancy. Inspection of the cervix might reveal amniotic fluid draining through the cervical os. Digital examination in the presence of ruptured membranes is likely to increase the risk of ascending infection and is, therefore, usually avoided unless there are regular uterine contractions. Exclusion of cervical pathology is important in the presence of APH, although care must be taken because, in the presence of placenta praevia, bleeding might be exacerbated.

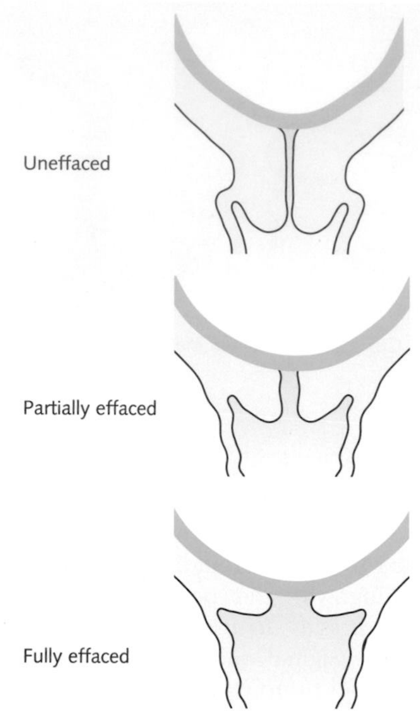

Fig. 3.10 Effacement of the cervix.

Vaginal examination

This should be performed under aseptic conditions in the presence of ruptured membranes. Once the cervix has been identified, the following characteristics should be determined:

- Dilatation
- Length
- Station of presenting part
- Consistency
- Position.

Cervical dilatation

Cervical dilatation is assessed in centimetres using the examining fingers. One finger-breadth is roughly 1–1.5 cm. Full dilatation of the cervix is equivalent to 10 cm dilatation.

Cervical length

When not in established labour, the normal length of the cervix is about 3 cm. Shortening occurs as the cervix effaces, becoming part of the lower segment of the uterus, in the presence of regular uterine contractions (Fig. 3.10).

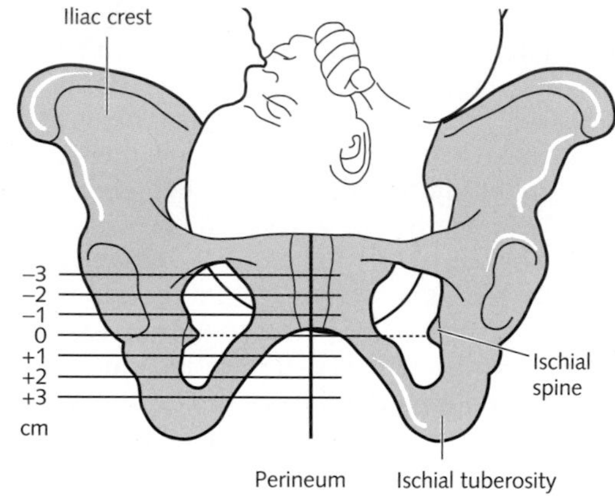

Fig. 3.11 The station of the presenting part.

Station of the presenting part

The station of the presenting part is determined by how much the presenting part has descended into the pelvis. The station is defined as the number of centimetres above or below a fixed point in the maternal pelvis, the ischial spines. This should equate to the engagement found on abdominal palpation (Fig. 3.11).

Fig. 3.12 The Bishop scoring system for the uterine cervix.

Cervical characteristic	Score 0	1	2	3
Dilalation (cm)	0	1–2	3–4	>4
Length (cm)	3	2	1	<1
Station (cm)	–3	–2	–1 or 0	+1 or +2
Consistency	firm	medium	soft	
Position	posterior	mid	anterior	

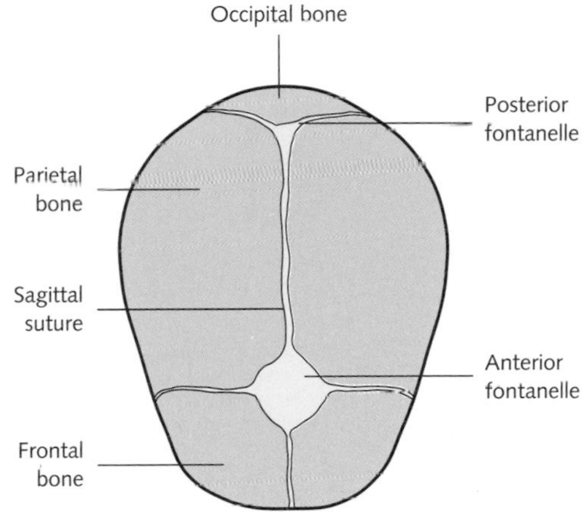

Fig. 3.13 The landmarks of the fetal skull including the anterior and posterior fontanelles.

Cervical consistency

Softening of the cervix occurs as pregnancy progresses aiding cervical effacement and dilatation. The consistency of the cervix can be described as firm, mid-consistency or soft.

Cervical position

This describes where the cervix is situated in the antero-posterior plane of the pelvis. As the cervix becomes effaced and dilated it tends to become more anterior in position.

The Bishop score

Using the above characteristics, Bishop devised a scoring system to evaluate the 'ripeness' or favourability of the cervix (Fig. 3.12). This system is used as an objective tool when inducing labour to assess the cervix. The higher the score, the more favourable the cervix and the more likely that induction of labour will be successful.

Defining the position of the presenting part

With a cephalic presentation, the anterior and posterior fontanelles and the sagittal sutures should be identified. The posterior fontanelle is Y-shaped and is formed when the three sutures between the occipital and parietal bones meet. The anterior fontanelle is larger, diamond-shaped and formed by the four sutures between the parietal and temporal bones meeting (Fig. 3.13). The position of the presenting part can be defined as shown in Figure 3.14. The presence of caput and moulding should also be assessed. Caput is the subcutaneous swelling on the fetal scalp that can be felt during labour and this increases if the labour is prolonged with failure of the cervix to dilate. Moulding is the term used to describe the overlapping of the skull bones that occurs as labour progresses.

HINTS AND TIPS

When assessing progress in labour one must always comment on engagement of head, cervical dilatation, cervical effacement, station of head in relation to ischial spines, position of head, moulding, caput and liquor colour (e.g. meconium staining).

HINTS AND TIPS

It has become increasingly recognized that the best test of a pelvis is the dynamic process of labour itself, so formal pelvic assessment is no longer performed as a routine. The Bishop score is used in the assessment of cervical favourability prior to induction of labour.

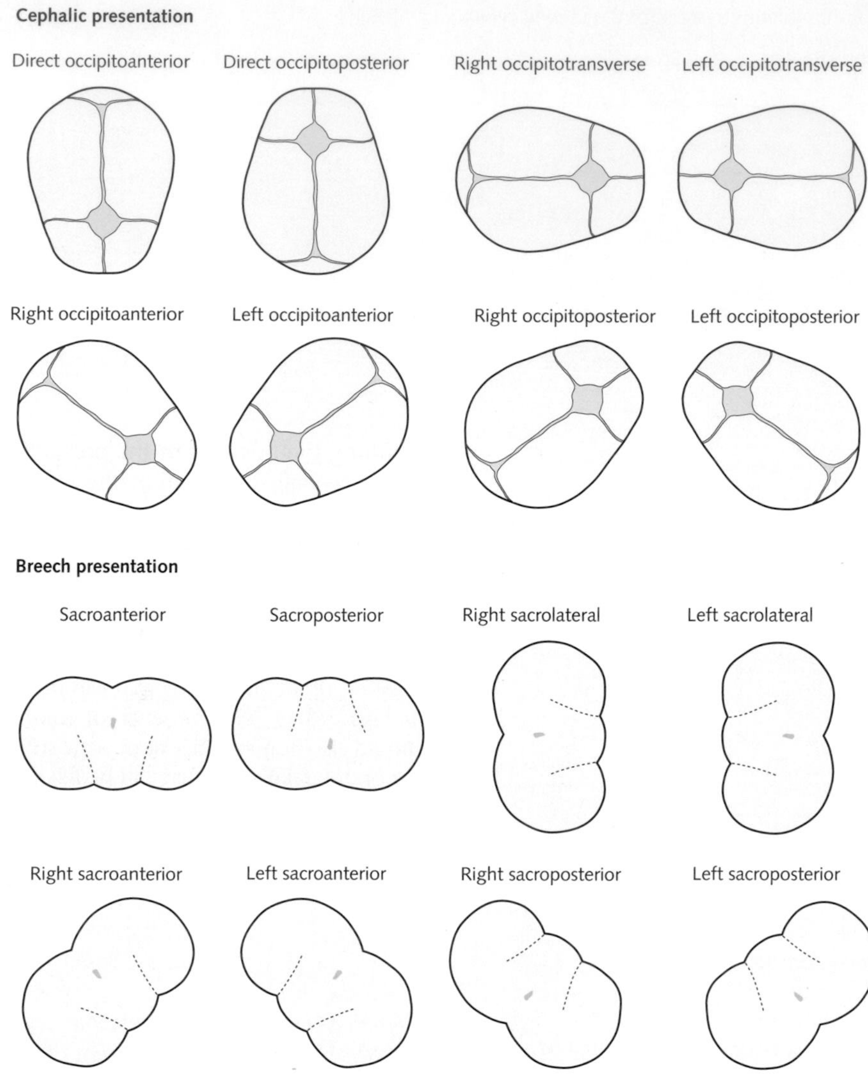

Fig. 3.14 Defining the position of the presenting part.

Further reading

RCOG, 2009. Female Genital Mutilation Management RCOG. Green-top Guideline No. 53. Royal College of Obstetricians and Gynaecologists, London.

Common investigations

Objectives

By the end of this chapter, you should be able to:

- Understand the indications, benefits and risks of the investigations commonly used in obstetrics and gynaecology.

A wide range of investigations are used for diagnosis and management in obstetrics and gynaecology. When considering investigations, always make sure you request the simplest investigations first, working your way to the more invasive and complex investigations only where necessary.

BEDSIDE TESTS

Urine

In patients presenting with pain or bleeding, always perform a urine dipstick to exclude haematuria or infection. If the urine dipstick is positive, send the urine for culture.

Swabs

In patients with signs and symptoms of infection (e.g. abnormal vaginal or wound discharge, pyrexia) take a:

- high vaginal swab to exclude Candida infection
- endocervical swab to exclude chlamydia and gonorrhoea
- consider a wound swab if the patient has had an operation and the wound looks inflamed and exudes pus.

Smears and colposcopy

The National Screening in Cervical Cytology Programme recommends performing a smear in women between the ages of 25 and 50 every 3 years, and 5 yearly after that until the age of 60 if smears are normal.

Smears must be taken **before** taking any swabs or performing a vaginal examination, as this can dislodge the cells on the surface of the cervix. Visualizing the cervix and sweeping the spatula 360° around the cervix at least five times for an accurate result.

CERVICAL CYTOLOGY

Squamous carcinoma of the cervix is amenable to screening because it exhibits a pre-invasive phase (see Chapter 10). Screening is carried out by cytological examination of cervical smears using the Papanicolaou test. Using a Cusco's speculum, the visible cervix is gently swept through 360° five times with a cervical cytobrush (Fig. 4.1). The sample is then placed into a fluid medium and sent for liquid-based cytology. This technique has effectively reduced the rate of inadequate smears and therefore the need to recall women for a repeat smear.

COLPOSCOPY

Women with smears suggestive of CIN or women with an abnormal-looking cervix are then referred for colposcopy. The colposcope is a binocular microscope enabling the surface epithelium of the cervix to be assessed under magnification and is usually performed in the outpatient setting. The patient is positioned in a modified lithotomy position and the cervix exposed using a Cusco's speculum. The cervix is then viewed through the colposcope to identify any lesions such as leucoplakia or frank invasive carcinoma. Two solutions are then applied:

- Acetic acid solution (5%) is applied to the entire surface of the cervix. Coagulation of proteins by the acetic acid in abnormal epithelial areas produces white changes, so called acetowhite changes. Areas of CIN appear as distinct acetowhite lesions with clearly demarcated edges and the associated abnormal vessel formation produces the typical mosaic and punctate patterns.
- Iodine is applied to the cervix to further highlight the squamocolumnar junction and areas of abnormalities, this time as an orange change.

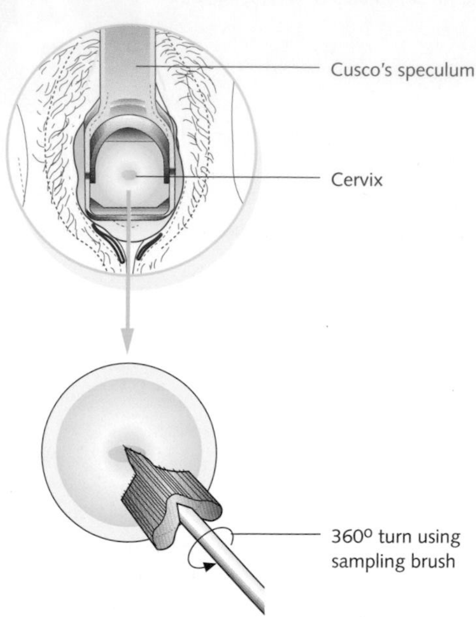

Fig. 4.1 Taking a cervical smear using a cytobrush. The cervix must be visualized and a 360° sweep must be performed.

The extent of the lesion should be noted, with particular regard paid to extension into the cervical canal. All abnormal-looking areas should be biopsied for histological assessment. If the histology shows severe cellular changes, the abnormal areas on the cervix should be removed using laser treatment.

HINTS AND TIPS

- **Smears** identify cytological cellular dyskaryosis. If these changes are moderate or severe, a biopsy should be taken.
- **Biopsies** identify histological cellular dysplasia – namely, CIN I, II, III or invasive disease.

Blood investigations

Consider the following investigations:

- FBC (to exclude infection, thrombocytopaenia and anaemia)
- U&Es (to check renal function in patients with benign fibroids or cysts or malignant masses which may press on the ureters)
- LFTs (to monitor liver function in pre-eclamptic and HELLP patients)
- Blood film (to exclude haemolysis in pre-eclamptic and HELLP patients)
- LH/FSH levels (to diagnose menopause or polycystic ovarian syndrome)
- Prolactin levels (to exclude a prolactinoma, associated with secondary amenorrhoea)
- TFTs (abnormal thyroid function can be associated with menorrhagia and miscarriage)
- Day 21 progesterone level (to confirm ovulation in those with a regular 28 day menstrual cycle; this date should be adjusted to the length of the woman's menstrual cycle)
- CA125 (in those with ovarian masses, to help characterize whether the mass is benign or malignant).

IMAGING TECHNIQUES

Imaging techniques are used widely in both obstetrics and gynaecology. Results of imaging tests should be interpreted carefully in the light of the history and clinical findings.

Ultrasound scanning

Ultrasound examination of the pregnant and non-pregnant pelvis is probably the most common investigation performed in obstetrics and gynaecology. Ultrasound waves passing through the pelvis are reflected in varying degrees depending on the density of the tissues present. For instance, bone is very reflective (or echogenic) and appears white on the monitor, whereas fluid is less echogenic and appears dark on the monitor. Interpretation of these echoes is the mainstay of diagnosis in ultrasound. There are two types of ultrasound scan:

- Transabdominal – this is non-invasive but requires a full bladder to obtain the best possible image of the ovaries and uterus. Limited views are obtained early in pregnancy and in those who are obese.
- Transvaginal – this requires an empty bladder and obtains a clear image of the pelvic organs, but is invasive and may be declined by women who have not had sexual intercourse.

While ultrasound examination of the female pelvis is common with few known side effects, it should not be requested unless necessary.

The non-pregnant pelvis

A full bladder is needed to examine the non-pregnant pelvis by abdominal ultrasound. This lifts the uterus from under the pubic bone, allowing a 'window' through which to view the pelvic contents and helps push the bowel out of the pelvis.

The uterus

The dimensions of the uterus can be measured and its position (e.g. retroflexed) recorded. Abnormal textures in the myometrium can suggest the presence of fibroids or adenomyosis. The midline echo corresponds to the endometrial thickness and will vary depending on the menstrual cycle. Pathology of the endometrial cavity, such as endometrial hyperplasia, endometrial polyps or submucous fibroids, might be detected. In some centres, this is aided by hysterosonography, where saline is instilled into the uterine cavity to outline abnormalities. Intrauterine contraceptive devices (IUCDs) will show up as very bright echoes.

The ovaries

The size and position of the ovaries can be assessed. In polycystic ovary syndrome (PCOS, see Chapter 16), the polycystic ovary is on average twice the normal volume with thickened central stroma and 10 or more peripherally sited follicles. Follicular tracking is possible in women trying to conceive.

Ovarian tumours can be identified ultrasonographically, but differentiation between benign and malignant tumours cannot be made with certainty. Figure 4.2 shows some of the ultrasound characteristics of benign and malignant ovarian tumours.

The fallopian tubes

The fallopian tubes are not normally visible by ultrasound. However, when they are blocked and distended with fluid (hydrosalpinx) they will appear as cystic structures that might be mistaken for ovarian cysts.

HINTS AND TIPS

Ultrasound has a central role in characterizing ovarian cysts and bleeding in post-menopausal women:

- If an ovarian cyst is 5 cm or more, the cyst should be monitored using repeat scans or surgically removed if the patient is symptomatic.
- If the endometrial thickness in a post-menopausal woman is 5 mm or more, an endometrial biopsy should be taken.

Fig. 4.2 Ultrasound features to distinguish benign and malignant tumours. Borderline tumours cannot be identified with certainty using ultrasound alone.

	Benign	Malignant
Size	<5 cm	>5 cm
Laterality	Unilateral	Bilateral
Cyst walls	Thin	Thick
Septa	Absent	Thick, incomplete
Solid areas	Absent	Present
Ascites	Absent	Present

Ultrasound and pregnancy

Early pregnancy ultrasound can be used to:

- check the fetal heartbeat – the fetal heart is detectable with ultrasound by 6 weeks' amenorrhoea
- confirm the number of fetuses – a gestation sac can be seen in the uterine cavity from as early as 5 weeks' amenorrhoea when using a transvaginal probe
- calculate the gestational age of the fetus – crown–rump length (CRL) is used to date the fetus up to 13+6 weeks' amenorrhoea (Fig. 4.3), after which time CRL measurement becomes inaccurate due to flexion of the fetus. After the first trimester, the biparietal diameter (BPD) is a more accurate measurement with which to date the pregnancy.

Early pregnancy complications

A delayed or missed miscarriage occurs if the embryo fails to develop or dies in utero (see Chapter 20). In the presence of an ectopic pregnancy, a thickened endometrium is usually seen with an adnexal mass. In about 5% of ectopic pregnancies a viable pregnancy can be seen outside the uterus with ultrasound.

The most important role of ultrasound in the management of a suspected ectopic pregnancy is to confirm or exclude a viable intrauterine pregnancy.

Anomaly scans

Most obstetric units offer routine anomaly scans between 18 and 22 weeks' gestation. Different fetal anomalies are best detected at different times throughout the pregnancy, but 18–20 weeks appears to be the optimum time for a screening scan. Apart from gross anatomical defects, certain 'markers', such as choroid plexus cysts and renal pelvi-caliceal dilatation, can be identified which are associated with chromosomal abnormalities.

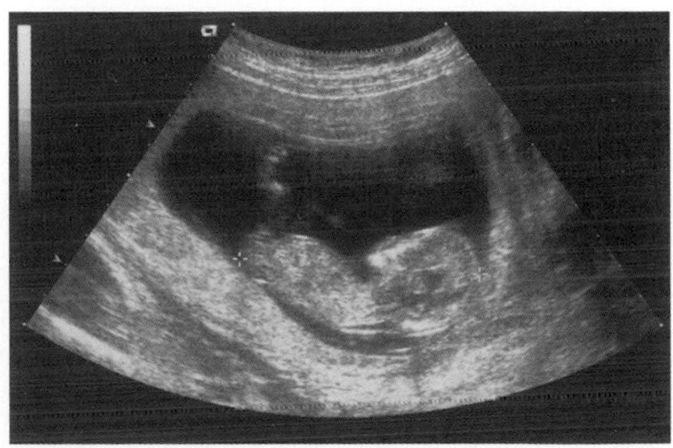

Fig. 4.3 Crown–rump length is used to date a singleton pregnancy in the first trimester. This must be measured carefully in the correct plane to ensure accurate dating.

Fetal growth

Fetal growth is assessed clinically in a normal singleton pregnancy. Where uterine size is not compatible with dates or clinical assessment is difficult, for instance in the presence of obesity or multiple pregnancy, objective measurements of fetal head circumference (HC), BPD and abdominal circumference (AC) are made using ultrasound and plotted on fetal growth charts. Scanning at regular intervals allows the growth of the fetus to be monitored.

Assessment of liquor volume

This is useful in the management of intrauterine growth restriction (IUGR) and postdates pregnancy. Reduced liquor volume can indicate the presence of placental insufficiency as the stressed fetus passes less urine, and might be an indication for delivery of the fetus depending on the clinical background. Reduced liquor might also be due to spontaneous rupture of the membranes (SROM).

Doppler studies

Doppler ultrasound assessment of the uteroplacental blood flow can be useful in the presence of fetal growth restriction due to placental insufficiency. Normally there is continuous flow through the umbilical artery to the placenta including during fetal diastole, known as end diastolic flow. Absent or reversed end diastolic flow in the umbilical artery suggests placental resistance to the returning blood. Such a compromised fetus diverts its blood flow to essential organs such as the brain and heart. This causes dilatation of the fetal middle cerebral blood vessels. Doppler studies need to be interpreted carefully with the clinical picture.

Safety of ultrasound scanning

Experimental evidence has not shown any harmful effects of ultrasound when used as a diagnostic test. However, more powerful modes of scanning such as colour flow Doppler should only be used if clinically indicated.

X-ray

The two most common X-ray procedures are:

1. hysterosalpingography (HSG): can be used to assess the uterine cavity and the patency of the fallopian tubes (Fig. 4.4). A catheter is inserted into the cervix and radiocontrast medium injected into the uterine cavity while X-rays are taken. It does not allow the exclusion of pelvic pathology as laparoscopy does, but is still useful in the presence of tubal blockage to assess whether the blockage is distal or proximal; it also allows excellent delineation of the uterine cavity. If there is clinical evidence of pelvic disease such as PID or endometriosis then a laparoscopy should be performed in preference to a HSG. Antibiotic prophylaxis should be given to reduce the complication of PID
2. erect lateral pelvimetry (ELP): can be used in situations where a contracted pelvis needs to be excluded, for instance in the management of a breech presentation. The inlet and outlet of the pelvis can be measured objectively as can the curve of the sacrum. This procedure can also be performed using CT scanning but is used infrequently.

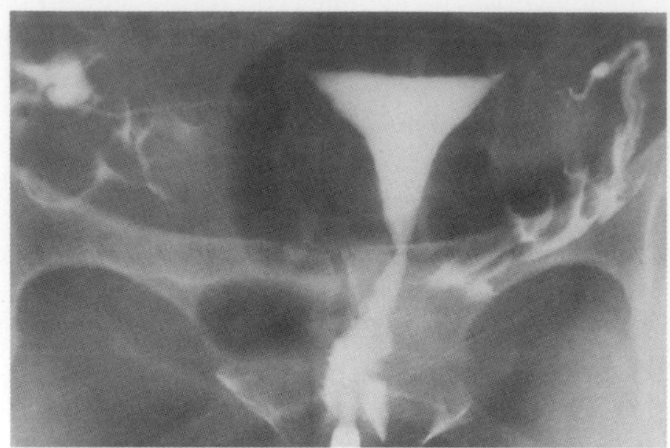

Fig. 4.4 Hysterosalpingography showing patent fallopian tubes with dye 'fill and spill'. In patients who have had previous surgery, a laparoscopy and dye test is recommended instead.

Wherever possible, X-rays should be avoided in pregnancy. However, the benefits to the women and the gestation of pregnancy must be considered when making this decision.

HYSTEROSCOPY AND PIPELLE BIOPSY

A hysteroscope is an endoscope that is inserted through the cervix to inspect the uterine cavity (Fig. 4.5). It is seen as the gold-standard investigation of abnormal uterine bleeding and can be performed in theatre under general anaesthetic or as an outpatient investigation. Diagnostic hysteroscopy is used to identify intrauterine pathology such as:

- endometrial polyps
- submucous fibroids
- endometrial carcinoma.

A distension medium is required to separate the uterine walls – most commonly, normal saline. Operative hysteroscopies use inert media such as glycine, to remove polyps and submucous fibroids. It is a relatively

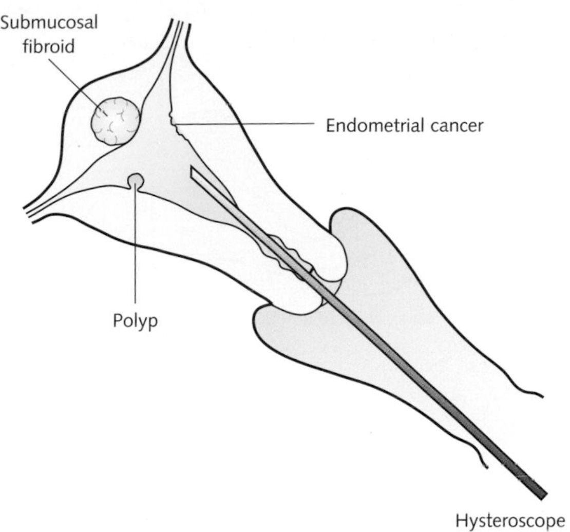

Fig. 4.5 A hysteroscope is used to visualize the endocervix and uterine cavity. This can identify polyps, fibroids or malignancy. Risks include uterine perforation, infection and bleeding.

safe procedure but complications include infection, perforation of the uterus and rarely gas embolism.

In some centres, first-line investigation for abnormal vaginal bleeding or menorrhagia may be a pipelle biopsy and transvaginal ultrasound. The pipelle consists of a plastic tube 1–2 mm in diameter which is inserted transcervically in the out-patient clinic. Withdrawing the plunger sucks in a sample of endometrium by negative pressure, which is sent for histological analysis.

LAPAROSCOPY

Laparoscopy is the mainstay of investigating pelvic pain. It is used to diagnose pelvic disease such as endometriosis and adhesions. The advantage of laparoscopy over imaging techniques is that the pelvic and other intra-abdominal organs can be visualized directly through an endoscope.

Technique

Most laparoscopies are performed under general anaesthesia. Having emptied the bladder, a Veress needle is inserted into the lower abdomen through a subumbilical incision. Carbon dioxide is pumped into the peritoneal cavity to produce a pneumoperitoneum (to a pressure of 20–25 mmHg) and then a trocar and cannula are inserted through the same incision into the pneumoperitoneum. A laparoscope can then be passed down the cannula and the pelvic organs visualized (Fig. 4.6). Complications of laparoscopy (and their rates per 1000) include:

- bowel injury (0.6)
- bladder injury (0.3)
- ureteric injury (0.3)
- vascular injury (0.1).

As well as diagnosing the cause of pelvic pain, laparoscopy can be used to treat it – for example, draining endometriomas or ablating endometriosis.

HINTS AND TIPS

In patients with a history of PID or previous surgery, the patency of fallopian tubes should be tested by injecting dye at the time of laparoscopy, rather than performing a hysterosalpingogram. This allows other causes of pathology to be identified and potentially treated.

URODYNAMICS

This term includes all the tests that assess the function of the lower urinary tract disorders, which include incontinence and voiding difficulties (see Chapter 14).

Flow studies

Using a flowmeter, the flow rate of urine can be measured. This should be above 15 mL per second and a low flow rate suggests either outflow obstruction or poor detrusor contraction.

Cystometry

The bladder is a reservoir designed to increase in volume at low pressure. Cystometry measures bladder pressure during filling or voiding. Pressure catheters are inserted into the bladder via the urethra and also the rectum to provide three measurements (Fig. 4.7):

- Intra-abdominal pressure
- Intravesical (bladder) pressure
- Detrusor muscle pressure.

The rectal catheter represents intra-abdominal pressure and is subtracted from the intravesical pressure to give the detrusor pressure. Detrusor pressure is measured during rapid filling of the bladder to detect the presence of detrusor instability. During voiding, detrusor contractility can be measured and outflow resistance and detrusor function assessed.

Videocystourethrography

Videocystourethrography (VCU) involves radiologically monitoring the bladder and urethra during cystometry. It can identify:

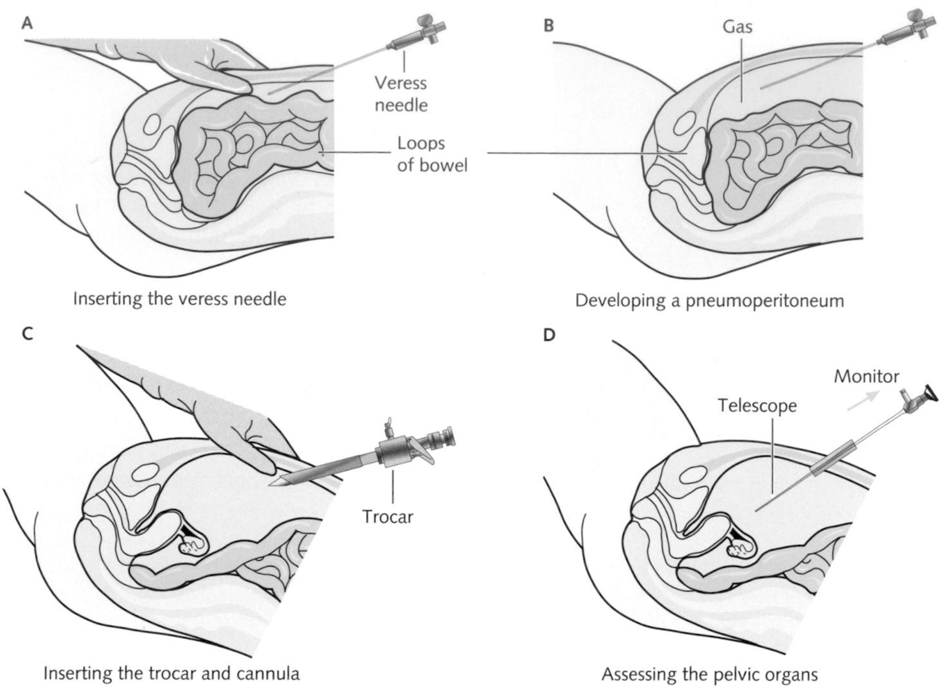

Fig. 4.6 Laparoscopic entry technique, using Veress needle insertion and gas insufflation. This is the gold standard for diagnosing endometriosis. Risks include bowel and blood vessel perforation.

Fig. 4.7 Cystometry. (A) Normal bladder: no increase in detrusor pressure with filling or contraction with cough. (B) Genuine stress incontinence – urine flow with cough seen. (C) Detrusor overactivity (DO) – detrusor contracts after cough and urine flows with detrusor contraction.

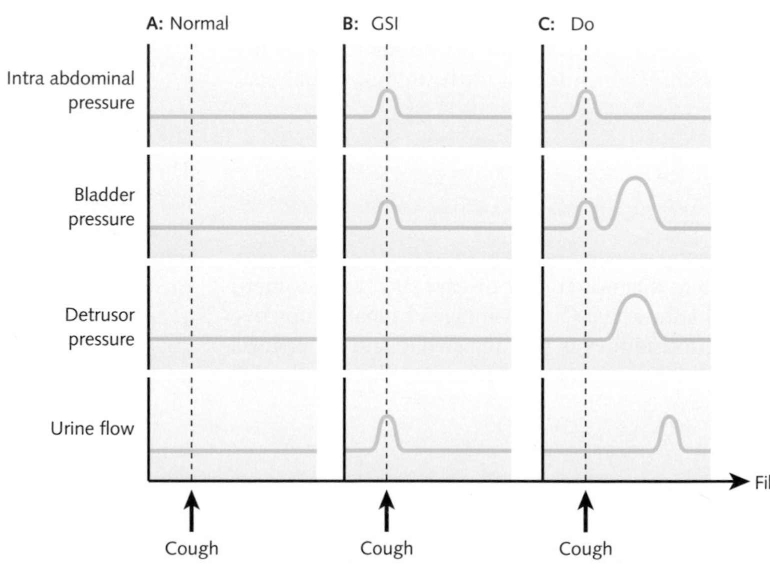

- congenital anomalies, diverticulae, fistulae and ureteric reflux – identified during the filling phase
- bladder neck descent and stress urinary incontinence – might be seen on coughing
- ureteric reflux, urethral fistulae and outflow pathology – can be seen on voiding.

Further reading

NICE. Available online at: www.nice.org.uk/CG40 (accessed 07.01.12).

RCOG. Available online at: www.rcog.org.uk (accessed 07.01.12).

Abnormal uterine bleeding

Objectives

By the end of this chapter, you should be able to:

- Understand the important points in the history for a patient presenting with abnormal uterine bleeding
- Perform an examination on a patient presenting with abnormal uterine bleeding
- Undertake appropriate investigations on a patient presenting with abnormal uterine bleeding in order to establish a diagnosis and treatment.

Abnormal uterine bleeding is a common problem experienced by most women at some time in their life. The causes can be physiological or pathological and, as long as serious pathology is excluded, might not require treatment. For normal menstruation to occur, the following are necessary:

- Hypothalamic function
- Pituitary function
- Ovarian function
- Endometrial function
- Patent cervix and vagina.

Abnormal uterine bleeding can be caused by malfunction or disease at any of these levels.

MENORRHAGIA

Menorrhagia (heavy menstrual bleeding) is defined as heavy cyclical periods, which interferes with physical, social and emotional quality of life. It can occur alone or in combination with other symptoms. Only about half of women complaining of heavy periods actually have menorrhagia, which is defined as more than 80 mL of menstrual blood loss (MBL) per period. This represents two standard deviations above the mean MBL, which is about 40 mL per period. Two-thirds of women with genuine menorrhagia will have iron-deficiency anaemia. Both local and systemic conditions can cause menorrhagia (Fig. 5.1).

Incidence

The incidence of menorrhagia is reported to be 9–15% of population samples in Western Europe; however, as many as one-third of women regard their menstrual loss as heavy. Early menarche, late menopause, reduction in family size with concurrent reduction in periods of lactational amenorrhoea have all contributed to an almost tenfold increase in the number of periods that women experience during their reproductive life. This has meant that excessive menstrual bleeding has become one of the most common causes of concern for health in women.

Diagnosis

Menorrhagia can be diagnosed using the following techniques:

- Subjective assessment
- Pictorial blood loss assessment charts (Fig. 5.2)
- Objective assessment.

Only half of women complaining of heavy periods will have menorrhagia, so relying on subjective assessment alone will mean that many women are treated for a condition that they do not have. A visual method of assessing menstrual blood loss using pictorial charts has been shown to be more effective at diagnosing menorrhagia than subjective assessment alone. This considers the degree to which each item of sanitary protection is soiled with blood as well as the quantity used, but, interestingly, the charts are not frequently used in practice.

Objective measurement of menstrual blood loss is rarely performed and usually only during clinical trials. This is because collecting and storing soiled sanitary protection for measurement of menstrual blood loss requires time and is inconvenient for most patients.

Aetiology

There are three categories for the aetiology of menorrhagia (Fig. 5.1):

1. Systemic conditions
2. Local pathology
3. Iatrogenic causes.

Fig. 5.1 Causes of menorrhagia.

Classification	Specific of cause of menorrhagia
Systemic disorders	Thyroid disease Clotting disorders
Local causes	Fibroids Endometrial polyps Endometrial carcinoma Endometriosis/adenomyosis Pelvic inflammatory disease Dysfunctional uterine bleeding
Iatrogenic causes	Intrauterine contraceptive devices Oral anticoagulants

Systemic conditions

The relationship between hypothyroidism and menorrhagia has not been confirmed because of insufficient objective data, although anecdotal individual cases have been reported.

Up to 90% of women with bleeding disorders have menorrhagia. Coagulation disorders are found in up to one-third of young women admitted to hospital with profound menorrhagia.

Local pathology

Fibroids increase menstrual loss in two ways:

1. They enlarge the uterine cavity, thereby increasing the surface area of the endometrium from which menstruation occurs
2. They may produce prostaglandins, which have been implicated in the aetiology of menorrhagia.

In a similar way, endometrial polyps increase the surface area of the endometrium and are also hormonally active.

Menstrual blood loss in the presence of pelvic pathology, such as endometriosis and PID, is variable and often in the normal range. Menorrhagia is therefore associated with, but not necessarily caused by, these conditions.

Dysfunctional uterine bleeding (DUB) is the most common cause of menorrhagia and is the term used when there are no apparent local or systemic causes for menorrhagia. It is therefore a diagnosis made by exclusion. Altered endometrial prostaglandin metabolism seems to have an important role in the aetiology of DUB. This is supported by the fact that prostaglandin inhibitors decrease menstrual blood loss in women with DUB.

Premalignant and malignant endometrium may present with menorrhagia and must always be excluded.

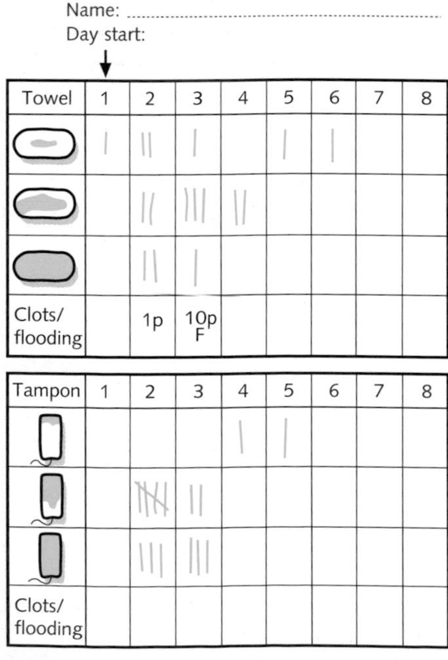

Fig. 5.2 Pictorial blood loss assessment chart.

Iatrogenic causes

The presence of an intrauterine contraceptive device (IUCD) may increase menstrual blood loss and is the most common iatrogenic cause of menorrhagia. Menorrhagia and iron deficiency anaemia are up to five times more common in IUCD users than with other forms of contraception.

Roughly one half of women taking oral anticoagulants have objective evidence of menorrhagia.

Of all the women complaining of heavy periods, only half will truly have menorrhagia. It is, therefore, important to use appropriate medical therapy for heavy periods and to counsel women effectively about surgical procedures. It is important that women with normal periods do not undergo unnecessary surgical intervention.

Complications

Apart from the effect on the quality of life and interference with both social life and work, which can be profound, the most common complication of menorrhagia is iron-deficiency anaemia.

History

A full gynaecological history should be taken. The length and frequency of menstruation should be noted, together with any intermenstrual and post-coital bleeding. Although subjective assessment does not quantify menorrhagia, the presence of clots and flooding, wearing double sanitary protection (internal and external), nocturnal soiling and interference with work or social events, all imply increased menstrual loss. Symptoms of iron deficiency anaemia might be present, including lethargy and breathlessness.

Menstrual pain, or dysmenorrhoea, is often associated with menorrhagia and usually occurs when the flow is heaviest. Premenstrual pain can indicate endometriosis (see Chapter 8). Fever, pelvic pain, dyspareunia and vaginal discharge are common symptoms of pelvic inflammatory disease (PID; see Chapter 13).

A history of PCOS increases the risk of endometrial hyperplasia and carcinoma. Symptoms of thyroid disease or clotting disorders can indicate a systemic cause of menorrhagia. Clotting disorders presenting with menorrhagia usually do so in the teenage years.

A contraceptive history is important. Normal periods experienced after stopping the COCP may appear heavier than the withdrawal bleeds associated with the COCP. Symptoms of heavy or painful periods dating from the insertion of an IUCD would suggest that it is the cause.

Examination

General examination aims to identify signs of iron deficiency anaemia, thyroid or clotting disorders. Abdominal examination might reveal a mass (e.g. fibroid uterus) arising from the pelvis.

Speculum examination may reveal vaginal discharge and cervical pathology, including cervicitis or frank malignancy. Occasionally, endometrial polyps or pedunculated fibroids will be seen prolapsing through the cervical os.

Bimanual examination might reveal an enlarged uterus due to fibroids, pelvic tenderness associated with endometriosis or PID and the presence of adnexal masses.

Investigations

Investigation (Fig. 5.3) is aimed at excluding the systemic and local causes of menorrhagia and includes:

- blood tests – a full blood count should be performed in all cases. Thyroid function and clotting studies should only be performed if clinically indicated
- ultrasound – a pelvic ultrasound will identify uterine enlargement caused by fibroids and adnexal masses. Endometrial polyps or submucous fibroids should be suspected if the endometrial thickness is excessive for the time of the menstrual cycle
- an endometrial biopsy – should be performed on all women aged over 45 years and in women under 45 years if there are risk factors in the history such as persistent intermenstrual bleeding or suspicious findings on ultrasound scan. This can be performed either in the outpatient clinic or under general anaesthesia. It might show endometrium inappropriate to the menstrual cycle secondary to anovulation, endometrial hyperplasia or carcinoma. A cervical smear should also be performed where this is due, or sooner if there is a history of intermenstrual or postcoital bleeding
- current methods of endometrial sampling – for example pipelle biopsy. These appear to be at least as accurate as D&C, have high levels of patient acceptability, lower complication rates and do not require inpatient admission or general anaesthesia. However, they may miss benign and malignant endometrial pathology and must therefore be considered inadequate for the further investigation of menorrhagia that has persisted despite medical therapy. In this instance, a hysteroscopy plus sampling should be performed either as an outpatient or under general anaesthesia depending on facilities and patient preference
- diagnostic hysteroscopy – the most effective way of excluding intrauterine pathology. This can be performed in the outpatient setting without analgesia and will identify endometrial polyps, submucous fibroids, endometritis and most endometrial carcinomas. Where appropriate, laparoscopy will be indicated to exclude pelvic pathology.

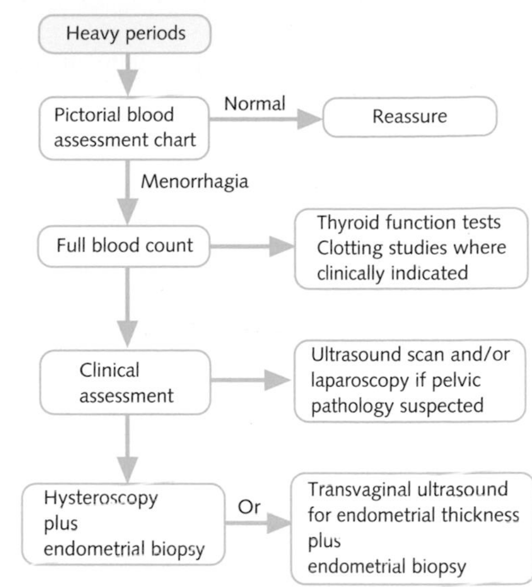

Fig. 5.3 Investigating menorrhagia.

N.B. Evidence suggests that a blind D&C, used as a diagnostic or therapeutic tool in the management of menorrhagia, is inadequate when used alone.

Abnormal bleeding before the age of 40 does not usually require endometrial sampling unless the patient is at high risk of endometrial hyperplasia, e.g. PCOS and increased BMI.

Treatment

Treatment of menorrhagia should be tailored to the patient's needs, fertility wishes and also to the findings of investigations. Practically, this includes:

- correcting iron-deficiency anaemia
- treating systemic disorders or focal pathology
- attempted control of menorrhagia by medical treatment and, if this fails
- surgical treatment.

Treatment of menorrhagia secondary to fibroids is considered in Chapter 7.

Medical treatment of menorrhagia

The two main forms of medical treatment for menorrhagia are:

- antifibrinolytics
- hormonal preparations.

The efficacy of medical treatment varies from individual to individual. The reduction of mean MBL for different medical therapies is shown in Figure 5.4.

Antifibrinolytics and haemostatics

Tranexamic acid is an antifibrinolytic that inhibits the activation of plasminogen to plasmin. It reduces the excessive fibrinolytic activity found in the endometrium of menorrhagic women. It is widely used for the treatment of heavy periods as it is effective for a substantial proportion of women. Its most important side effect is the risk of thrombosis, although uncommon. In women with menorrhagia, who have no history or family history of thrombosis, it should be regarded as the first line of medical treatment.

Prostaglandin inhibitors

Several non-steroidal anti-inflammatory drugs (NSAIDs), including aspirin, indomethacin and mefenamic acid, inhibit the cyclo-oxygenase enzyme system, which controls the production of cyclic endoperoxides from arachidonic acid. NSAIDs improve:

- MBL in 75% of women, with a mean reduction of 50%
- dysmenorrhoea
- menstrual headaches.

NSAIDS are taken during menstruation, so side effects are usually better tolerated than with drugs that are taken throughout the menstrual cycle.

Hormonal therapy

Progestogens

Oral progestogens used to be the most common drugs used to treat menorrhagia, but may not be the most effective. Early studies showed an improvement in subjective MBL but objective studies have shown no statistical improvement. They are most effectively used in anovulatory menorrhagia to gain cycle control.

Intrauterine systems

Intrauterine contraceptive systems with either progesterone or levonorgestrel dramatically reduce MBL as well as acting as contraception. The Mirena intrauterine system releases 20 μg of levonorgestrel every 24 h into the endometrium from a silicone barrel. As a result of minimal systemic absorption, side effects are usually limited to irregular spotting in the initial year of use.

Amenorrhoea occurs in up to 50% of long-term users because of endometrial atrophy. Contraceptively, it is as effective as sterilization, although fertility returns almost immediately once it is removed. Since it was granted its license in the UK for the treatment of menorrhagia for up to 5 years per system the use of the Mirena IUS for the treatment of heavy periods has increased dramatically.

HINTS AND TIPS

The most effective medical therapy for menorrhagia is either anti-fibrinolytics for women wanting to conceive or the levonorgestrel intrauterine system (Mirena IUS) for those who don't. The Mirena IUS's contraceptive efficacy is as good as sterilization.

Fig. 5.4 Mean per cent reduction in measured menstrual blood loss in women with menorrhagia treated with medical therapy.

Drug	Mean % MBL reduction
Non-steroidal anti-inflammatory drugs (NSAIDs):	
Mefenamic acid	47
Antifibrinolytics	
Tranexamic acid	54
Hormonal therapy	
COCP	50
Danazol	60
Levonorgestrel IUS	97
Luteal phase progestogen	15

The combined oral contraceptive pill

When taken in a cyclical fashion, the COCP inhibits ovulation and produces regular shedding of a thin endometrium. This makes it an effective long-term medical treatment for some women with menorrhagia. Thrombogenic side effects should be discussed with older women and smokers who are considering using COCP for therapeutic reasons.

Danazol

Danazol is a testosterone derivative producing a number of effects on the hypothalamic-pituitary-ovarian axis. It is not commonly used. The optimum dosage in the treatment of menorrhagia appears to be 200 mg daily, significantly reducing mean MBL as well as reducing dysmenorrhoea. The androgenic properties of danazol produce unacceptable side effects in some women.

Gonadotrophin-releasing hormone agonists

GnRH agonists suppress pituitary–ovarian function and effectively produce a temporary, reversible menopausal state. Because of the subsequent bone density loss their long-term use as a primary medical treatment for menorrhagia is limited unless add-back hormone therapy is given. This relegates their clinical use to that of preoperative aid, allowing:

- correction of iron-deficiency anaemia
- reduction in the size of fibroids
- reduction in surgical blood loss.

Medical management of menorrhagia should be tailored to the patient's individual needs. Guidelines for managing menorrhagia are shown in Figure 5.5.

Surgical treatment of menorrhagia

The exact surgical procedure used to treat menorrhagia depends on the diagnosis:

- Intrauterine pathology such as endometrial polyps and submucous fibroids should be removed hysteroscopically. This reduces MBL by 75%.
- Open myomectomy may be required for large fibroids, where the uterus is to be conserved.
- Endometrial ablative methods are becoming increasingly popular due to rapid recovery and the possibility of outpatient treatment.
- Hysterectomy – this is reserved for women who continue to experience menorrhagia despite trying other treatments and is discussed below in detail.

Endometrial ablation

Endometrial ablation is a day-case procedure which reduces menstrual blood loss by producing an 'iatrogenic' Asherman's syndrome. Endometrium is destroyed using laser, resection, thermal or microwave ablation techniques and the ensuing intrauterine adhesions reduce endometrial regrowth from deep within crypts or glands. It is therefore not suitable for women wishing to conceive.

Although this does not guarantee amenorrhoea as hysterectomy does, advantages include speed of surgery, quicker recovery, rapid return to work and the use of local as opposed to general anaesthesia. Following endometrial ablation, MBL has been shown to be reduced by up to 90%.

Complications of endometrial ablation

The most common operative complications are:

- uterine perforation – this commonly occurs where the uterine wall is thinnest, such as the cornual regions and the cervical canal. It is associated with fluid overload, trauma to the gastrointestinal and genitourinary tracts and major blood vessels resulting in peritonitis or haemorrhage.

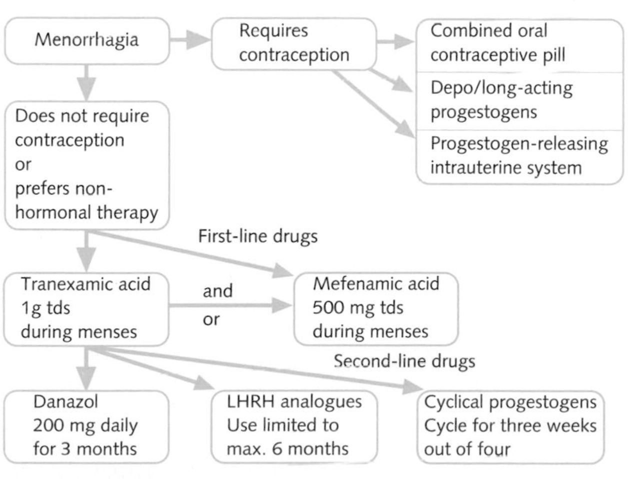

Fig. 5.5 Algorithm for investigating and managing menorrhagia.

- fluid overload – the use of non-electrolytic solutions, such as 1.5% glycine, for electrosurgery and the pressures needed to distend the uterine walls predispose to the absorption of large quantities of fluid, which can result in hyponatraemia due to dilutional effects of the irrigating fluid. Congestive cardiac failure, hypertension, neurological symptoms, haemolysis and coma occur.
- haemorrhage – this can occur if the myometrium is resected too deeply or if the uterus is perforated.
- infection – the true incidence of pelvic infection following endometrial ablation is difficult to quantify. Infection can be overwhelming and might cause long-term pelvic pain.

Rarely, deaths have occurred after endometrial ablation; these have been due to air embolism during laser ablation, toxic shock following endometrial resection, sepsis from bowel perforation and from haemorrhage following major pelvic vessel transection.

Hysterectomy

Hysterectomy was one of the most commonly performed operations in the UK. In 1993–4, 73 517 hysterectomies were performed in NHS hospitals and approximately two-thirds of these were performed for menorrhagia. By 2002, the number of hysterectomies had fallen to 44 000 due to better diagnostic abilities, better medical treatment and the development of focal and ablative hysteroscopic techniques.

Hysterectomy can be vaginal, laparoscopic or abdominal, depending on the uterine findings. Total abdominal hysterectomy is useful for women with large uteri, multiple large fibroids, adenomyosis, pelvic adhesions and endometriosis.

Hysterectomy can be a 'subtotal' procedure, where the cervix is left behind and can include removing the ovaries, to reduce the risk of ovarian cancer (oophorectomy). If the cervix is left behind, cervical smears must be continued.

Complications of hysterectomy

Almost half the women undergoing abdominal hysterectomy and one-quarter of those undergoing vaginal hysterectomy experience a complication. Although conditions such as thromboembolic disease should not be forgotten, the following are some of the more likely complications to be encountered:

- Short term complications:
  - Fever
  - Haemorrhage requiring transfusion
- Unintended major surgery because of:
  - Urinary tract damage
  - Bowel damage
- Long-term complications, e.g. pain, regret.

The mortality rate following hysterectomy for benign disease is very low — approximately 6 per 10 000 — and is usually a consequence of cardiovascular disease and sepsis.

Fever

This is the most common complication following hysterectomy, with one in three women experiencing this following the abdominal approach. In one-quarter of cases the source of infection is not identifiable; the most common identifiable infection is urinary tract infection, followed by wound or vaginal cuff infection. The use of prophylactic antibiotics is associated with a lower rate of infection of the urinary tract, abdominal wound and vaginal cuff.

Urinary tract damage

Damage to the ureter occurs in approximately 1 in every 200 hysterectomies. The ureter is likely to be damaged at the infundibulopelvic ligament, beneath the uterine artery and adjacent to the cervix. Predisposing factors to ureteric damage include congenital anomaly of the renal tracts and distortion of normal anatomy from pelvic inflammatory disease, endometriosis and malignancy.

Trauma to the bladder occurs in approximately 1 in 100 hysterectomies and is much higher following vaginal hysterectomy. Predisposing factors include previous surgery and obesity.

Bowel damage

The incidence of bowel trauma is approximately 1 in 200 hysterectomies. Risk factors predisposing to bowel damage are obesity, previous laparotomy, adhesions, intrinsic bowel problems (e.g. chronic inflammatory bowel disease) and irradiation.

Bowel dysfunction following hysterectomy is well documented, with constipation occurring in up to half the patients during the first 2 weeks of the abdominal approach. One in five patients will continue to experience constipation in the first three postoperative months.

Long-term complications of hysterectomy

When the uterus is removed, the pelvic floor and its nerve supply are disrupted. This can predispose to pelvic floor laxity with subsequent prolapse, as well as bladder and bowel dysfunction. Even when the ovaries are conserved, disruption of their blood supply can interfere with their function, and might even predispose to premature ovarian failure, a risk factor for cardiovascular disease and osteoporosis.

INTERMENSTRUAL AND POSTCOITAL BLEEDING

Intermenstrual and postcoital bleeding are common symptoms that can indicate serious underlying pathology.

Fig. 5.6 Causes of intermenstrual and postcoital bleeding.

Affected region/system	Specific cause
Cervical	Ectopy Polyps Malignancy Cervicitis
Intra-uterine	Polyps Submucous fibroids Endometrial hyperplasia Endometrial malignancy Endometritis
Hormonal	Breakthrough bleeding

Intermenstrual bleeding occurs between the menstrual periods and can be caused by local lesions of the cervix or intrauterine cavity (Fig. 5.6).

Postcoital bleeding is precipitated by intercourse and is caused by similar conditions.

History and examination

History taking, examination and investigation are similar to menorrhagia and should aim to exclude local causes and cervical pathology.

Investigation

In women with unexplained symptoms, the following should be considered:

- HVS, ECS – to exclude sexually transmitted infections
- Cervical smear – to exclude CIN or cervical cancer
- Pelvic ultrasound – to identify uterine polyps or fibroids
- Hysteroscopy – to obtain an endometrial biopsy in women with persistent intermenstrual bleeding.
- Laparoscopy – to identify pelvic pathology such as endometriotic nodules which may cause post-coital or intermenstrual bleeding.

Treatment

Treatment may involve:

- antibiotics for sexually transmitted infections
- cautery to the cervical surface
- removal of uterine polyps/fibroids.

HINTS AND TIPS

Intermenstrual and post-coital bleeding can be a sign of cervical malignancy, so a history of cervical smears and STIs must be taken. Clinical inspection of the cervix and an up-to-date smear are essential (see Chapter 4 for taking a smear).

POSTMENOPAUSAL BLEEDING

Postmenopausal bleeding (PMB) is vaginal bleeding occurring more than 12 months after the menopause. In clinical practice, the menopause is a retrospective diagnosis and it is therefore important to keep in mind, and exclude, causes of secondary amenorrhoea such as pregnancy. PMB is a common disorder and requires prompt investigation to exclude malignancy. Of all women in the UK with PMB 9% will be found to have a malignancy.

Figure 5.7 shows the causes of PMB using the anatomy of the female genital tract as a guide. Atrophic changes to the genital tract are the most common cause but must not be assumed to be the cause until other pathology, especially malignancy, have been excluded.

HINTS AND TIPS

Always investigate PMB promptly to exclude malignancy. Uterine malignancy is often detected early because it presents with abnormal uterine bleeding. Cervical malignancy can present with intermenstrual and post-coital bleeding, or smear abnormalities.

Aetiology

There are many causes of PMB (Fig. 5.7), but the most important causes to exclude are malignancy of the endometrium, cervix and ovary.

Fig. 5.7 Causes of postmenopausal bleeding.

Affected structure	Cause of postmenopausal bleeding
Ovary	Carcinoma of the ovary Oestrogen-secreting tumour
Uterine body	Myometrium:submucous fibroid Endometrium: atrophic changes polyp hyperplasia: simple or atypical carcinoma
Cervix	Atrophic changes Malignancy: squamous carcinoma adenocarcinoma
Vagina	Atrophic changes
Urethra	Urethral caruncle Haematuria
Vulva	Vulvitis Dystrophies Malignancy

Atrophic changes to the lower genital tract due to oestrogen deficiency can cause bleeding and, in fact, are the most common cause of PMB. Atrophic changes can occur to the endometrium, cervix and vagina. Urethral caruncle (prolapse of the urethral mucosa) is also associated with oestrogen deficiency.

Submucous fibroids or uterine polyps can cause PMB, although these are likely to have existed from before the menopause. The endometrium should be inactive in the postmenopausal years and atrophic endometritis is a common consequence. Endometrial polyps might be benign, contain areas of atypical hyperplasia or be malignant.

Endometrial hyperplasia can arise de novo, or be secondary to oestrogen stimulation. Exogenous unopposed oestrogens and endogenous oestrogens arising from peripheral conversion of precursors in adipose tissue, or from oestrogen-secreting ovarian tumours, can result in endometrial hyperplasia and adenocarcinoma.

Adenocarcinoma of the endometrium is an important cause of PMB and must always be considered in the differential diagnosis.

Cervical carcinoma and squamous carcinoma of the vulva can present with PMB and, although the non-neoplastic epithelial disorders of the vulva (vulval dystrophies) do not themselves usually cause PMB, scratching because of pruritus vulvae may.

Disease of the ovary in postmenopausal women is uncommon but can present with PMB. An oestrogen-secreting tumour causes PMB by stimulating the endometrium in the absence of progesterone. This can cause hyperplasia and even carcinoma of the endometrium. Ovarian carcinoma usually causes PMB by direct invasion through the uterine wall.

HINTS AND TIPS

There are several causes of PMB, but the easiest way to remember them is to consider the causes anatomically – atrophic vaginitis, cervical abnormalities/malignancy, uterine polyps/fibroids/malignancy, ovarian malignancy (rare).

History

Atrophic changes to the genital tract usually present with small amounts of bleeding. Local symptoms of oestrogen deficiency include vaginal dryness, soreness and superficial dyspareunia. Pruritus vulvae can indicate the presence of non-neoplastic disorders of the vulva (traditionally known as vulval dystrophies) and the presence of a lump, whether painful or painless, can suggest a vulval neoplasm.

Profuse vaginal bleeding or the presence of a blood-stained offensive discharge is an ominous sign and can indicate cervical or endometrial malignancy. PMB is usually the only presenting symptom of other endometrial cavity pathology, such as endometrial polyps or submucous fibroids.

Some ovarian tumours can stimulate endometrial proliferation and therefore cause bleeding.

Family history, drug history (including the use of HRT) and smear history are particularly important. Medical comorbidities such as obesity and coagulation disorders should also be noted.

Examination

Inspect the patient for signs of iron-deficiency anaemia.

Abdominal examination might reveal ascites or a mass arising from the pelvis.

Vulval lesions should be evident on vaginal examination. The vagina and cervix should be inspected using a speculum, to exclude atrophic vaginitis and a bimanual examination performed. Postmenopausal ovaries should not be palpable on bimanual examination.

Investigation

The following investigations should be performed on all women with PMB:

- Ultrasound examination of the pelvis
- Hysteroscopic examination of the uterine cavity
- Endometrial biopsy.

Intrauterine pathology is best excluded by hysteroscopic examination of the uterine cavity with endometrial biopsy, although ultrasound estimation of the endometrial thickness combined with endometrial sampling can be used. The endometrial thickness in a postmenopausal woman should be less than 5 mm. Although a negative endometrial sample is reassuring, the commonest method of taking the sample in the outpatient setting is by using the 'pipelle' endometrial sampler, which samples only 4% of the uterine cavity. Ultrasound with biopsy can, therefore, miss early focal pathology. The ovaries can be assessed using ultrasound and if an oestrogen-secreting tumour is suspected, circulating oestradiol levels should be measured.

When indicated the following investigations should also be performed:

- Vulval biopsies
- Cervical cytology or colposcopy
- Cystoscopy
- Sigmoidoscopy
- Oestradiol levels.

Occasionally, it is not always obvious whether the bleeding is vaginal, rectal or from the bladder, and in

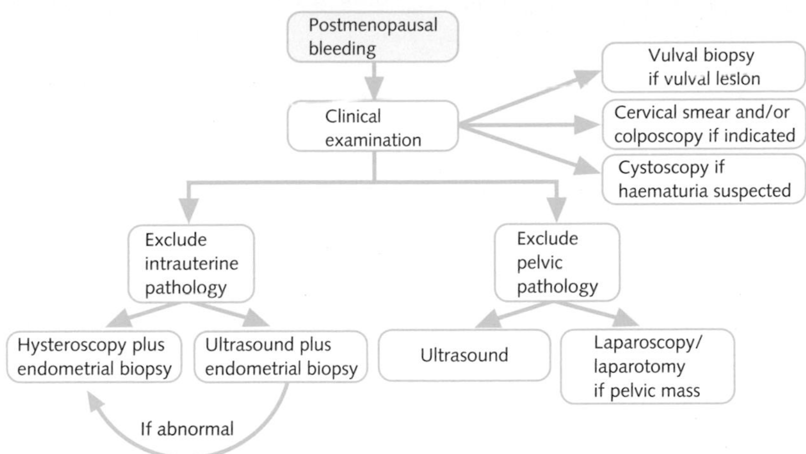

Fig. 5.8 Algorithm for postmenopausal bleeding.

these cases cystoscopy and sigmoidoscopy as well as hysteroscopy should be performed. In the very elderly, bimanual examination might not be possible, in which case examination under anaesthesia is indicated. However, elderly frail women are not always ideal candidates for general anaesthesia and less invasive investigations, such as ultrasound, are therefore, first-line.

Figure 5.8 provides an algorithm for the diagnosis and investigation of PMB.

Treatment

Treatment depends on the pathology. The most common cause of PMB is atrophic change and, therefore, oestrogen replacement is indicated not only to prevent a recurrence of PMB, but also to treat other symptoms associated with oestrogen deficiency (e.g. dyspareunia). Most women in this situation prefer to use topical oestrogen. The newer 17β oestradiol-releasing creams, rings and vaginal tablets avoid the risk of endometrial hyperplasia by minimizing systemic absorption. If systemic HRT is requested then oestrogen therapy must be combined with a progestogen in women who have a uterus.

The treatment of urethral caruncle is by surgical excision of the prolapsed urethral mucosa and is a painful and unpleasant procedure. It should, therefore, be reserved for those cases in which recurrent PMB or pain occur. Small caruncles might recede with oestrogen cream.

The treatment of vulval, cervical and ovarian malignancy is discussed in detail in Chapter 10, and fibroids are discussed in Chapter 7.

Further reading

Lethaby, A.E., Cooke, I., Rees, M., 2005. Progesterone or progestogen-releasing intrauterine systems for heavy menstrual bleeding. Cochrane Database Syst. Rev. (4): CD002126.

Lethaby, A., Farquhar, C., Cooke, I., 2000. Antifibrinolytics for heavy menstrual bleeding. Cochrane Database Syst. Rev. (4): CD000249.

Lethaby, A., Irvine, G., Cameron, I., 2008. Cyclical progestogens for heavy menstrual bleeding. Cochrane Database Syst. Rev. (1): CD001016.

Lethaby, A., Augood, C., Duckitt, K., 2013. Nonsteroidal anti-inflammatory drugs for heavy menstrual bleeding. Cochrane Database Syst. Rev. (1): CD000400.

Llewellyn-Jones, D., 2010. Fundamentals of Obstetrics & Gynaecology, 9th ed. Mosby, London.

McKay Hart, D., Norman, J., 2000. Gynaecology Illustrated, fifth ed. Churchill Livingstone, London.

NICE, 2007. Heavy Menstrual Bleeding: Investigation and Treatment. Clinical Guideline 44. National Institute for Health and Care Excellence, London. Available online at: www.nice.org.uk/guidance.

Nieboer, T.E., Johnson, N., Lethaby, A., Tavender, E., Curr, E., Garry, R., van Voorst, S., Mol, B.W., Kluivers, K.B., 2009. Surgical approach to hysterectomy for benign gynaecological disease. Cochrane Database Syst. Rev. (3):CD003677. doi:10.1002/14651858.CD003677.pub4.

Oehler, M.K., Rees, M.C., 2003. Menorrhagia: an update. Acta Obstet. Gynecol. Scand. 82, 405–422.

Reid, P.C., Mukri, F., 2005. Trends in number of hysterectomies performed in England for menorrhagia: examination of health episode statistics, 1989 to 2002–3. BMJ 330, 938–939.

Shaw, R.W., Soutter, W.P., Stanton, S.L., 1997. Gynaecology, 2nd ed. Churchill Livingstone, London.

Pelvic pain and dyspareunia

Objectives

By the end of this chapter, you should be able to:

- Understand the important points in the history for a patient presenting with pelvic pain or dyspareunia
- Perform an examination on a patient presenting with pelvic pain or dyspareunia
- Undertake appropriate investigations on a patient presenting with pelvic pain or dyspareunia in order to establish a diagnosis.

DIFFERENTIAL DIAGNOSIS

Pelvic pain, as for any type of pain, can be either:

- acute, or
- chronic.

Chronic pelvic pain is defined as pelvic pain that lasts 6 months duration or more. Often associated with 'dyspareunia', the term used to describe painful sexual intercourse. This is classified as superficial or deep, depending on whether it is experienced superficially at the area of the vulva and introitus or deep within the pelvis.

Figures 6.1 and 6.2 show the differential diagnoses that should be considered when the patient presents with these symptoms.

HISTORY

Because the differential diagnosis is so diverse, a thorough history is important.

Presenting complaint

A detailed history of the pain is essential to distinguish between pain of acute onset and chronic pain. The following characteristics should be elicited:

- Is it continuous or intermittent?
- Duration of the pain
- Nature of the pain – is it sharp or dull?
- Exacerbating or relieving factors – if needing opiates
- Site of the pain – is it unilateral or bilateral?
- Radiation to the back or legs
- Relationship of the pain to the menstrual cycle
- Relationship to bowel habit
- Associated symptoms, such as nausea and vomiting, vaginal discharge, vulval irritation.

For example, the pain related to torsion of an ovarian cyst is typically of acute onset, worse on one side of the pelvis than the other, associated with nausea and vomiting, and radiating to the upper thighs. It is important to make this diagnosis promptly because an operation to relieve the torsion might save the ovary from irreversible ischaemia.

Mittelschmerz is an acute pain associated with ovulation. To make this diagnosis, it is, therefore, essential to know the timing of the pain in relation to the patient's menstrual cycle. Endometriosis is also related to menses, typically starting up to 2 weeks before the period and usually being relieved when the bleeding starts. Deep dyspareunia is commonly associated with this condition.

Pelvic inflammatory disease (PID) may or may not be associated with vaginal discharge. The pain is typically felt across the whole of the lower abdomen and there might be a history of fever.

In relation to bowel habit, appendicitis can be associated with nausea and vomiting. Diverticulitis is more likely to be associated with constipation and to affect the older population.

Past gynaecological history

The date of the patient's last menstrual period (LMP) is important to exclude current pregnancy and the possibility of a miscarriage or ectopic pregnancy. It may also be relevant if symptoms such as superficial dyspareunia are consistent with the perimenopause. The date and result of the last cervical smear test should be checked, as well as a history of irregular or postcoital bleeding, which might be associated with malignancy.

Recent gynaecological procedures that involve instrumentation of the uterus could put the patient at risk of developing PID (e.g. insertion of an IUCD, termination of pregnancy or hysteroscopy).

Fig. 6.1 Differential diagnosis of pelvic pain.

Acute	Chronic
Pelvic inflammatory disease (see Chapter 26) **Tubo-ovarian abscess** post-termination of pregnancy post-insertion of IUCD post-hysteroscopy	**Adenomyosis** (see Chapter 22) **Endometriosis** **Adhesions** gynaecological operation pelvic inflammatory disease appendicitis
Early pregnancy complications (see Chapter 32) miscarriage ectopic pregnancy	
Gynaecological malignancy (see Chapter 24)	**Gynaecological malignancy**
Ovarian cyst (see Chapter 23) rupture haemorrhage torsion	**Gastrointestinal pathology** diverticulitis irritable bowel syndrome
Fibroid necrosis (see Chapter 21)	
Ovulation pain (Mittelschmerz)	
Abscess Bartholin's cyst labial	
Urinary tract infection **Renal calculi**	
Appendicitis	

Fig. 6.2 Differential diagnosis of dyspareunia.

Superficial	Deep
Congenital vaginal atresia vaginal septum	**Congenital** incomplete vaginal atresia vaginal septum
Infection vulvovaginitis (see Chapter 3)	**Infection** PID (see Chapter 26)
Postsurgery relating to childbirth pelvic floor repair	**Postsurgery** relating to childbirth pelvic floor repair
Vulval disease Bartholin's cyst vulval dystrophies carcinoma of vulva	**Pelvic disease** endometriosis fibroids ovarian cyst/tumours
Psychosexual vaginismus	**Psychosexual** vaginismus
Atrophic changes postmenopausal	

A history of sexually transmitted disease, previous PID or pelvic surgery could result in adhesion formation. This is more likely to result in a picture of chronic pain, and can be difficult to treat. Pelvic floor repair can alter the vagina in such a way as to cause deep dyspareunia. Recent childbirth is a common cause of superficial dyspareunia, particularly if suturing of vaginal lacerations or episiotomy was necessary.

Congenital malformations of the genital tract are rare and are likely to present before the patient is sexually active and experiencing dyspareunia. There might be a history of previous operations to restore normal anatomy.

Past medical/surgical history

A history of appendicectomy excludes one of the common differential diagnoses of pelvic pain. Find out if any contraindications to non-steroidal anti-inflammatories (NSAIDs), e.g. peptic ulcer disease.

Drug history

The type of analgesia and frequency of use is helpful to determine the severity of pelvic pain. A postmenopausal patient who has not been using hormone replacement therapy may have superficial dyspareunia secondary to atrophic changes.

Sexual history

Current use of contraception must be checked, both to exclude pregnancy and to determine the risk of PID. A recent change of partner increases the risk, particularly if no barrier contraception has been used.

With regard to dyspareunia, there may be a history of difficulty with intercourse, suggesting vaginismus. This might be a difficult subject for the patient and care should be taken to broach it in a sympathetic manner.

A sexual history must be taken in a sensitive manner with particular attention to a new partner, possible relationship issues or a history of abuse.

Social history

A useful guide to the severity of symptoms in patients presenting with chronic pelvic pain is how it affects activities of daily living, for example, going to school or taking time off work.

A history of sexual abuse has been shown to be relevant to presentation with chronic pain. Again, a sensitive approach is essential in questioning.

EXAMINATION

- General examination
- Abdominal palpation
- Vulval/vaginal/cervical inspection
- Bimanual pelvic examination.

General examination

Pyrexia and tachycardia are associated with PID. Rupture of an ovarian cyst can cause intraperitoneal bleeding and, subsequently, hypotension with tachycardia. A ruptured ectopic pregnancy would also present with these signs. It should be noted that hypotension is a late sign in an otherwise healthy patient and its absence does not exclude these diagnoses.

Gynaecological malignancy is more likely to present with symptoms other than pelvic pain, more commonly in the older age group. However, signs such as abdominal distension (pelvic mass, ascites or abscess), cachexia and anaemia should be excluded.

Abdominal palpation

The site of the pain should be elicited, as should the presence of guarding or rebound tenderness, which suggest peritonism. An abdominal mass arising from the pelvis, such as an enlarged fibroid uterus, may be present. This could give symptoms of acute pelvic pain, if there is fibroid necrosis, or of deep dyspareunia.

Vulval/vaginal/cervical inspection

Figure 6.3 shows the diagnoses responsible for both pelvic pain and superficial dyspareunia that might affect the vulva and vagina. A speculum examination should be performed to look for discharge.

Bimanual pelvic examination

Tenderness

Generalized tenderness, including uterine, is more common with PID. This condition is also associated with cervical excitation (cervical motion tenderness) which indicates peritonism. The tenderness may be unilateral with an ovarian cyst or an ectopic pregnancy. A common site for endometriosis is the pouch of Douglas, and tender nodules can be palpated in the posterior fornix.

Mass

The following conditions may present with a pelvic mass:

- Tubo-ovarian abscess
- Ovarian cyst
- Endometriotic cyst

Fig. 6.3 Vulval/vaginal inspection.

Cause(s)	Symptoms and signs
Postmenopausal changes (see Chapter 29)	Vulval and vaginal skin appears thin and atrophic. This can cause superficial dyspareunia
Vulval dystrophies (see Chapter 25)	There might be patches of inflammation, leukoplakia and ulceration, which cause superficial dyspareunia
Episiotomy/lacerations (see Chapter 40)	Injury secondary to childbirth commonly causes superficial dyspareunia
Abscesses	A Bartholin's abscess is an abscess of the gland situated towards the posterior fourchette; labial abscesses are commonly situated on the labia majora. Both types cause acute pain and need incision and drainage

- Fibroid
- Ectopic pregnancy.

The uterus is enlarged in pregnancy and the cervical os might be open if the patient is miscarrying. A fixed, tender, retroverted uterus could be a result of endometriosis or PID. The uterus typically feels tender and bulky with adenomyosis.

INVESTIGATIONS

A summary list of the investigations used in patients who present with pelvic pain and dyspareunia is shown in Figure 6.4.

Blood tests

A full blood count (to check haemoglobin) and group-and-save sample are necessary if there is an early pregnancy complication with vaginal or suspected intraperitoneal bleeding. A white blood cell count and a C-reactive protein (CRP) level will aid diagnosis of infection.

Pregnancy test

A urine pregnancy test is mandatory in a patient of reproductive age with acute abdominal pain. It must be performed regardless of the date of the LMP or if the symptoms suggest a gastrointestinal cause. The presentation of an ectopic pregnancy can be atypical and may be fatal if not diagnosed.

Always perform a pregnancy test on a patient of reproductive age who presents with acute abdominal pain in order to exclude an ectopic pregnancy.

Fig. 6.4 Investigation of patients who have pelvic pain and dyspareunia.

Investigation	Procedure
Blood tests Pregnancy test	FBC/G&S/CRP
Infection screen	Midstream urine sample Vulval/high vaginal swabs Endocervical/urethral swabs
Radiological investigations	Pelvic ultrasound scan Abdominal X-ray
Biopsy for vulval disease	
Laparoscopy to exclude: endometriosis ovarian cyst ectopic pregnancy adhesions PID	

Infection screen

A midstream urine (MSU) sample should be sent to exclude a urinary tract infection. Swabs for sexually transmitted infection should be sent whether the pain history is chronic or acute. Most importantly these should include a test for *Chlamydia* infection, either an endocervical swab or a urine sample.

Radiological investigations

A pelvic ultrasound scan is important in acute and chronic pain, as well as with deep dyspareunia. Pathology can include ovarian cysts, uterine fibroids, ectopic pregnancy or intrauterine pregnancy.

A plain abdominal X-ray might be appropriate if the patient gives a history suggesting diverticulitis.

Biopsy

If the appearances of the vulva are abnormal, biopsy is indicated. This can be performed under local anaesthesia, depending on the size of the lesion.

Surgery

Figure 6.4 shows some of the diagnoses that can be confirmed by diagnostic laparoscopy. The woman must be made aware of surgical risks and the possibility of finding no abnormality (negative laparoscopy).

Figure 6.5 is an algorithm for the diagnosis, investigation and treatment of pelvic pain. Figure 6.6 provides the same information for dyspareunia.

Further reading

RCOG, 2008. Management of Acute Pelvic Inflammatory Disease. Green-top Guideline No. 32. Royal College of Obstetricians and Gynaecologists, London. Available online at:www.rcog.org.uk.

RCOG, 2012. Initial Management of Chronic Pelvic Pain. Green-top Guideline No. 41. Royal College of Obstetricians and Gynaecologists, London. Available online at:www.rcog.org.uk.

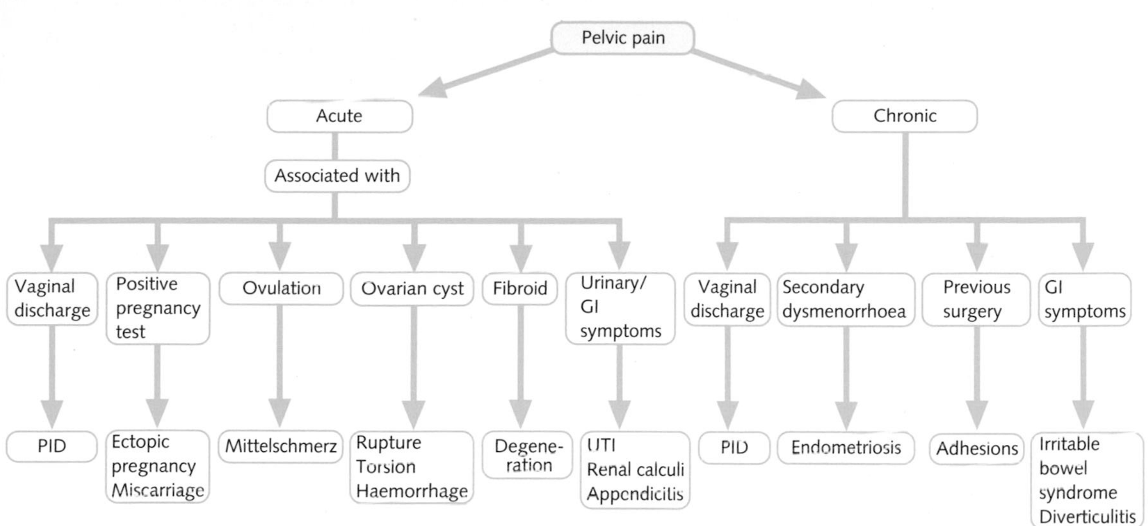

Fig. 6.5 Algorithm for pelvic pain.

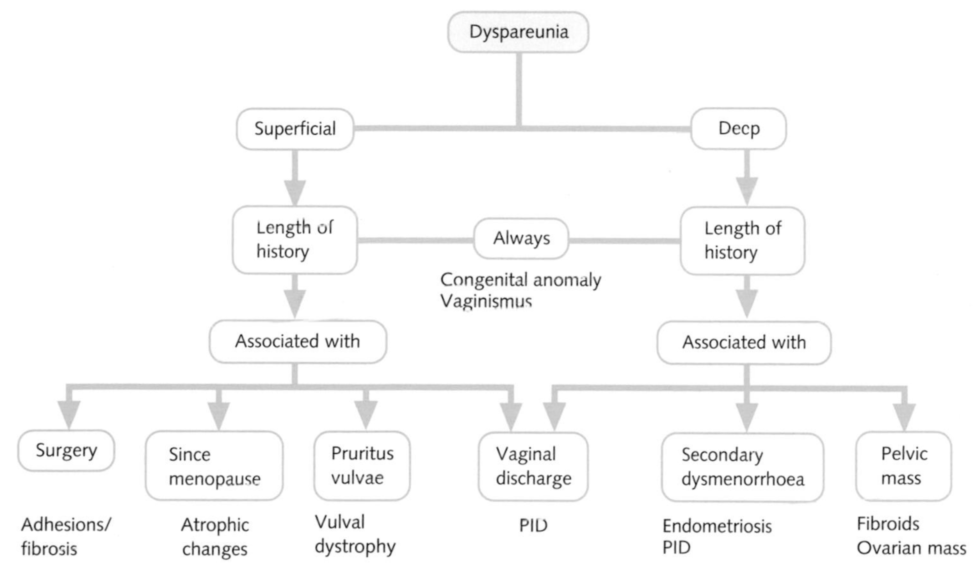

Fig. 6.6 Algorithm for dyspareunia.

Fibroids 7

Objectives

By the end of this chapter, you should be able to:
- Understand the prevalence and clinical impact of fibroids
- Outline where fibroids can occur and the impact location has on symptoms
- Discuss the medical, surgical and the newest treatments of fibroids.

Uterine fibroids are benign tumours of the myometrium. They are the most common benign tumours found in women, occurring in more than 50% of women over the age of 40 years. Histologically they are composed of whorling bundles of smooth muscle cells that resemble the architecture of normal myometrium.

Although their aetiology is unknown, fibroids are associated with exposure to oestrogens. Factors influencing the incidence of fibroids are shown in Figure 7.1. The hyperoestrogenic state of pregnancy can stimulate the growth of fibroids already present, whilst the hypoestrogenic state of menopause can reduce their size. Fibroids can be categorized by their position within the myometrium (Fig. 7.2).

SYMPTOMS OF UTERINE FIBROIDS

Symptoms associated with uterine fibroids are shown in Figure 7.3.

No symptoms

Approximately 50% of women with fibroids are asymptomatic. In these women, diagnosis is made during incidental clinical or ultrasound assessment of the pelvis, with little or no intervention necessary.

Menstrual abnormalities

Menstrual abnormalities occur in about one-third of women with fibroids, usually heavy periods. Submucous fibroids can also cause intermenstrual bleeding, postcoital bleeding, continuous vaginal bleeding or dysmenorrhoea. Increased menstrual blood loss due to fibroids is associated with:

- increased endometrial surface area
- prostaglandin production
- increased endometrial blood supply.

Abdominopelvic mass

Large fibroids growing into the abdominal cavity may cause abdominal swelling or distension. The fibroids can press on the ureters, affecting renal function.

Pain

Abdominopelvic pain can be caused by:

- degeneration of uterine fibroids
- the presence of associated pelvic varicosities
- stretching of the uterine ligaments.

Subfertility

Fibroids compressing the cornual region of the fallopian tubes may contribute to infertility. Submucous fibroids, especially those that are hormonally active, can affect implantation and might result in miscarriage. There is now evidence that even intramural fibroids that are not distorting the endometrial cavity can reduce embryo implantation and pregnancy rates following IVF, possibly because of interference with the endometrial blood supply.

Pressure symptoms

Urinary frequency, nocturia and urgency may be caused by pressure on the bladder from an enlarged uterus and incarceration of a pelvic fibroid may result in urinary retention. Pressure on the rectum and abdominal bloating might also be noticed.

COMPLICATIONS

Red degeneration occurring in pregnancy may present with acute pain and the subsequent massive release of prostaglandins may cause miscarriage or premature labour. Hyaline, cystic and calcified degenerative changes may also occur.

Fig. 7.1 Risk factors and protective factors for fibroids.

Increased incidence with:	Decreased incidence with:
African–Caribbean women	Cigarette smoking
Increasing age	Use of combined oral contraceptive pill
Nulligravidity	Full term pregnancy
Obesity	

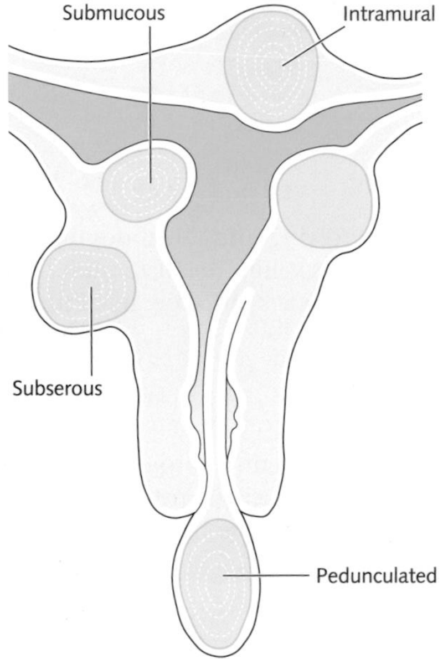

Fig. 7.2 Categorization of fibroids: subserosal fibroids impact on the endometrial cavity, intramural fibroids lie within the uterus wall, subserosal fibroids lie on the outer surface of the womb. Pedunculated fibroids are attached to the uterus through a stalk.

Fig. 7.3 Symptoms associated with uterine fibroids.

- Asymptomatic
- Menstrual abnormalities
- Abdominopelvic mass
- Subfertility
- Pressure symptoms
- Urinary symptoms secondary to pressure
- Pregnancy complications
- Pain

Pedunculated fibroids may undergo torsion and present with an acute abdomen.

Urinary retention might occur with impaction of a pelvic fibroid.

Sarcomatous (malignant) change, usually within very large or rapidly growing fibroids, is a rare (approximately 1:1000) but potentially fatal complication.

Fig. 7.4 Complications of fibroids.

Gynaecological complications
Degeneration – may include red degeneration or calcification Torsion – of pedunculated fibroids Malignancy – the risk of leiomyosarcoma is 0.1-0.5%
Pregnancy related complications
Infertility Obstructed labour Risk of PPH

In pregnancy, fibroids situated low in the uterus may result in malpresentation of the fetus and obstruct delivery. Fibroids may also restrict postpartum involution of the uterus and predispose to postpartum haemorrhage. Figure 7.4 summarizes the complications associated with fibroids.

HINTS AND TIPS

The main complications of fibroids are degeneration, torsion (if pedunculated) and malignancy. In pregnancy, fibroids may lead to a malpresentation, obstructed labour or PPH.

EXAMINATION

Fibroids can be palpated during abdominopelvic examination; classically the uterus feels enlarged, firm and irregular. If a fibroid is mobile on bimanual examination the uterus moves with it, although this can also occur with an ovarian mass adherent to the uterus.

INVESTIGATIONS

Relevant blood tests include full blood count (FBC) (to exclude anaemia in patients with menorrhagia) and U&Es (in patients with large fibroids which may compress the ureters or bladder).

Pelvic ultrasound is the main initial investigation and is used to:

- identify the location of individual fibroids
- measure the size of each fibroid.

However, it may be difficult to distinguish some fibroids from ovarian masses, particularly if the fibroid is located in the broad ligament. MRI has become the gold standard imaging method for differentiating fibroids from other pelvic masses. Laparotomy might be required to be 100% certain in some cases.

The most accurate method of excluding submucous fibroids is by hysteroscopy.

HINTS AND TIPS

In women with fibroids and menorrhagia, always request a FBC to exclude anaemia.

TREATMENT

Small, asymptomatic fibroids do not require intervention. Indications for treatment include:

- symptomatic fibroids
- rapidly enlarging fibroids
- fibroids that are thought to be causing infertility.

Medical therapy

Medical therapy is only useful as an adjunct to surgery and as an aid to correct anaemia prior to surgery. Fibroids regrow to their original size within 3 months of ceasing medical therapy without surgical intervention.

Gonadotrophin-releasing hormone analogues

Gonadotrophin-releasing hormone (GnRH) analogues produce a hypogonadotrophic hypogonadal state leading to a temporary, reversible, chemical menopause. This results in a reduction in fibroid volume by up to 50% with a maximum benefit within 3 months of starting therapy.

GnRH analogues have several different uses prior to surgery. They can:

- increase the likelihood of performing surgery through a transverse suprapubic incision rather than a midline incision. This reduces the patient's surgical morbidity
- reduce surgical blood loss and the need for blood transfusions
- reduce the risk of hysterectomy when myomectomy is planned.

The long-term use of GnRH analogues has been limited because of their side effects, which include menopausal symptoms and bone density reduction (osteoporosis). However, adding in low-dose hormone replacement therapy (HRT), used as 'add back', can avoid menopausal side effects and reduce loss of bone density while maintaining the benefits of the GnRH analogues. GnRH analogues are currently licensed for 6 months use. More data are required before GnRH analogues with add back are licensed for longer-term use.

Surgical treatment

Definitive surgery depends on the location of the fibroids. This includes:

- transcervical resection of fibroids (TCRF)
- myomectomy, or
- hysterectomy.

TCRF is suitable for submucous fibroids and involves removing them using an operative hysteroscope in the uterine cavity.

Myomectomy is the removal of pedunculated, subserosal and intramural fibroids with preservation of the uterus and can be performed either at laparotomy (open myomectomy) or laparoscopically. Complications include haemorrhage, which might require blood transfusion, and, potentially, hysterectomy. Adhesion formation may impair future fertility and is most common after open myomectomy, especially for posterior wall fibroids. Fibroid regrowth is likely to occur in 40% of patients with a reoperation rate of up to one-fifth of cases.

Hysterectomy is the surgical procedure of choice in women who have completed their families, although not all women wish to have their uterus removed. Surgical treatment by hysterectomy often causes less morbidity than myomectomy.

Uterine artery embolization

This is a newer less invasive alternative to surgery and involves the radiological embolization of fibroids. This is done with the patient under sedation, by inserting a catheter into the femoral artery. Small silicone microbeads are injected through the catheter into the arteries supplying the fibroids, causing thrombosis and fibroid infarction. It is performed by radiologists, who must see and assess the patient to determine their suitability for the operation. Complications include infection, pain and failed treatment. It is not suitable for women who wish to preserve their fertility.

Advances in fibroid treatment

Other techniques for the treatment of fibroids are being developed to reduce the need for laparotomy and the risk of postoperative adhesion formation and to avoid large uterine scars. These include:

- interstitial laser photocoagulation: laser probes are inserted into the fibroid laparoscopically to produce tissue degeneration and subsequent fibroid shrinkage
- laparoscopic diathermy
- directed high-energy ultrasound.

Further reading

Anderson, J., 1997. Gynaecological Imaging. Churchill Livingstone, London.

Llewellyn-Jones, D., 1999. Fundamentals of Obstetrics & Gynaecology, seventh ed. Mosby, London.

McKay Hart, D., Norman, J., 2000. Gynaecology Illustrated, fifth ed. Churchill Livingstone, London.

Monaghan, J.M., 1992. Bonney's Gynaecological Surgery, ninth ed. Bailliere Tindall, London.

NICE, 2010. Uterine Artery Embolisation for Fibroids: Interventional Procedure Guidance 367. National Institute for Health and Care Excellence, London. Available online at: www.nice.org.uk (accessed 07.01.12).

RCOG. Available online at: www.rcog.org.uk/guidelines.

Endometriosis

Objectives

By the end of this chapter, you should be able to:

- Understand the definition and aetiological theories of endometriosis
- List the common symptoms and sites of endometriosis
- Request the relevant investigations and treatments for endometriosis.

Endometriosis is the presence of endometrial tissue outside of the uterine cavity. Endometriosis occurring in the myometrium is known as adenomyosis. The true incidence of endometriosis is difficult to ascertain as not all women with endometriosis are symptomatic.

Endometriosis occurs in about 10% of the female population in their reproductive years but has been defined in up to 25% of women undergoing gynaecological laparoscopy. It is estimated to be the most common gynaecological condition after fibroids.

AETIOLOGY

The aetiology of endometriosis is unknown but several theories have been suggested (Fig. 8.1):

1. Retrograde menstruation/implantation theory

During menstruation, endometrial tissue spills into the pelvic cavity through the fallopian tubes: retrograde menstruation. This ectopic endometrium then implants and becomes functional, responding to the hormones of the ovarian cycle. This theory is supported by the association between endometriosis and increased menstruation occurring with a short menstrual cycle and prolonged periods, and by the fact that the most common sites for endometriosis are the ovaries and the uterosacral ligaments — areas in which retrograde menses spill. The implantation theory would also account for the rare cases of endometriosis found in the surgical incision following surgery on the uterus, for example, following open myomectomy or caesarean section. Imperforate hymen and other outflow obstructions that exacerbate retrograde menstruation are also associated with severe endometriosis.

However, this theory does not account for the existence of endometriosis at the distant sites in the body (e.g. lungs). There is growing laparoscopic evidence to suggest that most women experience retrograde menstruation, in which case the incidence of endometriosis would be expected to be higher. This theory may therefore be too simplistic.

2. Lymphatic and venous embolization

This theory hypothesizes that endometrial tissue is transported through the body by the lymphatic or venous channels and would explain the rare cases of distant sites for endometriosis. However, distant endometriotic deposits would be expected to be more common if the lymphatic and venous embolization theories were the only mechanism for the development of endometriosis.

3. Coelomic metaplasia

This theory relies on the principle that tissues of certain embryonic origin maintain their ability to undergo metaplasia and differentiate into other tissue types. This is certainly true of peritoneum of coelomic origin, which can undergo metaplasia and differentiate into functional endometrium. However, this does not explain the distribution of endometriosis within the peritoneal cavity itself (most common in the lower part of the peritoneal cavity) or the presence of endometriosis in sites of the body that are not of coelomic origin.

4. Genetic and immunological factors

The role of a genetic influence is supported by the strong family history seen in endometriosis sufferers, but its exact role has not yet been characterized. It is possible that women with a genetic predisposition to endometriosis have an abnormal response to the presence of

Fig. 8.1 Possible theories for the aetiology of endometriosis.

- Implantation/retrograde menstruation
- Genetic and immunological factors
- Lymphatic and venous embolization
- Coelomic metaplasia
- Composite theories

ectopic endometrium, which results in endometriosis developing. There is some evidence that an altered or defective cell-mediated response is implicated.

5. Composite theories

None of the above theories alone account for all cases of endometriosis, however, together all the theories could play a role. Whereas an abnormal response to the presence of ectopic endometrium might result in functioning endometrium responding to the ovarian cycle, this in turn could trigger coelomic metaplasia and further development or advancement of the disease process in response to the local release of endometrial hormones and/or the inflammatory response.

SITES OF ENDOMETRIOSIS

The most common sites for endometriosis are the ovaries and the uterosacral ligaments. These and other pelvic sites are shown in Figure 8.2. Although endometriosis has been reported in nearly every organ except the spleen, extrapelvic endometriosis is rare. The American Fertility Society Classification is used to assess the severity of pelvic endometriosis (Fig. 8.3). This takes into account the site and size of endometriotic lesions, and the presence and consequences of adhesions.

Endometriosis has been diagnosed in every organ in the body except the spleen. Symptoms are nearly always cyclical unless nerves or the intracranial cavity are affected.

HINTS AND TIPS

The most common sites of endometriosis are:
- Ovaries
- Pouch of Douglas
- Uterosacral ligaments.

SYMPTOMS

The main symptom of endometriosis is cyclical pain prior to menstruation. This occurs because the deposits of endometriosis, wherever their location in the body, respond to the ovarian cycle and bleeding from these deposits causes local irritation and inflammatory responses.

Although the cardinal symptom of endometriosis is cyclical pain, the classic 'quartet' of symptoms of endometriosis is:

- secondary dysmenorrhoea
- deep dyspareunia
- pelvic pain
- infertility.

The dysmenorrhoea associated with endometriosis typically starts prior to the beginning of the period and is exacerbated by menstrual flow. Endometriosis should be considered in any woman who presents with any of the symptoms shown in Figure 8.4.

Other common symptoms include:

- dyschezia (pain on opening bowels, particularly just before menstruation starts)

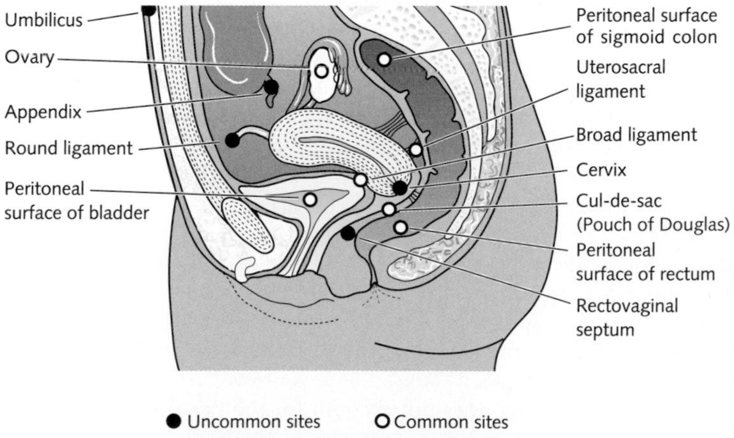

Fig. 8.2 Common sites of endometriosis.

Fig. 8.3 American fertility society classification of endometriosis.

Anatomical Site	Score	1	2	3	4	5
Peritoneum	Endometriotic lesion size	<1 cm	1–3 cm	>3 cm		
	Adhesions	Flimsy	Dense with partial pouch of Douglas occlusion	Dense with complete pouch of Douglas occlusion		
Ovary [points for each side involved]	Endometriotic lesion size		<1 cm		1–3 cm	>3 cm
	Adhesions		Filmy		Dense with partial ovarian coverage	Dense completely enclosing ovary
Fallopian tubes [points for each side involved]	Endometriotic lesion size		<1 cm		>1 cm	Tubal occlusion
	Adhesions		Filmy		Dense and distorting tubes	Dense and completely enclosing tubes
		Stage I (Mild) <5 Stage II (Mod) 6–15			Stage III (Severe) 16–30 Stage IV (Extensive) >31	

Scores are: Stage 1 (mild)<5, stage II (mod) 6–15, stage III (severe) 16–30, stage IV (extensive)>31.

- ovulation pain
- chronic fatigue
- chronic pelvic pain (worse just before periods).

Rupture of an ovarian endometrioma will cause acute, severe lower abdominal pain. The release of the very irritant 'chocolate' material from the cyst causes peritonism.

The site of ectopic endometrium dictates the location of the pain. If the endometriosis is severe, pain can be continuous, with exacerbations at the time of menstruation. Neural and intracranial endometriosis produces continuous pain.

Endometriosis of the lung, bladder, bowel or umbilicus will produce cyclical bleeding from these sites associated with menstruation.

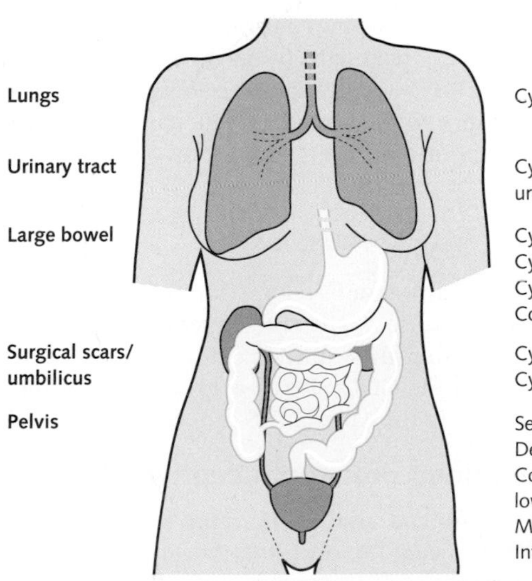

Fig. 8.4 Symptoms of endometriosis.

INFERTILITY

As many as one-third of infertile women are diagnosed to have endometriosis. Dense adhesions, tubal and ovarian damage and distortion caused by severe endometriosis can contribute to the lack of conception. The association with mild endometriosis, in which no mechanical damage has occurred, is more puzzling. Release of substances from the ectopic endometrium, such as prostaglandins, which can affect ovulation or tubal motility has been implicated. There is evidence that treating even mild endometriosis can improve fertility.

CLINICAL SIGNS

Abdominal inspection may reveal a slightly distended abdomen and palpation may be tender, particularly around the time of menses.

Pelvic examination may reveal a tender, retroverted, retroflexed, fixed uterus with thickening of the cardinal or uterosacral ligaments. Endometriotic nodules might be palpable in the posterior vaginal fornix and ovarian endometrioma might be evident on bimanual palpation. The pelvic anatomy might be normal with mild disease and a useful sign is to elicit pain on moving the cervix interiorly (cervical excitation). This stretches the uterosacral ligaments, which is painful in the presence of endometriosis. In the presence of adenomyosis, the uterus is typically smoothly enlarged (globular) and tender.

Deeply infiltrating rectovaginal nodules may be most reliably detected by vaginal examination during menstruation.

INVESTIGATIONS

Diagnosis and severity of pelvic disease can only effectively be assessed by laparoscopy. The classic 'powder-burn' lesions of endometriosis might be seen but these areas of haemosiderin pigmentation might represent 'burnt-out' endometriosis. Non-pigmented lesions can appear as opaque white areas of peritoneum, red lesions or glandular lesions. If there is doubt about the macroscopic appearance then a biopsy should be taken.

Ovarian endometrioma can be seen by ultrasound but differentiation from other ovarian pathology may be difficult without histological confirmation.

HINTS AND TIPS

Positive histology confirms endometriosis but a negative result does not exclude it as the biopsy may have been taken from the wrong place.

DIFFERENTIAL DIAGNOSIS

The differential diagnosis for endometriosis includes:

1. pelvic inflammatory disease
2. pelvic pain syndrome
3. submucous fibroids
4. ovarian accident
5. adhesions.

COMPLICATIONS

Complications of endometriosis are often due to the resultant fibrosis and scarring and can affect not only the reproductive organs but might cause colonic and ureteric obstruction.

Rupture of an endometrioma and the subsequent release of the very irritant 'chocolate' material contents can cause peritonism.

Malignant change within endometriotic lesions is rare and most commonly occurs in ovarian endometriosis.

TREATMENT

Treatment of endometriosis is indicated to:

- alleviate symptoms
- stop progression of disease and development of complications
- improve fertility.

Treatment depends on the severity of the disease and should be tailored to the woman's needs; it can be medical or surgical. Empirical treatment without a definitive diagnosis of endometriosis can be given by trialing medical treatment to see if this reduces symptoms.

Endometriosis is a recurring disease, with up to 40% of women developing recurring symptoms within 1 year of stopping treatment. Initial treatment should, therefore, be followed by maintenance therapy to reduce the chance of recurrence. Maintenance therapy is usually medical and aims to suppress or reduce the frequency of periods.

Medical treatment

Endometriotic lesions regress during pregnancy and after the menopause. Medical treatment is, therefore, aimed at mimicking these physiological processes (Fig. 8.5). Tricycling the COCP is the gold standard maintenance therapy, but the Mirena IUS can also be used.

Combined oral contraceptive pill

The combined oral contraceptive pill (COCP) suppresses ovulation and the normal cyclical ovarian production of oestrogen and progesterone. Mild

Fig. 8.5 Summary of medical treatment of endometriosis.

Drug	Mode of action	Side-effects
Progestogens	Pseudopregnancy	Break-through bleeding, weight gain, oedema, acne, abdominal bloating, increased appetite, decreased libido
Danazol	Pseudomenopause	Increase weight, break-through bleeding, muscle cramps, decreased breast size, hot flushes, emotional lability, oily skin, acne, hirsutism, headache, increased libido, hoarseness or deepening of the voice
Gestrinone	Pseudomenopause	Similar to Danazol
LHRH-analogues	Pseudomenopause	Hot flushes, break-through bleeding, vaginal dryness, headaches, decreased libido, bone density loss

symptoms of endometriosis may be controlled by using the COCP, but it is more often used as maintenance therapy following initial treatment.

Progestogens

Continuous progestogen therapy effectively induces a 'pseudopregnancy' state, causing endometriotic deposits to decidualize and then regress. Progestogens can be taken orally or as depot preparations, and treatment should be for 6 months.

Mirena coil

The Mirena coil releases small amounts of progesterone into the uterus and can be used for up to 5 years. Its advantages include the fact that it simultaneously acts as contraception and minimizes systemic side effects. Drawbacks are the impact on fertility and pain upon insertion. Studies have shown that it can reduce endometriosis-related pain.

GnRH analogues

This class of synthetic drugs is GnRH agonists. Continued administration desensitizes pituitary gonadotrophs, leading to a temporary, reversible state of hypogonadotrophic hypogonadism, in other words, a temporary chemical menopause. GnRH analogues are as effective as Danazol in reducing the symptoms and severity of endometriosis and are usually used for 3–6 months. Their menopausal side effects are often better tolerated than the androgenic side effects of Danazol and can be reduced by using 'add-back' continuous combined hormone replacement therapy (see Chapter 17).

Gestrinone

Gestrinone is a synthetic steroid that has mild androgenic, marked antioestrogenic and antiprogestogenic activity. It exhibits similar endocrine effects to those of Danazol without significantly reducing basal levels of gonadotrophins. Clinical response is also similar to Danazol.

Danazol

Danazol is a testosterone derivative and used to be first-line medical treatment for endometriosis. It is now rarely used. As well as its androgenic properties, Danazol produces a hypo-oestrogenic and hypoprogestogenic state, and it is this pseudomenopausal state that induces endometrial regression and atrophy.

The mechanism of action of Danazol is complex; it acts at pituitary, ovarian and target tissue levels. It should be taken for 6–9 months and the dose should be titrated to the patient's response and presence of side effects. Patients should be warned to stop treatment if they develop deepening of the voice, as this could be irreversible.

Surgical treatment

This can be conservative or radical and depends on the patient's:

- age
- symptoms
- fertility requirements
- response to medical treatment.

Conservative surgery

Conservative surgery can be performed through laparoscopy or at laparotomy and aims to:

- return the anatomy of the pelvis to normal
- destroy visible lesions of endometriosis
- improve fertility
- conserve ovarian tissue.

This includes division of adhesions, destruction of endometriotic lesions using diathermy or laser, and removing endometriomas, which do not respond well to medical therapy. Complications include damage to other pelvic structures including bowel, bladder and ureters. Recurrence of symptoms might occur because:

- endometriosis is a recurring disease
- endometriotic deposits not visible to the naked eye will not have been destroyed.

Diffuse peritoneal endometriosis might be better treated medically. Pregnancy rates following conservative surgery are directly related to the severity of the disease.

Radical surgery

Radical surgery for endometriosis is reserved for women who do not wish to maintain fertility and in whom other forms of treatment have failed. This may be performed in specialist centres in conjunction with bowel surgeons.

Total abdominal hysterectomy with bilateral salpingo-oophorectomy is the procedure of choice. This removes the ovaries, the main source of oestrogens, producing a hypo-oestrogenic state and effectively treating the endometriosis. As many of these women are relatively young, HRT is advised. Oestrogen replacement may cause a recurrence of endometriosis in a small percentage of women and should, therefore, be kept to a minimum. Continuous combined oestrogen and progesterone replacement might further reduce the rate of recurrence because of the effects of progestogens on endometriosis.

Further reading

Llewellyn-Jones, D., 2010. Fundamentals of Obstetrics & Gynaecology, ninth ed. Mosby, London.

McKay Hart, D., Norman, J., 2000. Gynaecology Illustrated, fifth ed. Churchill Livingstone, London.

RCOG, Endometriosis: Investigation and Management. Available online at: http://www.rcog.org.uk/guidelines (accessed 07.01.12.).

Shaw, R.W., Soutter, W.P., Stanton, S.P., 1997. Gynaecology, second ed. Churchill Livingstone, London.

Benign ovarian tumours

Objectives

After reading this chapter, you should be able to:

- Understand the embryological origins of the different types of ovarian cysts
- List the symptoms with which an ovarian cyst may present
- List the differential diagnoses for an ovarian cyst
- Discuss the management options with an ovarian cyst
- Consider how malignancy within an ovarian cyst can be predicted prior to surgery.

INCIDENCE

Benign ovarian cysts are common and often asymptomatic, resolving spontaneously. Therefore, despite being a frequent cause for admission to hospital, their exact incidence is unknown. Almost all ovarian masses and cysts are benign in premenopausal women with an incidence of malignancy of 1:1000 which increases to 3:1000 at the age of 50.

AETIOLOGY

Ovarian tumours can be physiological (functional) or pathological (benign or malignant). Classification depends on the ovarian tissue from which they arise (Fig. 9.1). Excluding the physiological group, a germ cell tumour is the more common diagnosis in a woman less than 40 years of age, whereas an epithelial cell tumour is more likely in an older woman.

Risk factors for ovarian tumours include obesity, infertility, hypothyroidism, early menarche and tamoxifen therapy.

Physiological cysts

These are often asymptomatic and occur commonly in younger women.

Follicular cysts

These are the result of either non-rupture of the dominant follicle during the normal ovarian cycle or failure of atresia of a non-dominant follicle. Smaller cysts might resolve spontaneously, but intervention could be necessary if the cyst causes symptoms (see below) or if ultrasound follow-up shows an increase in size.

Luteal cysts

Corpus luteal cysts are less common than follicular cysts. However, they are more likely to present with intraperitoneal bleeding secondary to rupture. This occurs more commonly on the right side and typically rupture occurs on day 20 to 26.

Theca lutein cysts

These are the least common of the functional ovarian cysts. They are usually bilateral and occur with pregnancy including molar pregnancy. They may be large, up to 30 cm, they are usually multicystic and regress spontaneously.

Benign epithelial tumours

The majority of ovarian cysts arise from the ovarian epithelium. They develop from the coelomic epithelium over the gonadal ridge of the embryo and are, therefore, derived from any of the pelvic organs or the renal tract.

Serous cystadenoma

This is the most common tumour in this group. They are bilateral in about 10% of cases and they contain thin serous fluid, usually within a unilocular cavity. Histologically, they appear to have a tubal origin.

Mucinous cystadenoma

These tumours are typically unilateral, larger in size compared with serous cystadenomas, and multilocular with thick mucoid fluid. The mucus-secreting cells are likely to indicate an endocervical derivation.

Fig. 9.1 Classification of benign ovarian tumours.

Type of tumour	Name
Physiological	Follicular cysts Luteal cysts
Benign epithelial tumours	Serous cystadenoma Mucinous cystadenoma Endometrioid cystadenoma Brenner
Benign germ cell tumours	Mature cystic teratoma (dermoid cyst) Mature solid teratoma
Benign sex cord stromal tumours	Theca cell tumours Fibroma Sertoli–Leydig cell tumour
Other Benign Ovarian tumours	Endometriotic cyst

Endometrioid tumours

These are mostly malignant tumours arising from endometrial cells.

Brenner tumours

The majority of these tumours are benign. They arise from uroepithelial cell lines and contain transitional epithelium. Between 10% and 15% are bilateral, they are usually small in size, and some secrete oestrogen, causing irregular vaginal bleeding.

Benign germ cell tumours

These tumours are among the most common in women under the age of 30. Such tumours arise from totipotential germ cells and thus can contain elements of all three layers of embryonic tissue — ectodermal derivatives such as teeth and hair, endodermal tissue such as intestine and mesodermal structures such as bone.

Mature cystic teratoma

Also known as a dermoid cyst, this common type of tumour has a median age of presentation of 30 years with about 10% being bilateral. Most are asymptomatic but they can undergo torsion (up to 10%) or, rarely, rupture.

Mature solid teratomas

Much less common than a dermoid cyst, these tumours must be distinguished from an immature solid teratoma, which is malignant.

Benign sex cord stromal tumours

Such tumours account for only about 4% of benign ovarian tumours. Many secrete hormones and thus present at any age with hormonally mediated symptoms.

Theca cell tumours

These cysts are nearly always benign solid tumours presenting over the age of 50 years (in contrast, granulosa cell tumours are always malignant). Many secrete oestrogen and thus have systemic effects such as postmenopausal bleeding.

Fibroma

These tumours are rare and can be associated with ascites. Most are derived from stromal cells. Meigs syndrome is seen in 1% of cases. It is characterized by a solid ovarian tumour, usually a fibroma (could be thecoma, a cystadenoma or granulosa cell tumour), accompanied by ascites and pleural effusion. Treatment of Meigs' syndrome consists of thoracocentesis and paracentesis to drain off the excess fluid, and unilateral salpingo-oophorectomy to correct the underlying aetiology.

Other benign ovarian tumours

Women with endometriosis may develop ovarian endometriomas (chocolate cysts) which can enlarge to 6 to 8 cm in size (see Chapter 22). They tend to have a typical ultrasound appearance and may need treatment depending on the symptoms with which they present. A mass that does not resolve with observation may be an endometrioma.

HISTORY

Benign ovarian tumours can be asymptomatic, detected by routine bimanual palpation during a cervical smear test or on routine antenatal ultrasound scan, for example.

The presenting symptoms include:

- pain secondary to torsion/rupture/haemorrhage/infection
- abdominal swelling
- pressure effects on bowel or bladder
- hormonal effects secondary to secretion of oestrogens or androgens.

Figure 9.2 shows the differential diagnoses that need to be considered for the history, examination and investigations. The history must include the date of the LMP

Fig. 9.2 Differential diagnoses for ovarian tumours.

Symptom	Differential diagnosis
Pain	Ectopic pregnancy Spontaneous miscarriage Pelvic inflammatory disease Appendicitis Diverticulitis
Abdominal swelling	Pregnancy Fibroid uterus Full bladder
Pressure effects	Constipation Urine frequency Vaginal prolapse
Hormonal effects	Menstrual irregularily Postmenopausal bleeding Precocious puberty

and the regularity of the menstrual cycle, as well as current contraception, if appropriate. Any history of gastrointestinal symptoms might be important, for example, a patient with an ovarian torsion might present with sudden onset of right-sided abdominal pain associated with nausea and vomiting, and appendicitis must be excluded.

HINTS AND TIPS

Benign ovarian cysts that undergo an accident (rupture or torsion) can present as an acute abdomen. Always exclude an ectopic pregnancy in a woman of childbearing age.

Ask about risk factors for ovarian malignancy and family history of ovarian and breast cancer.

EXAMINATION

Initial examination must include the pulse and blood pressure; rupture of an ovarian cyst can result in intraperitoneal bleeding that leads to hypovolaemia. In a young patient, this might present at first with tachycardia and cold peripheries, with hypotension developing as a relatively late sign.

Distension might be seen on abdominal inspection, resulting from the cyst itself or from ascites if the cyst is malignant. Look for any other signs of malignancy including cachexia. Determine the size, tenderness, mobility and nodularity of the cyst. If the cyst has undergone torsion, or if there is haemorrhage into the cyst so that the capsule stretches, abdominal palpation will elicit tenderness. This is typically in the iliac fossa and may be associated with signs of peritonism. A large ovarian tumour can rise up out of the pelvis and be palpated in the abdomen; this should be excluded by moving the left hand distally from the xiphisternum towards the pelvis (see Chapter 3). Ascites should be excluded by testing for shifting dullness.

Bimanual palpation of the pelvic organs, as described in Chapter 3 is essential. If the tumour has presented acutely with abdominal pain then adnexal tenderness or an adnexal mass will assist in excluding gastrointestinal aetiology. Assessing the size of the uterus will help to exclude a fibroid uterus or intrauterine pregnancy. If there seems to be an adnexal mass, then its approximate size, consistency and the presence of any tenderness should be elicited.

INVESTIGATIONS

In line with the list of differential diagnoses in Figure 9.2, investigations include:

- haemoglobin
- white blood cell count
- CRP
- HVS/endocervical swabs
- urine pregnancy test and/or serum β-hCG level
- pelvic ultrasound scan (transvaginal scan more sensitive than abdominal)
- serum CA125 level which is an epithelial tumour marker. However, this may be raised with other gynaecological pathology such as fibroids, or with pregnancy
- chest X-ray/intravenous urogram/CT scan if malignancy is suspected (see Chapter 10)
- serum alpha fetoprotein (alphafetoprotein) and human chorionic gonadotrophin (hCG) if germ cell tumour suspected in woman under 40 years with complex ovarian masses on USS.

MANAGEMENT OF A BENIGN OVARIAN TUMOUR

The patient's management depends on the:

- severity of presenting symptoms
- patient's age
- future fertility needs
- risk of malignancy.

Asymptomatic cysts

Ovarian cysts can be managed conservatively if they are asymptomatic. This depends on the patient's age and the size of the cyst (Fig. 9.3). In a younger woman (usually taken as less than 40 years of age), the risk of the

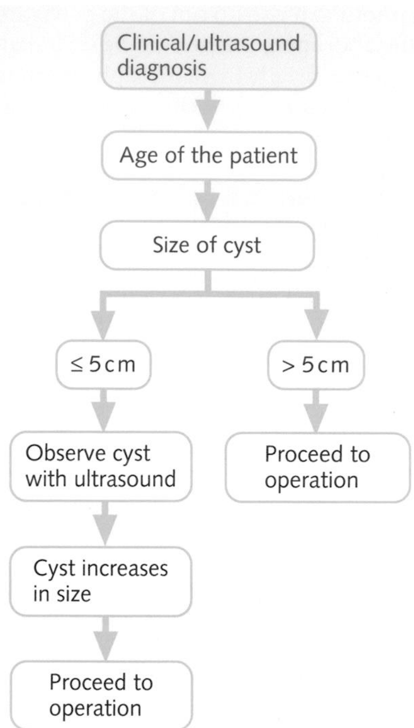

Fig. 9.3 Management of an asymptomatic benign ovarian tumour in a premenopausal woman.

tumour being malignant is reduced and, therefore, the cyst can be monitored with pelvic ultrasound scans. A physiological cyst is likely to resolve spontaneously, but, if it persists or increases in size, then a laparoscopy or laparotomy might be indicated.

The combined oral contraceptive pill is thought to be effective in preventing formation of functional tumours, but its effectiveness in shrinking or resolving cystic tumours has not been proven.

The risk of malignancy index (RMI) is used in both pre- and postmenopausal women to estimate risk of malignancy:

$$\text{RMI} = \text{U (ultrasound score) x M (Menopausal score)} \\ \text{x CA} - 125\ (\text{IU/ml})$$

Ultrasound scans are scored 1 point for each of the following characteristics: multilocular cyst; evidence of solid areas; evidence of metastases; presence of ascites; bilateral lesions:

$$\text{U} = 0\ (\text{no points});\ \text{U} = 1\ (1\ \text{point});$$
$$\text{U} = 3\ (2 - 5\ \text{points})$$

Menopausal score reflects the menopausal women:

$$\text{M} = 1 \text{ for premenopausal women;}$$
$$\text{M} = 3 \text{ for postmenopausal women}$$

The higher the RMI the greater the risk of ovarian cancer:

$$<25 = \text{low risk } (<3\%);$$
$$25 - 250 = \text{moderate risk } (20\%);$$
$$> 250 = \text{high risk } (30\%)$$

Once the RMI is calculated, follow-up investigations, laparoscopic assessment or laparotomy is advised in an appropriate centre.

Symptomatic cysts

If the patient presents with severe acute pain, an emergency laparoscopy and/or laparotomy is appropriate. With chronic symptoms, a procedure can be planned electively.

Thus the appropriate treatment for an ovarian tumour depends on many factors. A woman in whom a selective cystectomy is attempted must be advised of the risk of oophorectomy if haemostasis cannot be achieved or if the cyst cannot be isolated. Ovarian cystectomy and oophorectomy (removal of ovary) can be performed either laparoscopically or by laparotomy. The choice depends on:

- operator skills
- risk of malignancy
- the patient's BMI
- previous surgery.

An ovarian cyst thought to be benign can be managed by observation, laparoscopic or open ovarian cystectomy. If the patient is young, with minimal risk of malignancy, a laparoscopic procedure might be an option. In suspected malignancy, it may be more appropriate to perform a laparotomy, possibly including bilateral oophorectomy, hysterectomy and infracolic omentectomy (see Chapter 10).

Further reading

RCOG, 2003. Ovarian Cysts in Postmenopausal Ovarian Cysts in Postmenopausal Women, Green-top Guideline No. 34. Royal College of Obstetricians and Gynaecologists, London.

RCOG, 2011. Management of ovarian masses in premenopausal Women, Green-top Guideline No. 62. Royal College of Obstetricians and Gynaecologists, London.

Gynaecological malignancies

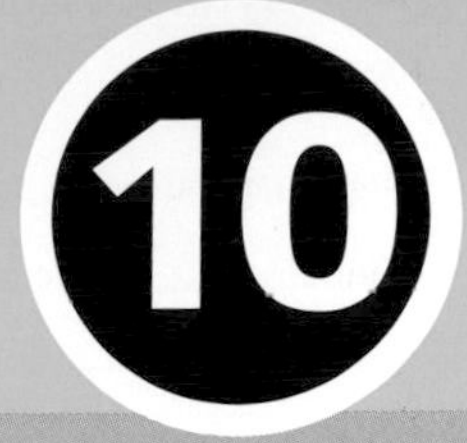

Objectives

By the end of this chapter, you should be able to:

- Understand what the common gynaecological cancers are and how common they are
- Understand how to take a focused history from a patient and the relevant examinations/investigations
- Understand the aetiology of each type of gynaecological cancer
- Understand the approaches to treatment and management

INTRODUCTION

Gynaecological malignancies include cancers affecting the ovary, uterus, cervix, vagina, vulva and fallopian tubes. This chapter aims to give you an overview of how common these cancers are, how they may present, how to diagnose and how to treat them.

OVARIAN CANCER

In the UK ovarian cancer is the fifth most common cancer in women (behind breast, bowel, lung and uterus) with around 6700 new cases being diagnosed each year. It has a peak incidence between the ages of 60 and 64 and it is the leading cause of death in women with a gynaecological cancer. The staging, treatment and survival rates are shown in Figure 10.1.

There are different types of ovarian cancers depending upon which cell they arise from. Most commonly tumours are from the epithelial cells but others can arise from germ cells, ovarian stroma, ovarian mesenchymal cells or, indeed, be metastatic from other sites.

Aetiology

The aetiology of ovarian cancer is not completely understood, although various risk factors have been identified. Women with a familial predisposition to ovarian cancer probably account for around 10% of cases, and most of these will have either the BRCA1 or BRCA2 mutations (chromosomes 17 and 13), or Lynch II syndrome (an autosomal dominant inherited disorder that predisposes to breast, endometrial, colon and ovarian cancer).

Risk factors

Increasing age, nulliparity, early menarche, late menopause, smoking and obesity are all risk factors for ovarian cancer. Pregnancy, breast feeding and exercise are thought to be protective factors (see Fig. 10.2).

Signs and symptoms

Ovarian cancer is often labelled the 'silent killer' as it may not have symptoms. There should be a high index of suspicion of even vague symptoms especially in at-risk groups (women over 50 years or with a family history).

Patients presenting with abdominal pain, bloating, distension, an abdominal mass, urinary frequency, post-menopausal bleeding or loss of appetite need careful assessment to rule out ovarian cancer.

Investigations

The most common first-line investigation for women suspected to have ovarian cancer is a pelvic ultrasound. This can be performed both trans-abdominally and trans-vaginally and can identify both ovarian and uterine pathology.

Suspicious features such as multilocular cysts, solid areas, metastases, ascites and bilateral lesions should be noted as this will help with further management.

Tumour markers are also used in the investigation of ovarian cancer, especially CA125, which is often raised in patients with epithelial cell tumours. Younger patients (i.e. <40 years old) suspected of having ovarian cancer should have serum alpha-fetoprotein (AFP), beta human chorionic gonadotrophin (βhCG) and CA125 levels measured to identify other tumour types.

Fig. 10.1 Staging of ovarian carcinoma.

Stage	Description	Treatment	Survival rates at 5 years (%)
I A B C	Limited to the ovaries: One ovary, capsule intact, no ascites Both ovaries, capsules intact, no ascites Breached capsule(s) or ascites present	Surgery	80
II A B C	Presence of peritoneal deposits in pelvis: On uterus or tubes On other pelvic organs With ascites	Surgery then chemotherapy	60
III	Peritoneal deposits outside pelvis: Microscopic deposits Macroscopic < 2 cm diameter Macroscopic > 2 cm diameter	Surgery then chemotherapy	25
IV	Distant metastases	Surgery for palliation only	5–10

Fig. 10.2 Risk factors for ovarian carcinoma.

Increased risk	Reduced risk
Hormone replacement therapy Few or no pregnancies Treatment with ovulation-induction drugs White Caucasian Blood group A Higher socioeconomic status Late age of first conception Family history	Pregnancies Treatment with the combined pill Black/Asian Blood group O

Patients suspected of having ovarian cancer (see below) will also have a computed tomography (CT) scan of their pelvis, abdomen +/- chest to establish the extent (or stage) of the disease.

Risk of malignancy index

Ovarian cysts are very common (especially in premenopausal women) and, therefore, distinguishing between benign and malignant cysts can be difficult. In order to identify women with a high risk of ovarian cancer the risk of malignancy index has been devised.

The risk of malignancy index (RMI) uses ultrasound features as well as the patient's menopausal status and CA125 level to give a risk score (see Fig. 10.3). Those with a score of >250 should be referred to a specialist multidisciplinary team.

Management

Surgery is the main modality of treatment in ovarian cancer and can be both diagnostic and curative (in early stage disease). It is performed by a gynaecological oncologist in a tertiary centre and involves a midline laparotomy, peritoneal washings, a total abdominal hysterectomy with bilateral salpingo-oophorectomy, omentectomy and biopsy of any suspicious areas. In addition, those patients who are suspected of having a mucinous tumour also undergo an appendicectomy. In patients with advanced disease the objective is to remove all visible tumour tissue. This allows accurate staging which will then dictate further management.

Chemotherapy may be needed following surgery based on the staging and type of tumour. In patients with low-risk stage I disease (grade 1 or 2, stage 1a or 1b) chemotherapy is not recommended. Patients with high-risk stage I disease (Grade 3 or stage 1c) or greater are recommended to have chemotherapy.

The choice of chemotherapy depends upon the individual patient. Most commonly a combination of a platinum-based agent and paclitaxel are used for six cycles.

Common side effects of chemotherapy agents include, nephrotoxicity, nausea, alopecia, mucositis, hypersensitivity reactions and neurotoxicity.

Screening

The rationale for screening for ovarian cancer is to reduce the late presentation that currently results in poor survival. Unfortunately, screening for this condition is difficult, partly because there is no premalignant

Fig. 10.3 Calculating an RMI

RMI = U x M x CA125

- **U = Ultrasound score**
  - 1 point for each of the following: multilocular cysts, solid areas, metastases, ascites and bilateral lesions
  - U = 1 If ultrasound score is 0-1
  - U = 3 If ultrasound score is 2-5
- **M = Menopausal status**
  - Pre-menopausal = 1
  - Post-menopausal = 3
- **CA125 = Serum CA125 level**

Example
Mary is 51 and went through the menopause aged 49. She was complaining of abdominal bloating and her GP organised an ultrasound. The ultrasound showed she has a large bilateral cyst which has solid areas. The GP also did a CA125 which came back as 104.

Mary's RMI
U = 3 x M = 3 (post menopausal) x CA125 = 104
3 x 3 x 104 = 936

stage, but also because there is no one test to diagnose ovarian cancer. Currently research is being carried out into screening to see which approach is more effective.

ENDOMETRIAL CANCER

In the UK endometrial cancer is the most common gynaecological cancer, with around 7700 new cases being diagnosed each year. Endometrial cancer predominantly occurs in postmenopausal women over the age of 50. These women may present with postmenopausal bleeding and it is essential they are appropriately investigated. A small number of cases occur in younger women (<40 years) who may have a genetic predisposition.

Risk factors

Obesity is a recognized risk factor for endometrial cancer, those with a body mass index of >29 are said to have a threefold increase in risk. Polycystic ovary syndrome (PCOS), nulliparity, unopposed oestrogen use, Tamoxifen use and genetic syndromes (HNPCC) are also risk factors.

Endometrial hyperplasia

Endometrial hyperplasia is a premalignant condition which if left untreated can progress to cancer. It is divided into simple hyperplasia and complex hyperplasia and can be treated with progesterone to encourage regression. The presence of atypia has a high likelihood of progression to cancer, and in many cases might indicate that a carcinoma is already present in another part of the uterus.

HINTS AND TIPS

Remember that women with atypical hyperplasia of the endometrium have a 30% chance of progression to endometrial cancer (if left untreated) so the option of definitive surgery, i.e. hysterectomy, should be discussed.

Pathology and spread

Endometrial cancer is an adenocarcinoma, the most common type being endometrioid. Other subtypes are serous, clear cell, mixed and small cell.

Spread initially involves local myometrial invasion and then transperitoneal. Lymphatic spread occurs to the para-aortic nodes. Staging is shown in Figure 10.4.

Investigation

Women with postmenopausal or suspicious perimenopausal bleeding should be investigated with a pelvic ultrasound to measure the endometrial thickness and also endometrial sampling. Endometrial cancer causes thickening of the endometrium and in the postmenopausal state should be less than 5 mm.

The endometrium in an outpatient setting can be sampled using a Pipelle biopsy. It involves the passage of a thin plastic tube through the cervix into the uterine cavity and uses aspiration to obtain an endometrial biopsy. This technique, however, only samples 4% of the endometrial surface area and may miss the cancer if present. More commonly patients are advised to undergo a hysteroscopy and endometrial biopsy (gold standard). This allows direct visualization of the endometrial cavity and a more representative sample to be taken. The procedure can be done under local or general anaesthetic.

Once a tissue diagnosis is obtained, an MRI scan is performed to assess the extent of myometrial invasion and thus differentiate between stages Ia, Ib and those above (see Fig. 10.4). Stages Ia and Ib can be treated locally; higher stages should be treated in a regional cancer centre. The decision as to where to treat should be discussed in a multidisciplinary team meeting.

Management

Surgery is the mainstay of treatment for patients with endometrial cancer. In stage I disease complete surgical staging is recommended. This includes a laparotomy (or laparoscopy) with peritoneal washing being taken for cytology, inspection of the pelvis and abdomen and a total abdominal (or laparoscopic) hysterectomy plus bilateral salpingo-oophorectomy. Stage II

Fig. 10.4 Staging of endometrial cancer.

Stage	Structures involved	% survival rates at 5 years
I	Body of uterus:	85
A	Endometrium only	
B	Extension into inner half of myometrium	
C	Extension into outer half of myometrium	
II	Extension from body of uterus to cervix:	60
A	Endocervical glands only	
B	Cervical stroma	
III		40
A	Spread to adnexae, or positive peritoneal cytology	
B	Metastases in vagina	
C	Pelvic or para-aortic lymphadenopathy	
IV		10
A	Involvement of bladder or bowel mucosa	
B	Distant metastases	

or high-risk disease is treated by a midline laparotomy and stage III disease is again surgically managed with the aim of debulking disease prior to radiotherapy. In stage IV disease a combination of surgery, radiotherapy and palliation may be required depending upon individual circumstances. The role of routine lymphadenectomy in patients with endometrial cancer is a much debated topic, a study in 2009 failed to show any benefit of routine lymphadenectomy in patients with early disease.

Prognosis

The overall 5-year survival rates for all stages of endometrial carcinoma are around 83–86%. Those with disease confined to the uterus, however, have a much better prognosis with a 95–97% 5-year survival rate.

UTERINE SARCOMA

Uterine sarcomas are a rare group of cancers associated with an aggressive nature and poor prognosis. The sarcomas can be of various types and are discussed below.

Stromal sarcoma

Tumours of stromal cells can be divided into the following categories:

- Low-grade sarcomas: look like fibroids, are slow-growing. Treatment is TAH + BSO with wide excision of the parametria.
- High-grade sarcomas: aggressive tumours with less than 50% survival rates, treated with radiotherapy.
- Mixed Mullerian tumours: derived from the glandular cells within the stroma, these are aggressive tumours that commonly spread to cervix and lymph nodes. Treatment is TAH + BSO with postoperative radiotherapy.

Myometrial sarcoma

Leiomyosarcoma could be described as a 'malignant fibroid', although only 5–10% of them arise within an existing fibroid, they are macroscopically very similar, being tumours of smooth muscle cells. Often diagnosis is not made until a TAH specimen is examined histologically, but lymph node sampling and BSO must be performed.

Pre-malignant disease of the cervix and human papilloma virus

In the United Kingdom approximately 2700 new cases of cervical cancer are diagnosed each year. In terms of incidence there appear to be two peaks in ages with the first occurring between 30 and 34 years and the second between 80 and 84 years.

The natural progression of the disease means that squamous cell cervical cancers (accounting for >90% of cervical cancers) exist in a pre-malignant form, which can be detected by cervical cytology. This is why the United Kingdom has an established screening programme that invites women to have cervical smears performed on a 3 yearly basis between the ages of 25 and 49 and on a 5 yearly basis from the ages of 50–65 (in England). Patients with abnormal smears will be offered a colposcopy and may need more frequent smears depending upon findings and treatment.

Human papilloma virus

Human papilloma virus (HPV) is a virus belonging to the papovaviridae family and was first isolated in 1933 by Richard E. Shope. There are over 100 different types which are known to cause warts as well as other conditions. In the 1980s HPV was linked with cervical cancer and since then research has identified certain types responsible. HPV can be transmitted by sexual contact and, therefore, any female who is sexually active is at risk. HPV types 16, 18, 6 and 11 are all known to cause cervical cancer with the former (16 & 18) often referred to as high risk.

Based on this research in the United Kingdom a vaccination programme is in place to vaccinate young girls before their first sexual contact and prevent cervical cancer. Girls are invited to have the vaccination between the ages of 13 and 14, which involves a course of three injections. It should be noted, however, that vaccination does not replace screening.

Cervical intraepithelial neoplasia

As mentioned above squamous cell cervical cancers exist in a pre-malignant state which can be detected via cervical smears. Cervical intraepithelial neoplasia (CIN) grading is one type of system which describes the pre-malignant condition and is made up of three stages which are thought to represent a continuum. Nowadays they are often divided into low grade (CIN I) and high grade (CIN II – CIN III) (see Fig. 10.5).

Patients with an abnormal smear result will then be referred for a colposcopy and, in some cases, HPV testing. At colposcopy the cervix is washed with acetic acid and then with iodine. The cervix is inspected for suspicious features (Fig. 10.6). Abnormal areas can be biopsied, meaning that the patient will be invited back at a later date for treatment if appropriate, or treatment can be performed at this point.

Treatment consists of either excising or destroying the transformation zone. Excision techniques include LLETZ (large loop excision of transformation zone), NETZ (needle excision of transformation zone) and cone biopsy; these allow the tissue removed to be sent for histology and examined to confirm the diagnosis and to check the margins, ensuring complete excision. Destructive techniques include cold coagulation, diathermy or laser.

Initial treatment has 95% success rate. Patients are followed up with a smear.

CERVICAL CANCER

Cervical cancer is the second most common cancer in women (under the age of 35) and even though the UK has a very successful screening programme around 1000 women per year still die from the disease. Risk factors for cervical cancer are shown in Figure 10.7.

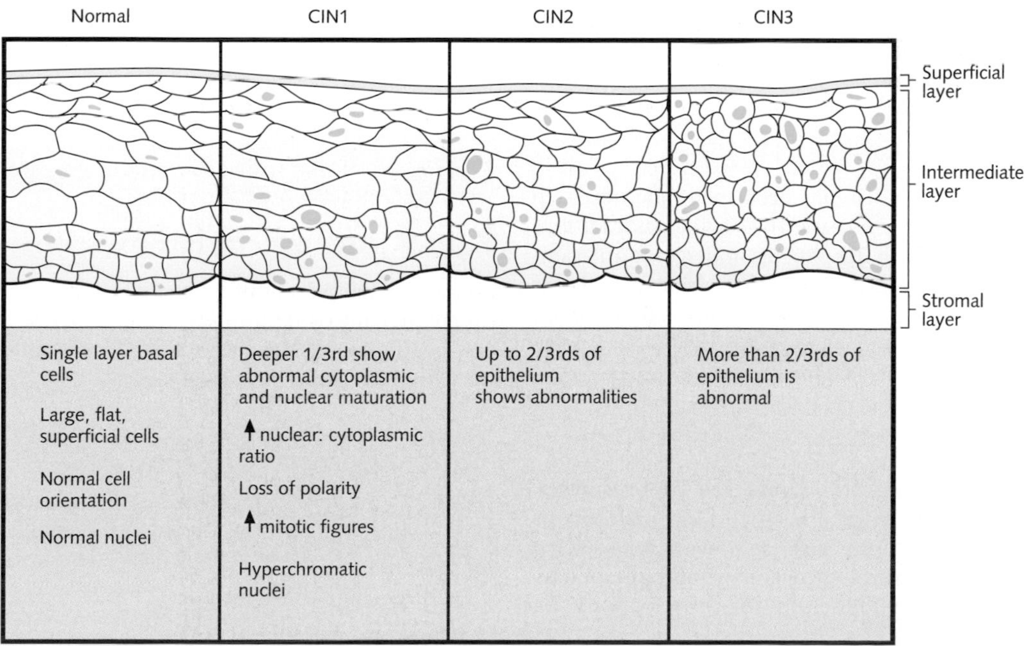

Fig. 10.5 Grades of cervical intraepithelial neoplasia.

Fig. 10.6 Suspicious features at colposcopy.

- Intense acetowhite, pale on iodine staining
- Mosaicism and punctation due to atypical vessel formation
- Raised or ulcerated surface

Fig. 10.7 Risk factors for cervical cancer.

- Early age of first intercourse
- Higher number of sexual partners
- HPV (human papilloma virus) infection
- Lower socioeconomic group
- Smoking
- Partner with prostatic or penile cancer

Fig. 10.8 Staging of cervical cancer.

Stage	Description
0	Carcinoma in situ
I	Confined to the cervix:
A	• Visible only under a microscope:
A1	• <3mm in depth
A2	• >3mm in depth
II	Beyond the cervix:
A	• No parametrial involvement
B	• Parametrial involvement
III	Spread to the pelvic side wall, or affecting the ureter, or spread to the lower third of the vagina
IV	
A	Involving the rectal or bladder mucosa
B	Beyond the true pelvis

As mentioned above HPV infection is a major risk factor for cervical cancer and it is hoped that the vaccination programme along with compliance with cervical screening will help to reduce the incidence of the disease.

Clinical presentation

Cervical cancer may be completely asymptomatic or may be identified by cervical cytology. Patients who present with post-coital bleeding, intermenstrual bleeding, persistent vaginal discharge (may be blood stained) or postmenopausal bleeding should all be examined to identify any abnormality on the cervix and any features of concern should prompt referral for colposcopic examination.

Investigations and staging

Once a tissue diagnosis has been made the next step would be to stage the disease. The staging has traditionally been clinical with the patients undergoing an examination under anaesthesia (plus cone biopsy, to assess depth of invasion, chest X-ray, intravenous urogram (IVU), cystoscopy and sigmoidoscopy), with a MRI. Figure 10.8 shows the staging of cervical cancer.

Treatment

The treatment of cervical cancer can be by surgery, radiotherapy and chemotherapy. Once all factors are taken into account such as patient age, staging and any other medical problems a multidisciplinary team will usually advise on the best options for treatment.

In stage I disease the treatment may need to be tailored to the patient's individual circumstances and desire for children. Stage Ia1 may be diagnosed on a LLETZ sample and if the lesion has been completely excised no further treatment may be necessary. In Stage 1a2 the incidence of lymph node involvement is 5% so lymphadenectomy is advised but in those wishing to preserve fertility a LLETZ or cone biopsy may be considered to remove the cancer.

Stages Ib – IIa can be treated with surgery or radiotherapy with equivalent results, generally fit and healthy patients will undergo surgery whilst older or medically unstable patients will be offered radiotherapy.

Stages IIb and above are treated with radiotherapy combined with chemotherapy.

VULVAL CANCER

Vulval intraepithelial neoplasia

Similar to CIN, vulval intraepithelial neoplasia (VIN) is a premalignant condition which can progress to invasive carcinoma. If VIN is present, CIN is often seen too with HPV being the causal factor.

Incidence and aetiology

Vulval tumours are rare, with an incidence of around 3 in 100 000 women per year. The peak incidence is from the ages of 63 to 65.

Predisposing factors include:

- history of CIN, VIN or HPV
- immunosuppression
- lichen sclerosus (see Fig. 10.9).

Fig. 10.9 Lichen sclerosus information box.

Lichen sclerosus is a benign skin condition, with white plaques and atrophy seen in a figure-of-eight pattern around the vulva and anus. Extragenital plaques on the trunk and back might be seen. It is associated with autoimmune disorders, e.g. vitiligo. It can be classed as premalignant, as around 4% will go on to develop vulval squamous cell carcinoma

Pathology

Around 90% of vulval tumours are squamous cell carcinomas. Non-squamous cell tumours include melanoma, sarcoma, adenocarcinoma and basal cell tumours. Paget's disease of the vulva is a malignant change in cells of the epidermal layer, which have a characteristic appearance. The presence of vulval Paget's disease is associated with an adenocarcinoma elsewhere in the body in one in four cases, with the most common sites being breast, urinary tract, rectum and genital tract.

Presentation

The most common presenting symptoms are:

- pruritus
- lump/ulcer
- bleeding
- pain
- discharge

Urinary symptoms may be a feature or, indeed, there may be no symptoms at all. The most common sites are shown in Figure 10.10. The tumour may be multifocal.

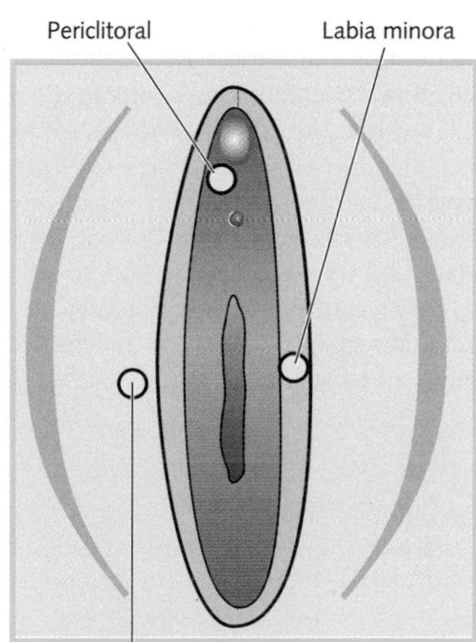

Fig. 10.10 Squamous cell carcinoma of the vulva.

It should be noted that some elderly patients who are embarrassed to seek help may present late with advanced disease.

Spread

- Local spread occurs to the vagina, perineum, clitoris, urethra and pubic bone.
- Lymphatic spread is to the superficial inguinal, deep inguino-femoral and iliac nodes. Unless the tumour is central (i.e. within 1 cm of the midline) only the nodes on the affected side are involved.

Investigations

A tissue diagnosis is obtained by taking a biopsy, and at the time of biopsy the vagina and cervix are thoroughly inspected for signs of involvement. Positive nodes may be detected by CT or MRI scan. Stages are shown in Figure 10.11.

Management

As vulval cancers are rare it is best practice for them to be managed in specialist centres. The aim of treatment is to excise the cancer and minimize the risk of recurrence while preserving as much function as possible. The management plan depends on the stage; early tumours are treated by wide local excision. If the initial biopsy showed the depth of invasion to be more than 1 mm, the nodes on the affected side must be dissected, if less than 1 mm nodal dissection is unnecessary.

Radiotherapy is necessary if histology reveals the nodes to be positive. Chemotherapy has not been shown to be helpful.

Complications of treatment are shown in Figure 10.12. Due to the large area involved, wound breakdown is, sadly, relatively common. With the en bloc method it occurs in up to 80% of cases, whereas rates for the butterfly incision are between 5 and 50%. Some surgeons advocate performing skin grafts at the time of initial surgery. Radiotherapy adds extra complications.

Fig. 10.11 Staging of vulval cancer.

Stage	Description
I A B	Confined to vulva: <1mm invasion <2cm diameter, no groin nodes
II	Confined to vulva, >2 cm diameter, no groin nodes palpable
III	Confined to vulva, suspicious nodes or beyond vulva with no suspicious nodes
IV	Obvious groin nodes *or* involving rectum, bladder, urethra or bone *or* pelvic or distant metastases

Fig. 10.12 Complications of treatment.

Type of treatment	Complication
Vulvectomy	Haemorrhage Thromboembolism Infection – wound, urinary tract Wound breakdown
Radiotherapy	Erythema Necrosis of the femoral head or pubic symphysis Fistula formation (urethrovaginal, vesiculovaginal or rectovaginal)

Prognosis

Stage I disease has a 92% 5-year survival rate, whereas advanced disease (Stage IV) has only a 13% 5-year survival rate.

VAGINAL TUMOURS

Vaginal tumours are rare and are usually either primary squamous carcinoma or spread from vulval or cervical squamous cancers. Even rarer tumours include endodermal sinus tumours, rhabdomyosarcoma (both seen in children, but the latter also seen in older women) melanoma, clear cell adenocarcinoma and leiomyosarcoma.

Aetiology

Associations are with CIN and HPV and with a history of another gynaecological malignancy in the past.

Presentation

The upper third of the vagina is the most common site, and women usually present at an early stage with abnormal bleeding.

Investigation

Staging is shown in Figure 10.13 and requires biopsy, examination under anaesthetic and assessment of the bladder and rectum either at operation or on MRI. Chest X-ray is performed as part of the evaluation.

Fig. 10.13 Staging of vaginal cancer.

Stage	Description
0	Vaginal intraepithelial neoplasia
I	Limited to the vaginal wall
IIA	Subvaginal tissue, but not the parametrium, involved
IIB	Parametrial involvement
III	Spread to the pelvic side wall
IV	Bladder/rectum involved or distant organ spread

Management

Treatment is a combination of external beam and intravaginal radiotherapy, with the complications being fistulae (as with vulval radiotherapy) and stenosis of the vagina and rectum.

Prognosis

Seventy per cent of women who present have stage I or II disease, with 5-year survival rates of around 70%.

Further reading

Arulkumaran, S., Regan, L., Papageorghiou, A., et al., 2011. Oxford Desk Reference Obstetrics & Gynaecology. Oxford University Press, Oxford.

Cancer Research UK, 2013. Cancer Statistics. Cancer Research UK, London. Available online at:www.cancerresearchuk.org.

NICE, 2011. Ovarian cancer: recognition and initial management of ovarian cancer. NICE clinical guideline No. 122. National Collaborating Centre for Cancer, Cardiff.

RCOG, 2003. Ovarian cysts in postmenopausal women. Green-top Guideline 34. Royal College of Obstetricians and Gynaecologists, London.

RCOG, 2006. Management of Vulval Cancer. Royal College of Obstetricians and Gynaecologists, London.

RCOG, 2011. Management of ovarian masses in premenopausal women. Green-top Guideline 62. Royal College of Obstetricians and Gynaecologists, London.

Vulval disease 11

Objectives

By the end of this chapter, you should be able to:

- Understand the importance of age at presentation in diagnosing the likely causes of pruritus vulvae
- Understand how to assess vulval disorders, including the important points in the history and examination
- Request the appropriate investigations on a patient presenting with vulval symptoms in order to establish a diagnosis
- Consider the treatment of the commonest vulval dystrophies.

The vulva extends from the mons pubis anteriorly to the perineum posteriorly and the labia majora laterally (Fig. 11.1). The whole surface of the vulva up to the inner aspect of the labia minora is covered by stratified, keratinized squamous epithelium with a superficial cornified layer. The cornified layer is absent in the vagina and there is a decreasing degree of keratinization (Fig.11.2).

SYMPTOMS

Common signs and symptoms include pain and pruritis. Itching or irritation of the vulval region is called pruritus vulvae. This is a common symptom and can be caused by a whole host of conditions (Fig.11.3):

- Vulval dystrophy
- Neoplasia
- Dermatological
- Infection.

Common skin changes include changes in texture and colour. Generalized dermatological conditions and systemic illness may present with vulval symptoms.

HISTORY

The age of the patient is important. Younger women are generally more likely to have an infectious cause, whereas vulval dystrophies and cancers are more likely in older women. Acute onset of symptoms occurs frequently with infection whereas other causes of pruritus vulvae can have a more chronic and insidious onset. Embarrassment often delays presentation. A history of postmenopausal bleeding is important to ascertain as this may indicate an underlying malignancy.

Exacerbating and relieving factors can give clues as to the aetiology. Symptoms of yeast and herpetic infection might worsen premenstrually. A recent change in soap or washing powder, or overzealous hygiene may suggest contact dermatitis. Self-treatment with emollients and antifungals is common and should be noted, as should the response.

Cervical intraepithelial neoplasia (CIN) and vulval intraepithelial neoplasia (VIN) are thought to share a common aetiology, so a history of CIN should be noted. Abnormal vaginal discharge can suggest infection and, if suspected, a detailed sexual history should be taken. The discharge of infection with *Trichomonas vaginalis* and bacterial vaginosis has a typically 'fishy' odour.

Dermatological conditions such as psoriasis and eczema can affect the vulva and a history of these conditions elsewhere on the body might be relevant. A history of atopy and symptoms suggestive of diabetes mellitus, renal and liver failure should be noted.

Drug history and family history of any autoimmune conditions are also important.

EXAMINATION

General examination of the patient includes assessment of skin surfaces prone to dermatological conditions: face, hands, wrists, elbows, trunk and knees. Signs of chronic renal failure and liver disease should be looked for.

Examination of the vulva, urethral meatus and perianal region in a good light is essential. The vagina and cervix should be inspected carefully using a speculum. Colposcopic examination of the vulva may also be useful, particularly with a history of abnormal smears.

Inguinal lymphadenopathy can occur secondary to infection or malignancy.

Fig. 11.1 The anatomy of the vulva.

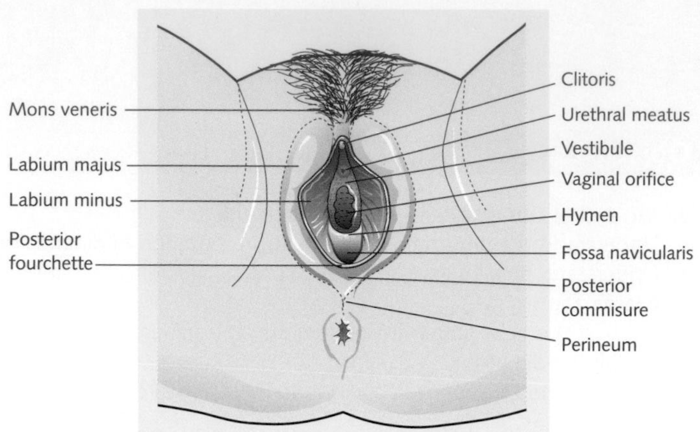

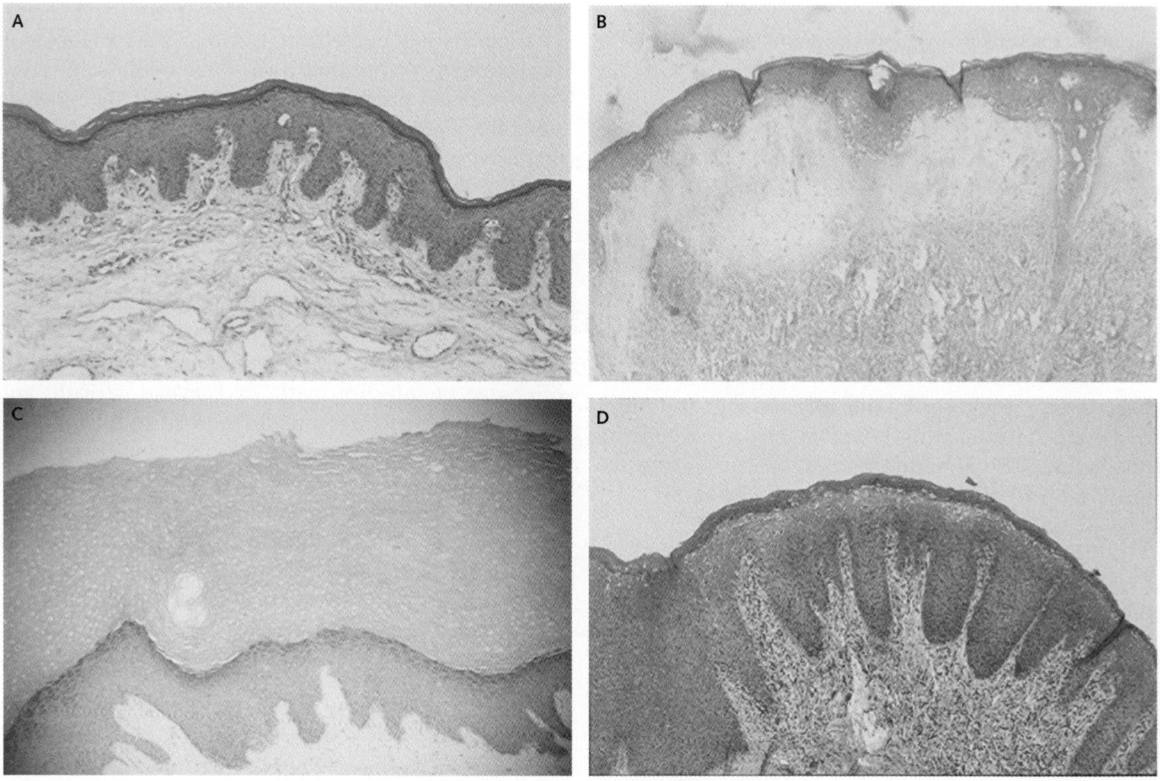

Fig. 11.2 Histology. (A) normal, (B) lichen sclerosus, (C) squamous hyperplasia and (D) dysplasia. From Llewellyn-Jones D, 2010. Fundamentals of Obstetrics and Gynaecology, 9th edn. London: Mosby, with permission.

Infection

Generalized vulvitis, vaginal discharge and ulcers suggest an infective cause, although ulceration should alert the examiner to the possibility of malignancy. Genital warts might be seen on the vulva, perianally, in the vagina or on the cervix.

Vulval dystrophies

Labial fusion, adhesions, stenosis of the introitus, leucoplakia (literally meaning 'white plaque') and atrophic changes are frequent signs of lichen sclerosus, the most common of the vulval dystrophies. The lesions of hyperplastic dystrophy can be localized or extensive, and

Fig. 11.3 Differential diagnosis of pruritus vulvae.

Type of cause	Description
Infection	Fungal *Candida* Tinea Parasitic *Trichomonas vaginalis* *Enterobius* (pinworm) *Pediculosis pubis* Bacterial Bacterial vaginosis /vaginitis Viral Herpes simplex virus Human papilloma virus
Vulval dystrophy	Lichen sclerosus Hypertrophic vulval dystrophy
Neoplastic	Vulval intraepithelial neoplasia (VIN) Squamous carcinoma Paget's disease of the vulva
Dermatological	Psoriasis Eczema Contact dermatitis

typically show thickening of the affected skin with variable colour change. Thickened plaques of leucoplakia might be present.

HINTS AND TIPS

When taking a history, ask about a history of autoimmune disease or allergy. Also check that there are no bowel or urinary symptoms. When examining, carefully inspect the anogenital area.

COMMON CAUSES

The most common local causes of vulval skin disorders are:

- lichen sclerosus
- lichen planus
- dermatitis
- vulval candidiasis.

Dermatological conditions which can affect the vulva include psoriasis and eczema.

Infective causes of vulval changes include sexually transmitted diseases (STDs), warts, herpes, scabies and threadworms.

Systemic causes include diabetes, renal failure and Crohn's disease.

INVESTIGATIONS

Where systemic disease is suspected, relevant investigations include thyroid and liver function, renal function and glucose tolerance. Urinalysis might reveal the presence of haematuria, proteinurea and glycosuria.

Bacteriological swabs should be taken to exclude yeast infection (Fig.11.4) and sexually active women should be screened for STDs.

Although certain vulval conditions have a typical appearance, many are difficult to distinguish with the naked eye. The mainstay of diagnosis of vulval dystrophies, dermatoses and neoplasms is histological. Punch biopsies of the vulva can be performed under local anaesthetic in the outpatient setting, with or without a colposcope. Discrete lesions can be excised in their entirety under general anaesthesia. Hysteroscopy may be needed to exclude endometrial pathology if there is a history of postmenopausal bleeding (see Chapter 4).

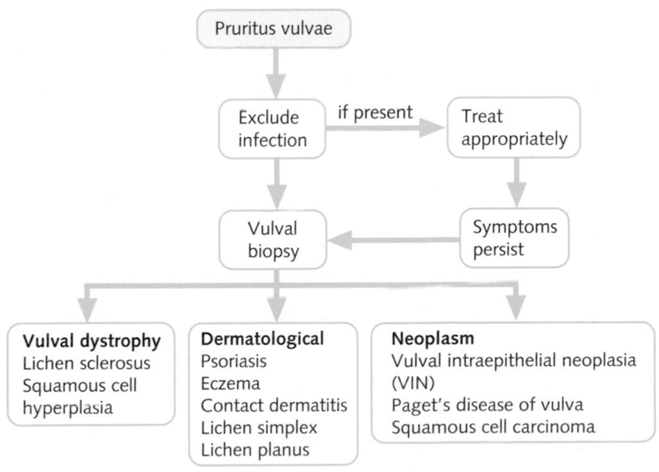

Fig. 11.4 Algorithm for the management of pruritus vulvae. From Llewellyn-Jones D, 2010. Fundamentals of Obstetrics and Gynaecology, 9th edn. London: Mosby, with permission.

VULVAL DYSTROPHIES

Histologically, the vulval dystrophies are divided into atrophic and hypertrophic or a mixed picture of both. Atrophic vulval dystrophy is better known as lichen sclerosus.

Any of the vulval conditions (including vulval carcinoma) may present simply as pruritis, so the symptom of pruritus vulvae should not be underestimated.

Lichen sclerosus

Lichen sclerosus is the most common of the vulval dystrophies. It usually develops in postmenopausal women, although any age group can be affected, including prepubertal girls (Fig. 11.5). The aetiology is unknown.

The whole of the vulva and perianal region may be affected. Affected skin is typically thin, shiny and can be white (leucoplakia) or red due to inflammation. Anatomical changes include shrinkage or loss of the labia minora and shrinkage of the introitus. Adhesions can fuse the labia together. Lichen sclerosus can affect the perineum and perianal region.

Symptoms include discomfort, dyspareunia and itching, leading to bleeding and skin splitting. The labia minora may fuse laterally and the introitus may narrow.

Diagnosis is made histologically from vulval biopsies, which classically show subepithelial haemorrhage (ecchymoses) and inflammation.

Treatment is aimed at relieving the itching and soreness and, as this is a chronic relapsing condition, is usually intermittent:

- Simple emollient creams can relieve mild symptoms.
- Short courses of potent topical steroids might be needed.
- The recommended second-line treatment is topical tacrolimus, with follow-up at a specialist clinic.
- Testosterone cream is sometimes used, but probably acts more as an emollient than hormonally.

Complications are unusual and include anatomical changes and the risk of malignancy. Anatomical changes can cause dyspareunia and, if fusion of the labia occurs in the midline, difficulty in micturition, which might require separation of the labia. Long-term follow-up of women with lichen sclerosus is important as up to 5% will develop squamous carcinoma of the vulva.

HINTS AND TIPS

Consider obtaining a biopsy if the patient does not respond to treatment, or VIN/cancer is suspected.

Lichen planus

This is a common skin condition which may occur anywhere on the body. It usually affects mucosal surfaces, most commonly seen in the mouth, and can affect all ages. Clinically, flat-topped purpuric plaques and papules are seen, with a fine white reticular pattern. It is more commonly associated with pain than with pruritis. The aetiology is unknown, but it may have an autoimmune component.

Treatment is aimed at managing symptoms and is predominantly based on topical or oral corticosteroids.

NEOPLASIA

Neoplastic conditions of the vulva include carcinomas-in-situ (see Chapter 10), VIN and Paget's disease of the vulva, and malignant squamous carcinoma.

Fig. 11.5 Characteristics of some important vulval diseases.

	Age at presentation	Incidence	Mode of treatment	Recurrence rate	Malignant potential
Vulval dystrophies					
Lichen sclerosus	Any age but usually postmenopausal	Common	Topical steroids and emollients	Frequent	<5% develop squamous carcinoma of the vulva
Neoplasias					
Vulval intraepithelial neoplasia	Any age but increasing in the young	Relatively uncommon, but increasing	Usually surgical more conservative in young women	Up to 80% will recur	Overall low, but higher in the elderly and immunosuppressed
Paget's disease of the vulva	Postmenopausal women	Rare	Surgical	Up to 33% will recur	Associated with adenocarcinoma in 25% Malignant change in lesion is rare

Vulval intraepithelial neoplasia

This is a relatively uncommon condition, although the incidence is increasing in young women. Human papilloma virus (specifically HPV 16) has been implicated in the aetiology. Histologically, neoplastic cells are contained within the basement membrane and the degree of dysplasia is divided into mild, moderate and severe (VIN 1, VIN 2 and VIN 3, respectively).

Symptoms include pruritus, pain, soreness and palpable lesions, but many are asymptomatic and found incidentally. VIN lesions are variable and can be papular (similar to genital warts) or macular with irregular borders. Pigmentation (brown or black) is common and leucoplakia and ulceration can occur. Invasive squamous carcinoma of the vulva usually appears as an exophytic tumour, often with surface ulceration. Lesions can be papular (like genital warts) or macular with irregular borders. They can be red, brown or black (pigmented), or white (leucoplakia) and ulceration might be present. Unifocal lesions are more common postmenopausally. The diagnosis is made histologically from vulval biopsies.

Treatment is usually surgical, either by ablating the lesion with laser or cryotherapy or by local excision. VIN will recur in up to 80% of treated women and as the risk of malignant change is small, especially in younger women, major mutilating surgery should be avoided. Surgical treatment is recommended when the risk of malignant change is increased:

- in excessively hyperkeratotic lesions
- in postmenopausal women
- in the immunosuppressed.

If the severity of dysplasia is seen to worsen on serial biopsy excision should be considered. Where conservative treatment is planned, topical steroids may give symptomatic relief.

HINTS AND TIPS

Women who have been treated for VIN are at risk of intraepithelial neoplasia at other sites. Colposcopy examination should be available at follow-up.

Squamous carcinoma of the vulva

Squamous carcinoma of the vulva is discussed in Chapter 10.

Paget's disease of the vulva

Paget's disease of the vulva is uncommon; it is usually seen in postmenopausal women. The aetiology is unknown, although the lesion is thought to be of glandular origin. In 25% of cases, there is an underlying adenocarcinoma (breast, urinary, genital or colonic).

Paget's disease of the vulva can be unifocal or multifocal and the lesions are typically clearly defined, scaly, erythematous plaques with varying degrees of ulceration and leucoplakia.

Lesions can be unifocal or multifocal and are typically clearly defined, scaly, erythematous plaques with varying degrees of ulceration and leucoplakia. The main symptom is pruritus and the diagnosis is made histologically. Treatment is surgical using laser ablation or local excision and up to one-third will recur. Although associated with adenocarcinoma, malignant change within the lesion is rare.

DERMATOLOGICAL CONDITIONS

Many dermatological conditions can affect the vulva often with a confusing clinical picture, especially if the vulva is the only area affected.

Psoriasis

The typical raised, erythematous, scaly lesions of psoriasis can occur on the vulva, although here they might appear smooth and without the scaling. The presence of psoriasis elsewhere on the body will suggest the diagnosis, which can be confirmed histologically. Treatment is with topical steroids, but the relapse rate is high.

Eczema

Eczema of the vulva is rare. More commonly, eczematous reactions occur due to contact with irritant substances such as soaps and detergents. Treatment is by identifying and removing the source of irritation and topical steroids.

Further reading

Llewellyn-Jones, D., 2010. Fundamentals of Obstetrics & Gynaecology, ninth ed. Mosby, London.

McKay Hart, D., Norman, J., 2000. Gynaecology Illustrated, fifth ed. Churchill Livingstone, London.

Monaghan, J.M., 1992. Bonney's Gynaecological Surgery, ninth ed. Bailliere Tindall, London.

Shaw, R.W., Soutter, W.P., Stanton, S.L., 1997. Gynaecology, second ed. Churchill Livingstone, London.

RCOG, 2011. Management of Vulval Skin Disorders. Available online at: www.rcog.org.uk/guidelines.

Vaginal discharge

Objectives

By the end of this chapter, you should be able to:

- Understand the important points in the history for a patient presenting with vaginal discharge
- Perform an examination on a patient presenting with vaginal discharge
- Undertake appropriate investigations on a patient presenting with vaginal discharge in order to establish a diagnosis.

DIFFERENTIAL DIAGNOSIS

Vaginal discharge can be either:

- physiological, or
- pathological.

Physiological discharge varies with the changing oestrogen levels associated with the luteal phase of the menstrual cycle and pregnancy. Once pathological causes have been excluded, the patient can be reassured that her symptoms are normal. Possible causes of physiological vaginal discharge are:

- vestibular gland secretions
- vaginal transudate
- cervical mucus
- residual menstrual fluid.

Don't forget to reassure the patient that vaginal discharge might simply be physiological, related to the menstrual cycle or to pregnancy. Pathological causes need to be excluded.

The differential diagnoses of pathological vaginal discharge are shown in Figure 12.1. The most common group is the infections.

HISTORY

Presenting complaint

The patient should be asked about the nature of the discharge. This includes:

- timing of onset
- colour
- odour
- presence of any blood
- irritation.

For example, candidal infection is associated with a thick, itchy, white discharge, whereas with bacterial vaginosis there is typically a grey, fishy-smelling discharge. An allergic reaction is usually associated with itching. Urinary symptoms, such as dysuria and frequency, might be present with a sexually transmitted infection.

Lower abdominal pain, backache and dyspareunia are suggestive of pelvic inflammatory disease (PID) (see Chapter 13), more commonly in a younger woman. In relation to malignancy, the patient age group is usually older than the infective group (see Chapter 10). General symptoms such as weight loss and anorexia should be excluded.

Past gynaecological history

The date of the menopause and the last cervical smear test are relevant, particularly if malignancy is suspected.

A ring pessary might previously have been sited to relieve genital prolapse (see Chapter 15). This should be changed every 6 months. Previous history of hysterectomy could be linked with development of a uretero- or vesicovaginal fistula. This results in constant vaginal loss that is actually urine. A history of obstructed labour, more common in developing countries, also puts the patient at risk of a vesicovaginal fistula.

Past medical history

A history of diabetes mellitus predisposes the patient to candida infection.

Generalized symptoms can be indicative of different pathologies, depending on the age of the patient. Lower abdominal pain, backache and dyspareunia suggest infection in a younger woman but malignancy in older age groups.

Fig. 12.1 Differential diagnosis of pathological vaginal discharge.

Diagnosis	Cause of discharge
Infective	Sexually transmitted infection *Chlamydia trachomatis* *Trichomonas vaginalis* *Neisseria gonorrhoea* Infection not sexually transmitted *Candida albicans* Bacterial vaginosis
Inflammatory	Allergy to soap/contraceptives etc Atrophic changes Postoperative granulation tissue
Malignancy	Vulval carcinoma Cervical carcinoma Uterine carcinoma
Foreign body	Retained tampon/condom Ring pessaries
Fistula	From bowel, bladder and ureter to vagina

Sexual history

The patient's current method of contraception is important with regards to the risk of a sexually transmitted infection, as is a recent new partner. The risk is increased with a non-barrier method of contraception (see Chapter 19).

Drug history

Recent antibiotic therapy can precipitate candida infection.

EXAMINATION

- General examination
- Abdominal palpation
- Speculum examination
- Bimanual palpation.

General examination should be aimed at identifying signs of systemic infection (tachycardia, pyrexia, local lymphadenopathy) or malignancy (cachexia, generalized lymphadenopathy).

Always remember to perform a general examination and abdominal palpation, and not simply vulval/vaginal examination.

Abdominal palpation should exclude localized tenderness, which may be present if the patient is developing PID, or an abdominal mass if malignancy is suspected.

The vulva and vagina should be inspected carefully. A speculum examination should be performed to check the cervix and to confirm or exclude:

- vaginal discharge
- inflammation
- ulceration
- foreign bodies
- local tumours.

Bimanual pelvic examination will reveal pelvic tumours. It might also elicit tenderness and cervical excitation, suggesting PID.

INVESTIGATION

- Microbiological swabs (vulval/high vaginal/endocervical/urethral)
- Blood test: full blood count (FBC), creatinine-reactive protein (CRP), cultures if signs of systemic infection, i.e. acute PID
- Mid-stream urine (MSU) specimen
- Cervical cytology/biopsy: only if cervical smear due or abnormalities noted on the cervix, opportunistic smears not recommended
- Pelvic ultrasound scan: transvaginal if not virgo intact
- Endometrial sampling/hysteroscopy can be done as an outpatient or under general anaesthetic
- Laparoscopy.

Figure 12.2 shows the relevant investigations for vaginal discharge. Figure 12.3 is an algorithm for the diagnosis and investigation of vaginal discharge.

Fig. 12.2 Investigations for vaginal discharge.

Investigation	Cause of discharge
Microbiological swabs	Vulval/high vaginal swab (HVS) *Candida albicans* *Trichomonas vaginalis*
	Endocervical/urethral swab *Chlamydia trachomatis* *Neiserria gonorrhoea*
Midstream urine specimen	Infection
Cervical cytology	Cervical disease
Endometrial sampling/hysteroscopy	Uterine disease
Pelvic ultrasound scan	Pelvic mass
Laparoscopy	Pelvic inflammatory disease Pelvic malignancy

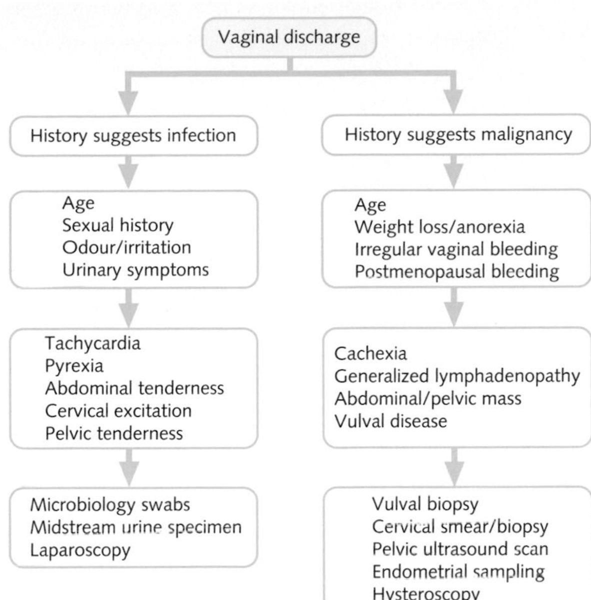

Fig. 12.3 Algorithm for vaginal discharge.

Further reading

Faculty of Sexual & Reproductive Healthcare (FSRH) and The British Association of Sexual Health and HIV (BASHH) Guidance (February 2012): Management of Vaginal Discharge in Non-Genitourinary Medicine settings. www.fsrh.org/pdfs/CEUGuidanceVaginalDischarge.pdf.

Pelvic inflammatory disease

Objectives

By the end of this chapter, you should be able to:

- List the differential diagnoses for pelvic inflammatory disease (PID)
- Describe the investigations necessary to exclude PID
- List the potential sequelae of PID
- Discuss the principles of treatment for PID
- Consider the issues in public health with respect to PID.

DEFINITION

Pelvic inflammatory disease (PID) is defined as the clinical syndrome associated with ascending spread of microorganisms from the endocervix to the endometrium, fallopian tubes and/or contiguous structures. It usually begins with an acute infection; this might resolve completely or develop a chronic course with repeated acute or subacute episodes.

INCIDENCE

The true incidence of PID is difficult to determine because of the lack of a precise clinical definition or a specific diagnostic test. However, the incidence is strongly correlated with the prevalence of sexually transmitted infections, and has increased in most countries. In the USA, the highest annual incidence is among sexually active women in their teenage years; 75% of cases occur in women under the age of 25. Figure 13.1 outlines risk factors for the development of PID.

AETIOLOGY

PID is caused by sexually transmitted infections such as *Chlamydia trachomatis*, *Neisseria gonorrhea* and *Mycoplasma genitalium*.

Chlamydia trachomatis is the most common cause of PID in the UK. Along with *Neisseria gonorrhoeae*, this microorganism is responsible for at least 60% of cases of PID. They are thought to act as primary pathogens, causing damage to the protective mechanisms of the endocervix and allowing endogenous bacteria from the vagina and cervix into the upper genital tract as secondary invaders. A variety of endogenous aerobic and anaerobic bacteria have been isolated from women with PID, such as *Mycoplasma* species, may have a causative role.

PID can also develop secondary to other disease processes, such as appendicitis. Rarely, it is part of more generalized disease such as tuberculosis.

DIAGNOSIS

The diagnosis of PID is sometimes difficult to make, since it does not rely on one particular sign or symptom or a specific diagnostic test. However, it is thought that the benefits of early diagnosis and appropriate treatment outweigh the possible overuse of antibiotics in a patient who might seem to have only mild disease.

The differential diagnoses (see Chapter 6) include:

- appendicitis
- ovarian cyst accident
- endometriosis
- early pregnancy complications including ectopic pregnancy
- urinary tract infection
- constipation.

HISTORY

The history may include one or more of the following symptoms:

- Pelvic pain/lower abdominal pain, usually bilateral
- Bilateral pelvic pain – sometimes radiating to the legs
- Deep dyspareunia
- Dysmenorrhoea
- Abnormal or increased vaginal discharge
- Fever.

Fig. 13.1 Risk factors for the development of pelvic inflammatory disease.

Risk factor	Description
Age	75% of patients are below 25 years of age
Marital status	Single
Sexual history	Young at first intercourse High frequency of sexual intercourse Multiple sexual partners
Medical history	Past history of sexually transmitted disease in patient or partner Past history of PID in patient Recent instrumentation of uterus, e.g. termination of pregnancy
Contraception	Use of intrauterine contraceptive device, especially insertion within 3 weeks

Sensitivity is essential when taking a sexual history. It should include age at first intercourse, timing of last intercourse, as well as number of recent partners. A menstrual history and the use of contraception, in particular barrier methods, should be assessed. Take care not to make assumptions about a patient, for example, with respect to age and sexual activity.

PID can also be asymptomatic (Fig. 13.2), presenting many years after the acute infection with subfertility.

EXAMINATION

At least three of the following signs should be present to make the diagnosis of acute PID:

- Raised temperature >38 °C
- Tachycardia

Fig. 13.2 An overview of pelvic inflammatory disease.

Organism	Symptoms	Diagnosis	Treatment
Chlamydia	• Asymptomatic (80%) • Post-coital or intermenstrual bleeding • Lower abdominal pain • Purulent vaginal discharge • Dysuria	Endocervical swab Urethral swab Vulvovaginal swab 1st catch urine less sensitive NAAT	Doxycycline 100 mg bd 7 days or Azithromycin 1 g PO stat or Erythromycin 500 mg bd 14 days if pregnant
Gonorrhoea	• Asymptomatic (50%) • Increased or altered vaginal discharge • Lower abdominal pain • Dysuria	Endocervical swab Urethral swab NAAT	Ceftriaxone 250 mg IM stat or cefixime 400 mg PO stat or Spectinomycin 2 g IM stat or Ciprofloxacin 500 mg PO stat
Anaerobes including Gardnerella and Mycoplasma	Asymptomatic (50%) Offensive fishy-smelling discharge	High vaginal swab for microscopy and culture +/– pH test >4.5 +/– fishy odour with10% KOH solution	Metronidazole 400 mg bd 7 days

NAAT = nucleic acid amplification test, see text.

- Abdominal tenderness
- Purulent vaginal discharge
- Cervical motion tenderness
- Adnexal tenderness
- Adnexal swelling.

INVESTIGATIONS

Appropriate investigations include:

- white blood cell count (WBC)
- creatinine-reactive protein (CRP)
- erythrocyte sedimentation rate (ESR)
- blood cultures, depending on the level of the pyrexia
- full screen for sexually transmitted infections, including high vaginal swab, endocervical swabs and urethral swabs
- mid-stream urine (MSU) specimen
- pregnancy test (urinary β-hCG)
- ultrasound scan, usually transvaginal, is appropriate to exclude an ovarian cyst complication or a tubo-ovarian abscess
- swabs (high vaginal, endocervical and low vaginal) taken to exclude sexually transmitted infections are now examined using nucleic acid amplification tests (NAATs). These are replacing enzyme-linked immuno-assays because of the improved detection rates (90–95% compared with 40–70%).

Laparoscopy is considered to be the gold standard to diagnose acute PID. However, in practice, it is only considered if there is doubt about the differential diagnoses, such as the presence of an ovarian cyst, or if the patient fails to respond to antibiotic therapy. In acute disease, the pelvis will appear generally inflamed, with pus seen around the Fallopian tubes. These may be distended. In chronic disease, there may be generalized pelvic adhesions or evidence of old tubal disease/hydrosalpinges. Fitz-Hugh-Curtis syndrome indicates previous chlamydia infection, when the typical bow-string perihepatic adhesions are seen.

COMPLICATIONS

The long-term morbidity associated with acute PID is considerable (Fig. 13.3) and thus the need for prompt appropriate treatment, especially to cover chlamydial infection, is important. Moderately severe disease is associated with inflammation and oedema in the fallopian tubes, with deposits of fibrin and subsequent adhesion formation between the pelvic and abdominal organs. Thus, tubal morphology and function are affected resulting in subfertility and an increased risk of ectopic pregnancy. Adhesions in the pelvis may lead to chronic pain, either as a sole feature, or in relation to menstruation or sexual intercourse.

Fig. 13.3 Complications of acute pelvic inflammatory disease.

Type of complication	Description
Short term	Pelvic abscess formation Septicaemia Septic shock
Long term	Infertility Ectopic pregnancy Chronic pelvic pain Dyspareunia Menstrual disturbances Psychological effects

Early diagnosis and treatment are essential to reduce the risk of long-term complications.

TREATMENT

There should be a low threshold for empirical treatment for PID in the absence of definitive diagnostic criteria. The principles are:

- antibiotic therapy
- contact tracing
- surgery. The aim of treatment is to prevent the long-term sequelae of PID. Out-patient administration of broad-spectrum antibiotics is indicated once the diagnosis of PID is suspected and should be started prior to obtaining the results of microbiology specimens (see Fig. 13.2). In-patient treatment with intravenous antibiotics is indicated for more severe clinical disease. Recommended antibiotics depend on local patterns of microbial sensitivity.

Antibiotic therapy must include treatment for *Chlamydia* because this microorganism is most commonly implicated in PID and its sequelae.

If a patient resumes sexual intercourse with a partner who is infected but untreated, there is obviously a high chance of re-infection. It is, therefore, important to trace all recent contacts so that they can be given treatment, either empirically or as a result of microbiology results. This can be done more effectively by referring the patient to a genitourinary medicine clinic. The patient should avoid intercourse until both have completed a course of treatment.

Apart from diagnostic laparoscopy, there is rarely a need for more invasive surgery in the management of PID. Laparoscopy or laparotomy may be necessary to drain a tubo-ovarian abscess.

PREVENTION

PID and its sequelae are responsible for a substantial amount of morbidity, both physical and psychological. There are also considerable financial implications, estimated at £100 million per year in the UK. Therefore, primary prevention of the disease is of great importance and needs the help of both the media and health-care professionals. Government educational programmes are currently in progress and national screening programmes are being evaluated:

- Health education activities to increase awareness of at-risk behaviour
- Opportunistic screening of those at risk, e.g. termination of pregnancy (TOP) clinic, patient having evacuation of the retained products of conception (ERPC)
- Knowledge of up-to-date treatment regimens with locally agreed protocols
- Understanding the importance of contact tracing.

Effective treatment for PID must include contact tracing and treatment of the patient's partners. Again this should be done in a sensitive manner and confidentiality is essential at all times.

Further reading

British Association of Sexual Health and HIV, 2012. Guidelines. Available online at: www.bassh.org.

RCOG, 2008. Management of Acute Pelvic Inflammatory Disease. Green-top Guideline No. 32. Royal College of Obstetricians and Gynaecologists, London. Available online at: www.rcog.org.uk.

Shaw, R.W., Luesle, D., Monga, A., 2010. Gynaecology, fourth ed. Churchill Livingstone, London.

Urinary incontinence

Objectives

By the end of this chapter, you will be able to:

- Take a history to distinguish between stress incontinence and detrusor overactivity
- Perform an examination on a female patient presenting with urinary incontinence
- Request and interpret the relevant investigations to diagnose the type of incontinence a patient has
- Consider the treatments available for incontinence.

Urinary incontinence is an objectively demonstrable, involuntary loss of urine that is a social or hygienic problem. The two most common causes of urinary incontinence are stress urinary incontinence (SUI) and detrusor overactivity (DO), which account for approximately 90% of incontinent women. These, and other causes, are shown in Figure 14.1 in order of frequency of occurrence.

INCIDENCE

Female urinary incontinence is a very common problem, with up to one quarter of women leaking urine occasionally. The prevalence of regular female urinary incontinence increases with increasing age:

- 8.5% of women under 65 years of age
- 11.6% over 65 years
- 43.2% over 85 years.

AETIOLOGY

The bladder has two major roles: the retention of urine and expulsion of urine. Failure to retain urine, or loss of normal voiding control, gives rise to two distinct aetiologies of incontinence:

- Stress urinary incontinence (SUI) – 50% of incontinence
- Detrusor overactivity (DO) – 40% of incontinence.

Urinary tract infection must always be excluded in the presence of urinary symptoms.

Stress urinary incontinence

The bladder acts as a low-pressure reservoir. As the volume of urine increases, the bladder pressure rises slightly. Urethral closure pressure, produced by the passive effect of elastic and collagen fibres and active striated and smooth muscle, causes the urethra to remain closed at rest. In the resting state the urethral closure pressure is higher than the relatively low bladder pressure and continence is maintained.

Intra-abdominal pressure is transmitted to the bladder and raised intra-abdominal pressure, such as during coughing or straining, increases the bladder pressure. Intra-abdominal pressure is also transmitted to the bladder neck and that part of the proximal urethra which is intra-abdominal (above the pelvic floor) maintaining the positive pressure gradient and hence continence (Fig.14.2B). If the bladder neck and proximal urethra are situated below the pelvic floor then the raised intra abdominal pressure is no longer transmitted to these structures, the positive pressure gradient is lost and incontinence occurs (Fig. 14.2C).

SUI increases with increasing age as maximal urethral closure pressure decreases. Also, older women are more likely to be parous and postmenopausal. SUI increases with increasing parity. Prolapse is commonly thought to be associated with SUI, although this is only true if the proximal urethra is below the pelvic floor (see above). Atrophic changes associated with the post-menopausal state and vaginal surgery to cure prolapse are also associated with SUI.

Detrusor overactivity

In women with DO, the urethra functions normally, but if the uninhibited detrusor activity increases bladder pressure above maximal urethral closure pressure, urinary leakage occurs.

The majority of women with DO have an idiopathic aetiology with no demonstrable abnormality. DO can be caused by surgery to the bladder neck and proximal urethra, especially following surgery for SUI, which involves dissection around these structures. Multiple sclerosis, autonomic neuropathy and spinal lesions lead

Fig. 14.1 The causes of female urinary incontinence in order of frequency of occurrence.

1. Stress urinary incontinence (SUI)	50%
2. Detrusor overactivity (DO)	40%
3. Mixed SUI and DO	5%
4. Sensory urgency	4%
5. Chronic voiding problems (chronic retention)	<1%
6. Fistula	<1%

to uninhibited detrusor contractions, causing detrusor hyperreflexia.

Increasing age and a history of nocturnal enuresis are associated with DO and diuretics will obviously exacerbate this condition.

Sensory urgency

Irritation of the bladder mucosa, due either to infection (cystitis), bladder stones or tumours, can cause sensory urgency. The aetiology of primary vesical sensory urgency is not well understood, but accounts for almost 4% of incontinent women.

Voiding disorders

Voiding difficulties can present as acute or chronic urinary retention with overflow incontinence. Chronic overdistension of the bladder is likely to exacerbate and can itself cause voiding difficulties due to detrusor ischaemia and denervation.

Central, spinal and peripheral neurological lesions can produce voiding difficulties (Fig.14.3). Approximately 25% of women with multiple sclerosis will present with acute urinary retention. Postoperative pain can cause reflex inhibition of micturition, as can severe inflammation of the bladder, urethra and vulva.

Drugs can cause voiding difficulties, epidural anaesthesia in labour being the most common encountered. Tricyclic antidepressants, anticholinergic agents, α-adrenergic agonists and ganglion blockers can all cause voiding difficulties.

Voiding difficulties can occur secondary to mechanical obstruction. Impaction of a pelvic mass, for instance the gravid uterus or fibroids, might obstruct the urethra, as can bladder polyps or malignancy. Oedema following bladder neck surgery causes voiding difficulties frequently enough to warrant prophylactic drainage of the bladder following these procedures. Surprisingly, it is rare for prolapse to cause retention.

Fistulae

The most common cause of fistula formation worldwide is obstructed labour. In the UK, avoiding prolonged labour has almost eradicated this complication. Although uncommon, fistulae are likely to be secondary to malignancy, surgery and radiation to the pelvis or a combination of these. Fistulae can occur from the ureter, bladder or urethra to the vagina.

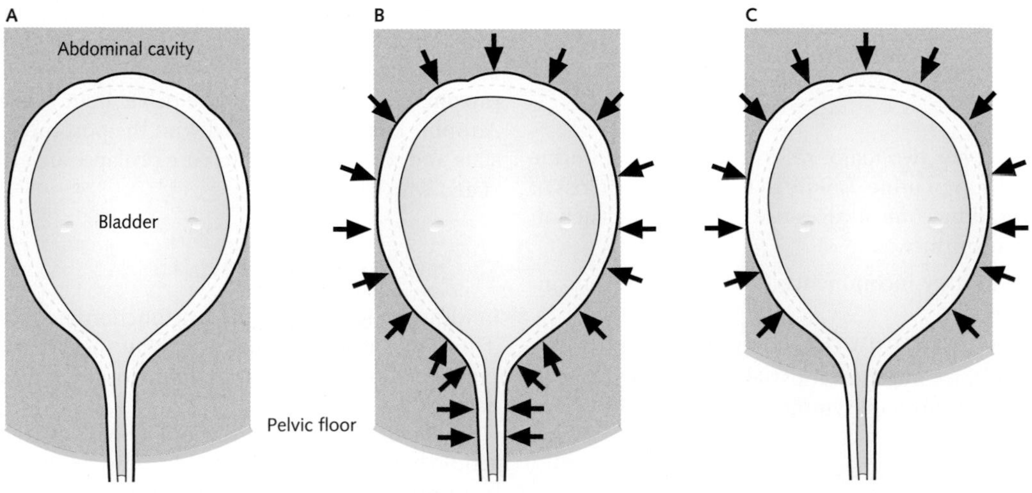

Fig. 14.2 Mechanism of stress urinary incontinence (SUI). (A) Bladder at rest. (B) Intra-abdominal pressure transmitted to bladder and urethra (normal). (C) Intra-abdominal pressure not transmitted to bladder/urethra (SUI).

Fig. 14.3 Neurological causes of voiding difficulties (acute and chronic retention).

Type of lesion	Neurological cause of voiding difficulty
Central (suprapontine)	Cerebrovascular accident Parkinson's disease
Spinal	Spinal cord injury Multiple sclerosis
Peripheral	Prolapsed intervertebral disc Peripheral autonomic neuropathies (e.g. diabetic)

COMPLICATIONS

Although incontinence itself is not life threatening, it does cause major psychosocial problems. Urgent referral is warranted in patients with:

- microscopic haematuria over the age of 50
- macroscopic haematuria
- recurrent UTI with haematuria
- suspected pelvic mass arising from the urinary tract.

Changes in lifestyle are common and occasionally symptoms are so severe as to render the woman housebound.

Excoriation and soreness of the vulva occurs secondary to continual dampness and chronic urinary tract infection can lead to long-term damage of renal function.

Acute and chronic overdistension of the bladder can cause denervation and necrosis of the detrusor muscle thereby causing further voiding difficulties.

HISTORY

A detailed history is mandatory because patients may present with multiple symptoms of varying degrees. The two symptoms stress incontinence and urge incontinence are commonly used synonymously with the conditions SUI and DO, respectively (see Fig.14.4 for definitions of common urogynaecological terms). This is inaccurate and can lead to inappropriate treatment. Many incontinent women will admit to both symptoms, but these may not correlate well with an underlying bladder condition. Objectively, only 5%

Fig. 14.4 Commonly used urogynaecological terms.

Term	Definition
Cystometry	The measurement of bladder pressure and volume
Detrusor overactivity	An overactive bladder is one that is shown objectively to contract spontaneously or on provocation during the filling phase while the patient is attempting to inhibit micturition
Frequency of micturition	Voiding more than seven times per day
Stress urinary incontinence	The involuntary loss of urine when the intravesical pressure exceeds the maximum urethral pressure in the absence of detrusor activity
Nocturia	Voiding more than twice per night
Nocturnal enuresis	The involuntary passage of urine at night
Stress incontinence	Involuntary loss of urine associated with raised intra-abdominal pressure
Urge incontinence	Urinary leakage associated with a strong and sudden desire to void
Urgency of micturition	A strong and sudden desire to void
Urinary incontinence	Involuntary loss of urine that is a social or hygienic problem and is objectively demonstrable
Uroflowmetry	The measurement of urine flow rate
Videocystourethrography	Combines radiological with pressure and flow studies

of women have both SUI and DO. A patient giving a history of stress incontinence may have detrusor overactivity as the underlying pathology.

Stress urinary incontinence

The most common symptom of SUI is usually small amounts of urinary leakage. However, one-third of women with SUI also experience urge incontinence and up to a half will experience urgency of micturition. Frequency of micturition and nocturia are also common symptoms.

SUI is associated with the following factors and these must be highlighted in the history:

- Increasing age
- Increasing parity
- Obesity
- Genital prolapse
- Postmenopausal status
- Previous pelvic floor surgery
- Constipation
- Smoking/chronic cough.

Detrusor overactivity

Women with DO present with urgency, urge incontinence, frequency and nocturia. However, up to one-quarter also complain of stress incontinence because raised intra-abdominal pressure can stimulate an unstable bladder to contract and produce the symptom of stress incontinence.

The following factors should be highlighted in the history:

- Age
- History of nocturnal enuresis
- Neurological history
- Previous incontinence surgery
- Drug history.

Sensory urgency

Sensory urgency differs from detrusor overactivity (motor urgency) because the urgency occurs in the absence of detrusor activity. The presenting symptoms are the same as for detrusor overactivity, although incontinence is not such a common feature.

Voiding disorders

Voiding disorders can result in chronic retention leading to overflow incontinence. As well as urgency and frequency, the classic symptoms include hesitancy, straining to void, poor flow and incomplete emptying. Large residual volumes of urine due to incomplete emptying predispose to urinary tract infection, which aggravates the symptoms of incontinence, urgency and frequency. Stress incontinence might be a presenting symptom.

Fistulae

Fistulae are rare in the UK, but should always be suspected when incontinence is continuous during the day and at night, particularly where there is a history of operative surgery.

EXAMINATION

Chronic dampness can cause excoriation of the vulva. The best way to demonstrate stress incontinence is to ask the patient to cough while standing with a moderately full bladder. Stress incontinence is not always demonstrable, especially with the patient in the supine position. Examination of the vaginal walls, using a Sims' speculum with the patient in left lateral position, will identify scarring from previous surgery and the presence of uterovaginal prolapse or a cystourethrocoele. Bimanual examination should identify a pelvic mass.

As neurological disease can present with urinary symptoms, including incontinence, a neurological examination should be performed.

HINTS AND TIPS

Uterine, urethral or vaginal wall prolapse should be excluded by examining the patient in left lateral position using a Sims speculum.

INVESTIGATIONS

Excluding a urinary tract infection (UTI), a common cause of sensory urgency, is important because the UTI might cause the presenting symptoms and infection could be exacerbated by further invasive investigations (Fig. 14.5).

Women should be asked to complete a bladder diary for at least 3 days, to cover variations in their normal activities.

HINTS AND TIPS

Incontinence surgery should never be considered without performing urodynamic studies, as surgery may not be necessary.

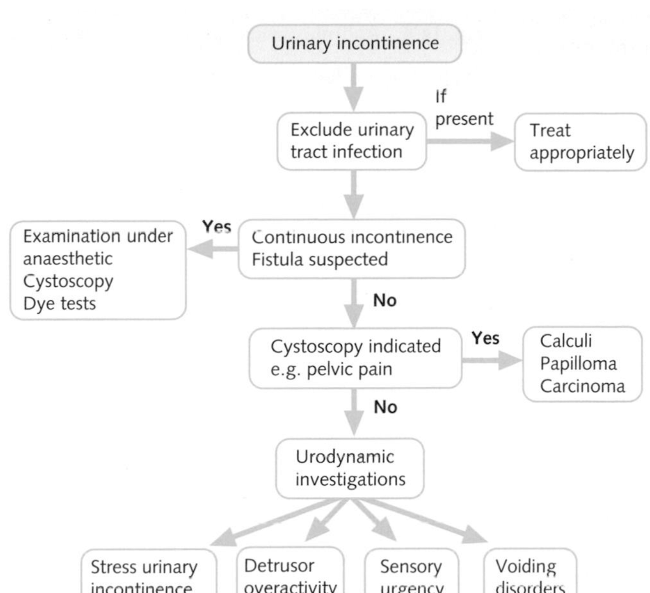

Fig. 14.5 Algorithm for diagnosis in urinary incontinence.

Urodynamics

Urodynamic studies are important for diagnosing the causes of incontinence, as symptoms are often multiple and do not correlate well with the underlying disorder. Uroflowmetry will identify low peak urine flow rates, which suggests a voiding disorder. Cystometry is probably the single most useful urodynamic investigation and will confirm or exclude DO. Cystometry will not diagnose SUI, but will suggest this diagnosis by exclusion of other disorders such as DO (see Chapter 4).

Videocystourethrography (VCU) combines radiological with pressure and flow studies and gives the most information about bladder function. VCU can positively identify SUI as well as DO and other disorders. It is a very useful test to perform prior to incontinence surgery, although not all units provide this service.

Cystoscopy

Although cystoscopy allows inspection of the anatomy of the bladder and bladder neck, it does not give information about their function. Anatomical assessment of the bladder neck is important to exclude polyps, calculi and malignancies will be obvious, as will trabeculation. True bladder capacity can be measured under general anaesthesia.

OTHER INVESTIGATIONS

Bimanual pelvic examination and pelvic ultrasound will identify pelvic masses.

Uretero-vaginal fistulae will require radiological investigations. Infusing coloured dyes into the bladder and observing vaginal leakage may confirm the presence of vesico- or urethro-vaginal fistulae.

TREATMENT

Treatment is determined not only by the underlying condition but also by the severity of the symptoms. Some women might be happy to undergo a trial of oral medication but not major abdominal surgery for the same degree of symptoms. Similarly, depending on lifestyle, some women can live with their symptoms whereas others find the same symptoms intolerable. A sympathetic approach and detailed counselling of the pros and cons of treatment are essential in treating women with incontinence.

Conservative management involves weight loss, reduction in caffeine intake and smoking, and treating constipation or chronic cough. These can all contribute to urinary symptoms.

Stress urinary incontinence

Conservative treatment of SUI involves physiotherapy. Women are taught pelvic floor exercises to achieve better urinary control and symptoms improve in up to 60%. Techniques include simple pelvic floor exercises or insertion of vaginal cones, which can be retained only by contraction of the relevant pelvic floor muscles.

Problems include return of symptoms if exercises are stopped and a spontaneous worsening of symptoms associated with the menopause. Oestrogen replacement can improve the symptom of stress incontinence in postmenopausal women, although long-term use is required to maintain the effect.

The majority of women with SUI can be cured by surgery. This is achieved by lifting and supporting the bladder neck and urethra, thereby restoring their intra-abdominal position. This also increases the urethral pressure by increasing outflow resistance. This is done by inserting a tension free vaginal tape (TVT) through a small vaginal incision over the mid-urethra. Long-term success rates are comparable with colposuspension, a more invasive abdominal procedure, achieving success rates of up to 90%. In the presence of poor detrusor activity, the bladder might not produce high enough pressures to overcome the relative outflow obstruction produced by abdominal procedures and self-intermittent catheterization might be necessary. Urodynamic studies will help to identify this group of women, although all women undergoing surgery for SUI should be warned of this complication.

Recently, a medical treatment for SUI has been introduced which may be offered as an alternative to surgical treatment. Duloxetine is an inhibitor of serotonin and noradrenaline re-uptake and it increases the tone of the urethral sphincter. It appears to be most effective when used in conjunction with pelvic floor exercises. Where SUI and DO coexist it is sensible to treat the DO in the first instance. A significant percentage of women will have a satisfactory enough response to simple medical treatment and thereby avoid major surgery.

HINTS AND TIPS

Physiotherapy should be the first-line treatment for women with SUI – 60% of women with SUI notice an improvement in their symptoms when taught to perform pelvic floor exercises.

Detrusor overactivity

DO is primarily treated medically using behavioural and drug therapy.

Behavioural therapy

Bladder re-training aims to increase the voiding intervals and may be successful in up to 80% of women with DO, although there is a significant relapse rate. Having explained how the bladder functions, subjects are taught to micturate by the clock rather than desire and encouraged to increase voiding intervals incrementally. Other techniques include hypnotherapy and acupuncture.

Fig. 14.6 Anti-muscarinic (atropine-like) side effects.

Type of side-effect	Description
Peripheral	Dry mouth Reduced visual accommodation Constipation Glaucoma
Central	Confusion

Drug therapy

There is a strong placebo effect in the drug treatment of DO. Drugs that are effective in treating DO rely on their antimuscarinic properties (less correctly termed 'anticholinergics'). Antimuscarinic drugs effectively increase bladder capacity by:

- delaying initial desire to void
- decreasing the strength of detrusor contractions
- decreasing the frequency of detrusor contractions.

Although improving symptoms in many women, the use of antimuscarinics is limited by their atropine-like side effects (Fig. 14.6). Oxybutynin is currently widely used, although Tolterodine has antimuscarinic properties that are highly selective for the bladder. Tolterodine shows good efficacy with fewer antimuscarinic side effects and now can be given as a once daily formulation. Newer antimuscarinic drugs licensed for the treatment of DO include Solifenacin and Trospium.

Tricyclic antidepressants also have antimuscarinic properties as well as a central sedative effect. They are useful for incontinent women who suffer from anxiety.

HINTS AND TIPS

Whilst medical management is important in DO, surgical management is more important in women with SUI. Surgical management should not be considered unless women have completed their family.

Sensory urgency

Removal of the source of bladder mucosal irritation (infection, bladder stones, tumours) is likely to relieve symptoms.

Voiding difficulties

The symptoms of urinary outflow obstruction, hesitancy, poor flow and incomplete emptying, can be treated by drug therapy but where retention has occurred catheterization is necessary.

In general, SUI is treated surgically (TVT), if medical management and physiotherapy fails, and DO is treated medically (antimuscarinics) which is why urodynamic investigation is so important in the management of urinary incontinence.

Drug therapy

Drugs used to treat the symptoms of voiding difficulties are often ineffective or have limited use due to side effects. They work in two ways:

- Relax the urethral sphincter mechanism
- Produce detrusor contractions.

The selective α-blocker indoramin increases the flow rate and improves obstructive symptoms by relaxing the sphincter mechanism. Side-effects include sedation, dizziness, tachycardia and hypotension and must be used with extreme caution in the elderly and in antihypertensive users.

The parasympathomimetics (bethanechol, carbachol and distigmine) exhibit muscarinic activity which improves voiding by increasing detrusor contraction. Side-effects include sweating, bradycardia and intestinal colic.

Catheterization

Acute urinary retention requires catheterization. If caused by a gravid uterus, the catheter may be required until the uterus is abdominally sited. If retention is due to an ovarian cyst or fibroid, this may need to be removed surgically, although disimpaction from the pelvis is sometimes possible as an interim or palliative measure.

Postoperative or postpartum retention usually resolves with free bladder drainage for 48 hours or so. If the bladder has been overdistended then normal bladder function is unlikely to occur immediately and free bladder drainage is required until normal function returns. Residual volumes can be measured to assess progress.

Chronic retention may require long-term indwelling catheters which has a significant risk of sepsis. Intermittent self-catheterization might be more appropriate in those who are able to perform this technique. Subclinical sepsis is common, although treatment is usually given only if symptoms are present.

Fistula

Small fistulae might close spontaneously by providing continuous free drainage of the bladder. This might require stenting the ureters or catheterizing the bladder. If spontaneous closure does not occur, or if the fistulae are large, then surgical closure by a surgeon experienced in such techniques is required.

Further reading

Cardozo, L., Staskin, D. (Eds.), 2006. Textbook of Female Urology and Urogynaecology, second ed. Informa Healthcare, Tampa.

Llewellyn Jones, D., 2010. Fundamentals of Obstetrics & Gynaecology, ninth ed. Mosby, London.

Stanton, S., Monga, A., 1998. Clinical Urogynaecology, second ed. Churchill Livingstone, London.

RCOG. Urodynamic Stress Incontinence, Surgical Treatment (Green-top 35). Available online at: http://www.rcog.org.uk/guidelines.

Urinary incontinence: the management of urinary incontinence in women. Clinical guidelines, CG40 – Issued: October 2006. NICE guidelines, http://publications.nice.org.uk/urinary-incontinence-cg40 (last accessed 15.08.13).

Genital prolapse

Objectives

By the end of this chapter, you should be able to:

- Understand the anatomy and causes of different types of prolapse
- Understand the important points in the history for a patient presenting with prolapse
- Perform an examination on a patient presenting with prolapse
- Undertake appropriate investigations on a patient presenting with prolapse in order to establish a diagnosis.
- Discuss the option of conservative management
- Understand the principles behind choosing the appropriate operation.

DEFINITION

A prolapse is the protrusion of an organ or a structure beyond its normal anatomical site. Genital prolapse involves weakness of the supporting structures of the pelvic organs so that they descend from their normal positions. In the female genital tract, the type of prolapse depends on the organ involved and its position in relation to the anterior or posterior vaginal wall (Fig. 15.1; see also Fig. 15.3).

INCIDENCE

Genital prolapse is common. A cystourethrocoele is the most common type, next uterine descent and then rectocoele. The incidence increases with increasing age. Prolapse is seen less commonly in Afro-Caribbean women than in Caucasian women.

PELVIC ANATOMY

Some knowledge of the pelvic anatomy, with particular reference to the pelvic floor muscles, fascia and ligaments, is necessary to understand the development of genital prolapse. Weakness of these tissues, either congenital or acquired, results in descent of the pelvic viscera.

Pelvic floor muscles

The pelvic floor consists of a muscular, gutter-shaped, forward sloping diaphragm formed by the:

- levator ani muscles
- internal obturator and piriform muscles
- superficial and deep perineal muscles.

The levator ani consists of two parts, the pubococcygeal part anteriorly and the iliococcygeal part posteriorly and is covered by pelvic fascia. The vagina and urethra pass through the urogenital aperture formed by the medial border of the levator ani. The rectum passes posteriorly with muscle fibres from the pubic bone uniting behind the anorectal junction. Thus, the muscles provide an indirect support for these structures (Fig. 15.2).

Pelvic ligaments

Condensations of the pelvic fascia form strong ligaments that act to support the upper part of the vagina, the cervix and the uterus. Those that support the uterus include the:

- transverse cervical or cardinal ligaments
- uterosacral ligaments
- round ligaments.

The transverse cervical and uterosacral ligaments consist of smooth muscle and elastic tissue. They attach to the pelvic side wall and the sacrum, respectively. The round ligaments pass from the cornu of the uterus through the inguinal canal to the labium majus. They contain smooth muscle and maintain flexion of the uterus with only minimal role in support.

AETIOLOGY OF GENITAL PROLAPSE

Congenital

Some women are born with a predisposition to genital prolapse, which is probably secondary to abnormal collagen production. Conditions associated with prolapse include:

- spina bifida
- connective tissue disorder.

Fig. 15.1 Differential diagnosis of prolapse.

Organ that has prolapsed	Name of prolapse
Bladder	**Cystocoele**: Prolapse of upper anterior wall of the vagina, attached to bladder by fascia.
Bladder and Urethra	**Cystourethrocoele:** A cystocoele extending into the lower anterior vaginal wall, displacing urethra downwards.
Rectum	**Rectocoele:** Weakness in the levator ani muscles causes a bulge in the mid-posterior vaginal wall which incorporates the rectum.
Small Bowel	**Enterocoele:** True hernia of the Pouch of Douglas. Prolapse of the upper third of the posterior vaginal wall and contains loops of small bowel.
Uterus and Cervix	**Uterine descent:** Uterus descends within the vagina and may even lie outside it (called procidentia). May be associated with a cystocoele and/or rectocoele. Graded according to the position of the cervix on vaginal examination: First degree: Cervical descent within the vagina Second degree: Cervical descent to the introitus Third degree: Cervical descent outside the introitus (Procidentia)
Vaginal Vault	**Vault descent:** After hysterectomy, the proximal end of the vaginal vault can prolapse within or outside the vagina.

Fig. 15.2 Anatomy of the pelvic floor muscles.

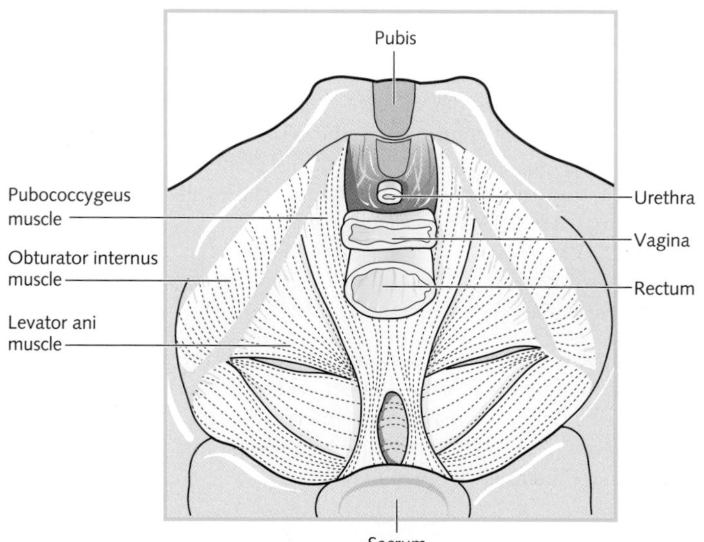

Acquired

Although most women with genital prolapse have a degree of congenital predisposition, the following factors are also important:

- Obstetric factors
- Postmenopausal atrophy
- Chronically raised intra-abdominal pressure
- Iatrogenic.

In terms of aetiology, obstetric factors are particularly important, and if prolapse is to be prevented, good intrapartum management of the patient is essential.

Obstetric factors

Figure 15.3 lists the factors that can cause prolapse secondary to denervation and muscular trauma of the pelvic floor.

Postmenopausal atrophy

The incidence of prolapse increases with age. This is due to atrophy of the connective tissues secondary to the hypo-oestrogenic state following the menopause.

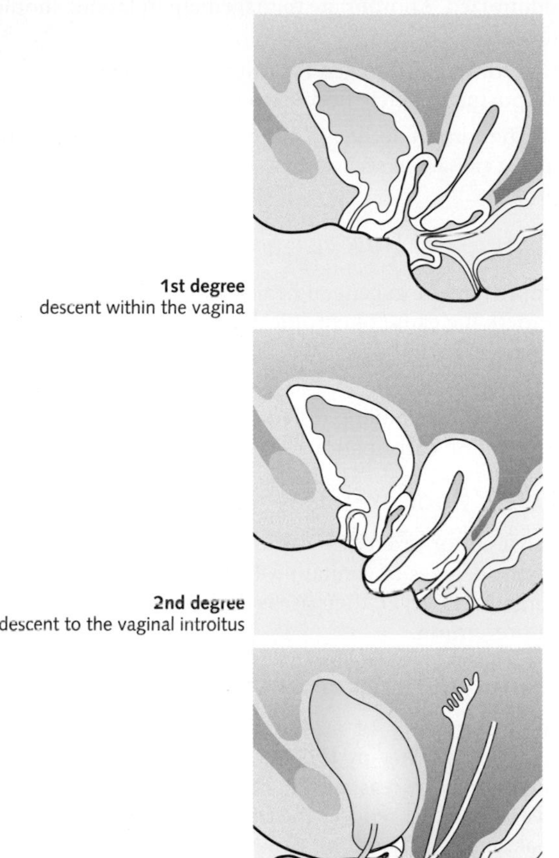

Fig. 15.3 Factors that predispose to prolapse.

Chronically raised intra-abdominal pressure

Any factors that raise intra-abdominal pressure in the long term can predispose to prolapse, including:

- intra-abdominal or pelvic tumour
- chronic cough
- constipation.

Iatrogenic

Hysterectomy predisposes to future prolapse of the vaginal vault. In order to remove the uterus, the transverse cervical and uterosacral ligaments have to be divided and the upper vaginal supports are weakened.

Colposuspension (see Chapter 14) predisposes to development of an enterocoele because the anterior vaginal wall is lifted anteriorly, which in turn pulls the upper posterior vaginal wall forwards.

HISTORY

Presenting complaint

Local discomfort or a feeling of 'something coming down' is a common symptom. This is usually worse with standing or straining (cough, defecation) and relieved by lying down. It may interfere with sexual function.

Remember that your history should exclude symptoms related to the urinary and bowel systems.

Uterine descent

Can give symptoms of backache. However, other causes of backache must be excluded, especially in the older patient. A procidentia causes discomfort as it rubs on the patient's clothing and can cause a bloody, sometimes purulent, discharge.

Other symptoms depend on the organ/organs involved.

Urinary symptoms

These occur with a cystocoele or a cystourethrocoele, such as frequency of micturition. The patient might notice incomplete emptying of the bladder, which predisposes her to urinary infection and even possibly overflow incontinence. Stress incontinence may be present if there is descent of the urethrovesical junction (bladder neck) associated with a cystocoele.

Bowel symptoms

A rectocoele can cause incomplete bowel emptying. This can be relieved if the patient pushes back the prolapse digitally.

Figure 15.3 shows factors that should be elicited in the history that may predispose the patient to prolapse in general.

EXAMINATION

- General examination
- Abdominal palpation
- Sims' speculum examination
- Bimanual pelvic examination.

Following abdominal palpation to exclude a mass, the patient should be examined in the left lateral position using a Sims' speculum in order to exclude a vaginal wall prolapse. With the posterior vaginal wall retracted, any anterior wall prolapse will be demonstrated if the patient is asked to bear down. Conversely, if the anterior vaginal wall is retracted, then an enterocoele or rectocoele will be seen.

Abdominal palpation and bimanual pelvic examination are mandatory to exclude a pelvic mass.

Uterine descent is assessed by examining the position of the cervix within the vagina, again usually in the left lateral position with the Sims' speculum. If the patient has a full bladder, stress incontinence can be demonstrated by asking the patient to cough.

INVESTIGATION

This is a clinical diagnosis so there are few relevant investigations. If the patient has urinary symptoms the following would be appropriate:

- Mid-stream urine specimen
- Urodynamics: only used in special circumstances, e.g. if surgical intervention contemplated, a mixed incontinence picture or failed medical management.

Figure 15.4 shows an algorithm for the further management of a prolapse (see Chapter 14).

MANAGEMENT

The aim is to replace the prolapsed organs to their normal anatomical site. The options can be categorized into:

- prevention
- conservative measures
- surgery.

Always remember to consider the patient's general health and other conservative measures, such as HRT, as well as the need for surgery.

Prevention

Because obstetric factors are most commonly involved in the development of a genital prolapse, it is important that damage to the supporting structures of the pelvis is minimized. Appropriate management of labour should include:

- avoiding prolonged first and second stages
- postnatal pelvic floor exercises.

The current decline in parity, as well as the increasing use of caesarean section may influence the incidence of prolapse.

Conservative measures

Improvement in general health should aim to treat the underlying cause of chronically raised intra-abdominal pressure, including:

- weight loss
- stopping smoking to reduce cough
- treating constipation.

Pelvic floor exercises

Pelvic floor exercises can improve symptoms with minor degrees of genital prolapse, sufficiently to avoid surgery. However, their use is probably more important in prevention.

Hormone replacement therapy

In the presence of atrophic pelvic tissues, hormone replacement therapy (HRT) can help minor degrees of prolapse by increasing skin collagen content. Preoperative use of HRT reduces the friability of atrophic tissues; making tissue handling easier during surgery.

Vaginal pessaries

The more commonly used pessary is the ring pessary, made of inert white plastic. The diameter is measured in millimetres and the appropriate size is assessed by vaginal examination. The pessary is passed into the

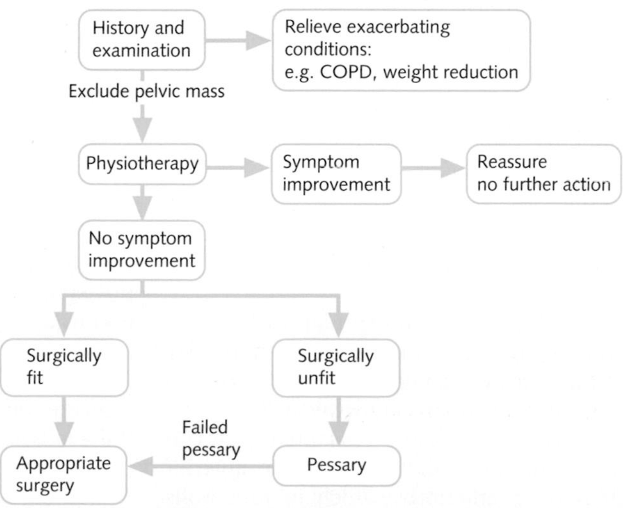

Fig. 15.4 Algorithm for prolapse.

vagina so that it sits behind the pubic bone anteriorly and in the posterior fornix of the vagina posteriorly, enclosing the cervix. The other type of pessary is the shelf pessary, used for larger prolapses.

The indications for the use of a vaginal pessary include the following:

- The patient has not completed her family.
- The patient prefers conservative management.
- The patient is medically unfit for surgery.

With major degrees of prolapse, especially where the introitus is lax and the perineal body deficient, the pessary may not be supported enough to stay in situ. It can also fall out if too small a size is fitted. The main complications of a pessary are vaginal discharge or bleeding, particularly if the pessary is not replaced every 6 months. Granulation tissue may develop, incarcerating the pessary, if it is not changed regularly. If the pessary is too large it will cause discomfort and may ulcerate the vaginal walls.

Surgical treatment

Surgery should be considered with a severe degree of prolapse or if conservative management fails. Prior to surgery it is important to know whether a woman is sexually active, because the vagina might be narrowed and shortened, potentially causing dyspareunia.

Surgery is not recommended in a woman who has not yet completed her family. In pregnancy, after pelvic floor repair, caesarean section is indicated to reduce soft tissue trauma and the risk of recurrent prolapse.

Anterior colporrhaphy

This operation, also known as an anterior repair, is indicated for the repair of a cystocoele or a cystourethrocoele. A portion of redundant anterior vaginal wall mucosa is excised and the exposed fascia is plicated to support the bladder. Postoperatively, there is a risk of worsening urinary symptoms.

Posterior colporrhaphy

Also known as a posterior repair, this operation is used to repair a rectocoele or a rectocoele combined with an enterocoele. Using a similar technique to the operation described above, a triangle of posterior vaginal wall mucosa – its apex behind the cervix and the base at the introitus – is removed. The underlying levator ani muscles are plicated to support the perineum. If an enterocoele is present, the pouch of Douglas is opened and the enterocoele sac of redundant peritoneum is excised.

Vaginal hysterectomy

This operation is performed for uterine prolapse, as well as for other gynaecological pathology. It can be combined with one or both of the operations above.

Manchester repair (Fothergill procedure)

This operation is rarely performed for uterine prolapse nowadays. It consists of amputation of the cervix and then apposing the cardinal ligaments to lift the uterus, followed by anterior and posterior colporrhaphy if necessary. It may be offered to a woman who wants to preserve the uterus.

Sacrospinous fixation

To treat the prolapsed vaginal vault, the apex is fixed to sacrospinous ligament using a transvaginal approach. This ligament runs from the ischial spine to the lower lateral aspect of the sacrum. Care must be taken to avoid the pudendal nerve and vessels, as well as the sacral plexus and the sciatic nerve.

Sacral colpopexy

This abdominal procedure involves suspending the vaginal vault from the sacrum or from the sacral promontory, using either strips of fascia or synthetic mesh. The main complications are intraoperative haemorrhage and infection of the mesh.

New procedures are currently being developed using synthetic mesh to relieve prolapsed vaginal walls or the vaginal vault. At present, follow-up data regarding success rates are limited.

Further reading

Lopes, T., Spirtos, N., Naik, R., et al., 2011. Bonney's Gynaecological Surgery, 11th ed. Wiley Blackwell, London.

RCOG, 2007. The Management of Post Hysterectomy Vaginal Vault Prolapsed. Green-top Guideline No. 46. Royal College of Obstetricians and Gynaecologists, London. Available online at:www.rcog.org.uk.

RCOG, 2009. Pelvic Floor Repair and Vaginal Hysterectomy for Prolapse: Consent Advice 5. Royal College of Obstetricians and Gynaecologists, London. Available online at:www.rcog.org.uk.

Shaw, R.W., Luesley, D., Monga, A., 2010. Gynaecolocy, fourth ed. Churchill Livingstone, London.

Gynaecological endocrinology 16

Objectives

By the end of this chapter, you will be able to:

- Identify the common causes of amenorrhoea, precocious and delayed puberty
- Request the relevant investigations and their treatments
- Understand some of the rarer endocrinological conditions which may present in gynaecology.

This chapter focusses on the aetiology and management behind amenorrhoea, delayed puberty and precocious puberty.

AMENORRHOEA

This describes the absence of menstruation. There are two types:

- Primary amenorrhoea – where menstruation has not started by the age of 16 years. This is relatively uncommon.
- Secondary amenorrhoea – where menstruation has occurred in the past, but has been absent for 6 months or more. This can be common, and causes may be physiological, most frequently pregnancy and the menopause.

The causes of amenorrhoea can be broken down into the following five major categories:

- Central nervous system
- Gonadal dysfunction
- Genital tract disorders
- Endocrine disorders
- Drug therapy.

A history of post-pill amenorrhoea is usually the result of pre-existing pathology that has been masked by the combined oral contraceptive pill (COCP).

Complications of amenorrhoea

Although amenorrhoea itself does not cause any complications, some of the underlying conditions do carry certain risks:

- Women who carry a Y chromosome (genotype XXY) have a 25% chance of developing gonadal malignancy, usually a gonadoblastoma or dysgerminoma.
- Low oestrogenic states, seen in hypothalamic amenorrhoea and premature ovarian failure, are associated with an increased risk of osteoporosis and ischaemic heart disease.
- Endometrial hyperplasia and endometrial carcinoma occur more frequently in women with polycystic ovary syndrome (PCOS) because of the unopposed oestrogen effect on the endometrium associated with chronic anovulation.
- Haematocolpos is associated with an increased risk of endometriosis due to retrograde menstruation.
- Amenorrhoeic women are usually subfertile.

History

There are so many causes of amenorrhoea that it is important to focus the history onto the relevant systems.

Gynaecological

A full gynaecological history is mandatory. By definition, menarche will not have occurred in women with primary amenorrhoea. The timing of pubertal development will establish whether this is normal, precocious or delayed.

Menstrual irregularity or oligomenorrhoea from the time of menarche may be due to polycystic ovary syndrome, especially if associated with obesity and hirsutism.

Cyclical pain might indicate congenital or acquired outflow obstruction to menstrual fluid, resulting in primary amenorrhoea.

Pituitary failure can occur after massive postpartum haemorrhage (Sheehan's syndrome) and so a full obstetric history should be taken. This should include early pregnancy loss with subsequent uterine curettage, which can lead to Ashermann's syndrome.

Relevant gynaecological surgery includes cervical surgery, which can cause stenosis and, more obviously, oophorectomy and hysterectomy.

Central nervous system

A history of head injury or recent symptoms of central nervous system (CNS) tumour such as headache and vomiting should be elicited. Visual field disturbance might indicate an expanding pituitary tumour and galactorrhoea could indicate hyperprolactinaemia.

General health

The general health of the patient should be assessed. Emotional stress, from any cause, can precipitate amenorrhoea, as can weight loss from dieting, anorexia nervosa or severe systemic illness. The reduced peripheral fat stores and body mass index (BMI) that are commonly seen in female athletes can cause amenorrhoea even though these women are fit and well. Patients undergoing chemotherapy or radiotherapy often undergo an iatrogenic menopause.

Endocrine disorders

Thyroid disease and diabetes mellitus may present with amenorrhoea and symptoms of these disorders should be elicited. Hirsutism and virilism may be due to congenital adrenal hyperplasia (CAH), PCOS or an androgen-secreting tumour of the ovary or adrenal.

Drugs

Many prescribed drugs can cause amenorrhoea by producing either hyperprolactinaemia or ovarian failure, and a detailed drug history should be taken (see Fig.16.1)

Examination

A general examination should be performed, with particular emphasis on looking for signs of thyroid disease and diabetes mellitus. The BMI should be calculated (kg/m^2). Anosmia (absent sense of smell) is associated with Kallmann's syndrome. The typical appearance of Turner's syndrome should be apparent; short stature, webbing of the neck, increased carrying angle at the elbow and coarctation of the aorta. The presence of galactorrhoea should be noted.

A full gynaecological examination is mandatory. Assessment of secondary sexual development must be made, using Tanner's system (see Fig.16.2). Absent secondary sexual characteristics might constitute delayed puberty. Incongruous pubertal development might also suggest underlying pathology. For example, normal breast development in the absence of pubic or axillary hair is typically found in women with androgen insensitivity. Poor breast development with normal pubic and axillary hair or hirsutism, virilism and obesity can be signs of raised circulating androgens secondary to PCOS, and more rarely congenital adrenal hyperplasia (CAH), adrenal tumours or androgen-secreting ovarian tumours.

Pelvic examination should assess the patency of the vagina. If a haematocolpos is present it often causes a blue-coloured bulge at the introitus. An enlarged uterus might represent a pregnancy, and ovarian masses might be palpable.

Investigations

Physiological causes such as pregnancy, lactation or the menopause must first be excluded.

Primary amenorrhoea

In general, primary amenorrhoea should be investigated from the age of 16 years. However, if pubertal development has not started by the age of 14 years then investigation is warranted (see Fig.16.3).

When no pubertal development has occurred by the age of 14 years then investigation should be as for delayed puberty.

Where pubertal development is normal, genital tract anomalies, such as an absent uterus or vagina, should be excluded by clinical examination or ultrasound scanning. If normal then investigation should be as for secondary amenorrhoea (see below).

Incongruous pubertal development can be caused by chromosomal abnormality or increased circulating androgens. For instance, women with testicular feminization often have normal breast development in the absence of axillary and pubic hair. Poor breast development in the presence of normal or excessive axillary or pubic hair is compatible with increased circulating androgens commonly associated with PCOS, and less

Fig. 16.1 Prescribed drugs that can cause hyperprolactinaemia.

Types of drug	Drug class
Antipsychotic drugs	Phenothiazines Haloperidol
Antidepressants	Tricyclic antidepresssants
Antihypertensive drugs	Methyldopa Reserpine
Oestrogens	Combined oral contraceptive pill
H_2-receptor antagonists	Cimetidine Ranitidine Metoclopramide and domperidone

Note: Don't forget chemotherapy for malignancy or immunological disorders.

Fig. 16.2 Tanner staging of puberty.

Acute	Chronic
Pelvic inflammatory disease (see Chapter 13) **Tubo-ovarian abscess** post-termination of pregnancy post-insertion of IUCD post-hysteroscopy	**Adenomyosis** **Endometriosis** (see Chapter 8) **Adhesions** gynaecological operation pelvic inflammatory disease appendicitis
Early pregnancy complications (see Chapter 20) miscarriage ectopic pregnancy	
Gynaecological malignancy (see Chapter 10)	**Gynaecological malignancy**
Ovarian cyst (see Chapter 9) rupture haemorrhage torsion	**Gastrointestinal pathology** diverticulitis irritable bowel syndrome
Fibroid necrosis	
Ovulation pain (Mittelschmerz)	
Abscess Bartholin's cyst labial	
Urinary tract infection **Renal calculi**	
Appendicitis	

commonly with CAH or androgen-secreting tumours of the ovary or adrenal.

The following group of investigations should be performed as indicated:

- Chromosomal analysis
- Hormone profiles
- Imaging studies.

Chromosomal analysis

Chromosomal analysis should be performed on women with primary amenorrhoea where a chromosomal abnormality (e.g. Turner's syndrome) is suspected. Buccal smears or blood samples can be taken for this purpose.

Secondary amenorrhoea

The most common cause of secondary amenorrhoea in women of childbearing age is pregnancy, and this should be excluded before further investigation is commenced. A urinary pregnancy test detects the presence of β-human chorionic gonadotrophin (hCG) and can be performed quickly in the outpatient setting.

Having excluded physiological causes of secondary amenorrhoea, further investigation includes measuring:

- serum gonadotrophins – levels of follicle stimulating hormone (FSH) and luteinizing hormone (LH) are greatly raised with ovarian failure, whereas with 'hypothalamic' amenorrhoea or hypogonadotrophic hypogonadism the levels will be at the lower limits of normal. In PCOS the LH: FSH ratio is usually greater than 2.5
- androgen levels – serum testosterone levels might be normal or raised with PCOS, although free testosterone is usually raised. If serum testosterone levels are very high then an androgen-secreting tumour of the ovary or adrenal should be suspected
- prolactin – serum prolactin levels are important to exclude hyperprolactinaemia. Thyroid stimulating hormone and free thyroxine levels should be tested if there is clinical suspicion of thyroid dysfunction or if hyperprolactinaemia is confirmed.

Other useful investigations include:

- pelvic ultrasound scan – this will identify the typical ultrasound appearances of polycystic ovaries (enlarged ovaries with increased central stroma associated with multiple peripherally sited follicles).

Fig. 16.3 Algorithm for primary amenorrhoea.

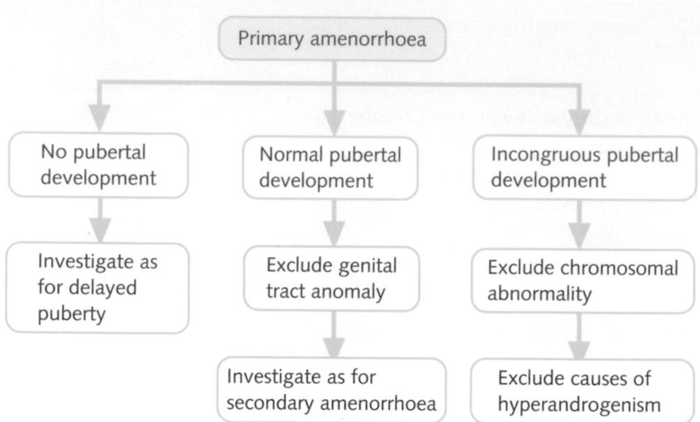

The presence of an intrauterine pregnancy, haematometra or haematocolpos can also be identified

- lateral skull X-ray, CT or MRI scan of the head – this identifies a pituitary or CNS tumour (Fig.16.4)
- analysis of chromosome in women under 30 years of age who have ovarian failure.

HINTS AND TIPS

Chromosomal analysis is mandatory in the investigation of unexplained primary amenorrhoea or primary ovarian failure.

Treatment of amenorrhoea

Certain conditions cause primary and secondary amenorrhoea, depending on the age at which the condition presents. Their treatment is discussed under secondary amenorrhoea.

Treatment of primary amenorrhoea

Gonadal dysgenesis

Apart from the management of the psychosexual aspects of gonadal dysgenesis, these women require HRT to protect against cardiovascular disease and osteoporosis. This will also stimulate secondary sexual development in those who have not yet been exposed to oestrogens (e.g. Turner's syndrome). Women who carry a Y chromosome should have both gonads removed, because of the risk of malignancy, followed by long-term HRT.

Genital tract anomaly

- Women with a congenitally absent vagina should be referred to a tertiary centre and offered the option of vaginal construction to enable sexual activity. If the uterus is present, this will allow drainage of a haematometra.
- Women with a haematocolpos can be treated by surgical excision of the persistent vaginal membrane, thereby draining the build-up of menstrual blood.

Treatment of secondary amenorrhoea

In young women who have no pathology, the condition may be temporary and might not require treatment.

Hypothalamic amenorrhoea (or hypothalamic hypogonadism)

Here, the main causes of amenorrhoea are usually weight loss or stress. A return of BMI to the normal range (20–25) usually results in spontaneous menstruation, as does the removal of stressful situations or treatment of systemic illness.

Polycystic ovary syndrome

One of the key treatments for PCOS is weight loss. As the BMI approaches the normal range spontaneous ovulation and regular menstruation often occurs. Infrequent periods can lead to endometrial hyperplasia in the long-term, so this should be treated with progestogens. Long-term protection of the endometrium can be provided using cyclical progestogens, the COCP or the levonorgestrel intra-uterine system. The COCP Dianette (Schering®) is ideal for those with hirsutism because the anti-androgenic and progestogenic effect of cyproterone acetate will reduce symptoms of hyperandrogenism and protect the endometrium from hyperplasia. Yasmin (Schering) is another COCP with a progestogen (drospirenone) which has both a weak anti-androgenic and antimineralocorticoid activity.

Metformin is now increasingly being used in clinical practice for the treatment of PCOS as insulin resistance is an important factor in the disease process. Some women with PCOS on Metformin find weight loss targets easier to achieve and some will start to spontaneously ovulate without the need for ovulation induction agents.

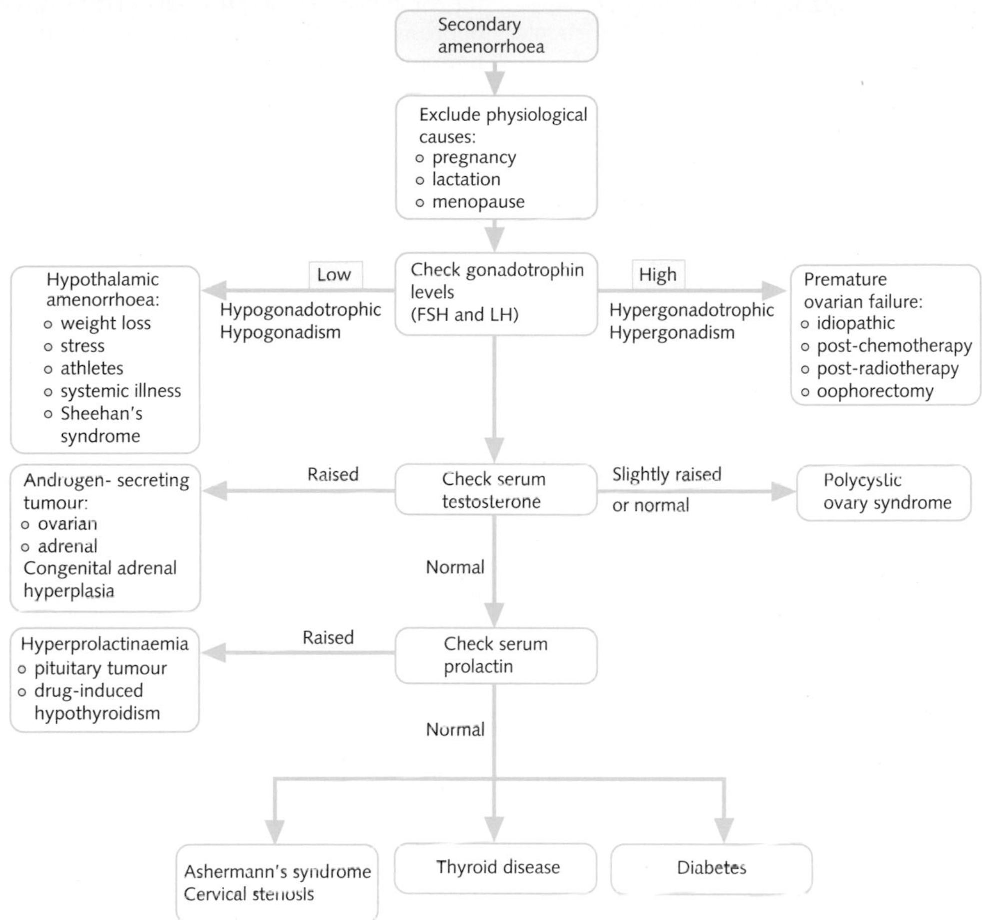

Fig. 16.4 Algorithm for secondary amenorrhoea.

HINTS AND TIPS

PCOS is diagnosed by two of the three criteria: oligo/anovulation, clinical or biochemical signs of hyperandrogenism, polycystic ovaries (12+ peripheral follicles or increased ovarian volume). Long-term consequences of PCOS include type II diabetes, endometrial hyperplasia and cancer, hirsutism, acne.

Hyperprolactinaemia

The treatment of hyperprolactinaemia includes the following:

- Dopamine agonists for microadenoma
- Dopamine agonists or surgery for macroadenoma
- Cessation of drugs, where possible, in drug-induced hyperprolactinaemia
- Correction of hypothyroidism.

Treatment is advisable for pituitary microadenoma to reduce the risk of osteoporosis. Dopamine agonists such as bromocriptine and cabergoline should be used to reduce the serum prolactin levels. Side-effects include nausea, dizziness, hypotension, drowsiness and headaches, and are less common with cabergoline, which can be given once weekly. Cessation of therapy usually results in recurrence of hyperprolactinaemia but is recommended if pregnancy occurs.

Transphenoidal removal of pituitary macroadenoma carries a risk of diabetes insipidus, cerebrospinal fluid leakage, panhypopituitarism and recurrence of the tumour. Shrinkage of the tumour and resolution of symptoms might occur with medical treatment, as for microadenoma.

Where hyperprolactinaemia is drug induced (Fig.16.1), stopping the drug results in a fall of serum prolactin levels to normal levels. However, cessation of drug treatment is not always advisable, depending on the condition being treated. If the drug treatment is likely to be long term, oestrogen replacement might be advisable to prevent osteoporosis. Hypothyroidism should be corrected with thyroxine replacement.

Asherman's syndrome

Cervical stenosis can be treated by dilating the cervix. Intra-uterine adhesions should be divided hysteroscopically. Insertion of an intra-uterine contraceptive device is advisable for at least 3 months to prevent redevelopment of adhesions. Stimulation of endometrial re-growth using exogenous oestrogens, i.e. hormone replacement therapy is sometimes necessary.

Hormone-secreting tumours

Ovarian and adrenal hormone secreting tumours should be surgically removed. As much ovarian tissue as possible should be preserved, especially in younger women given the implications to their fertility.

Sheehan's syndrome

Sheehan's syndrome is postpartum infarction of the pituitary gland due to massive obstetric haemorrhage. This requires oestrogen replacement in the form of the combined contraceptive pill or HRT to prevent osteoporosis. In addition, replacement of other pituitary hormones might be necessary.

PRECOCIOUS AND DELAYED PUBERTY

Precocious puberty

Precocious puberty occurs when sexual maturation takes place before the age of 9 years.

Aetiology

The conditions that may cause precocious puberty and their approximate incidence are summarized in Figure 16.5 and an algorithm for identifying the most common causes is shown in Figure 16.6. Although it is important to exclude androgen-secreting tumours in the ovary and adrenal glands, most cases are constitutional.

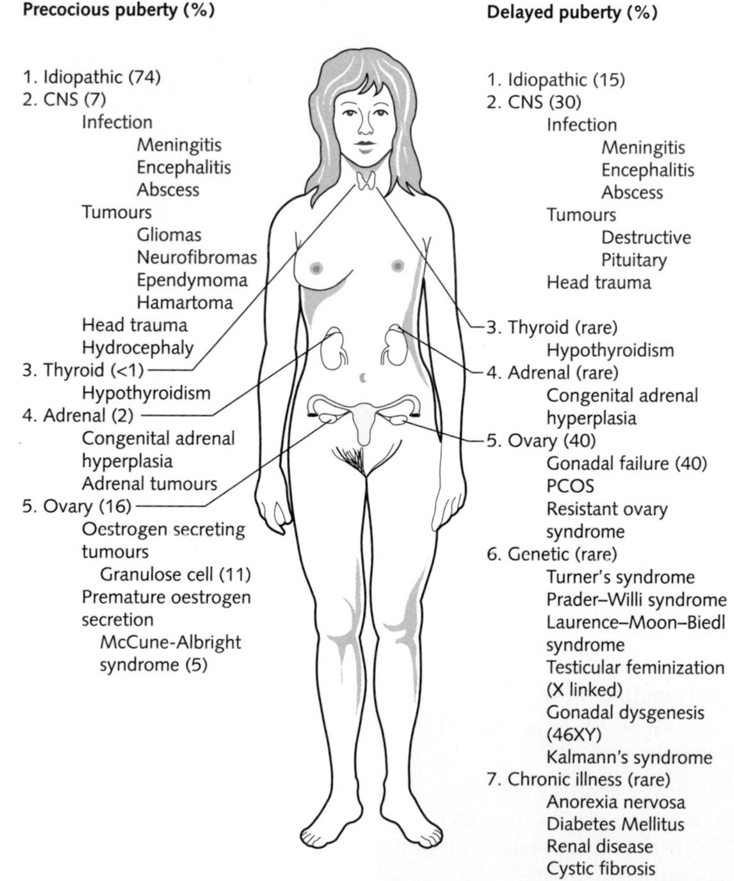

Fig. 16.5 Causes of precocious puberty and delayed puberty.

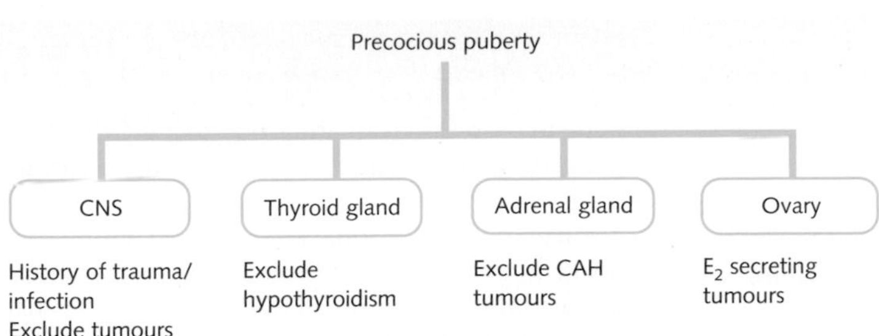

Fig. 16.6 Aetiology for precocious puberty.

Investigations

- Full history and physical examination
- Full endocrine profile (oestradiol, FSH, LH, testosterone, sex hormone binding globulin (SHBG), androstenedione, dehydroepiandrosterone sulphate (DHEAS), 17-OH progesterone)
- Bone age studies
- Imaging: ultrasound scanning of the gonads and adrenals should be performed as first line, but CT or MRI is the gold-standard investigations for excluding tumours.

Management

- Endocrinological: the mainstay of endocrine support is suppression of oestrogen and androgen production by GnRH analogues to reverse the physical changes. This can either be given as a daily sniff or monthly depot preparation.
- Psychological support: this is vital, together with counselling, because the affected girl will see herself as being different from her friends.
- Surgical: if a tumour is discovered then this must be dealt with, usually surgically.

HINTS AND TIPS

Don't forget the effects on growth in patients with precocious puberty – a growth spurt may start prematurely, but may also be completed early.

Delayed puberty

Puberty is defined as being delayed when there are no signs of pubertal development by 14 years of age, when it is expected that more than 95% of normal females will have shown some signs of pubertal development.

Aetiology

Some of the causes of delayed puberty and their approximate incidence are shown in Figure 16.5 and an algorithm for identifying the commoner causes shown in Figures 16.6 and 16.7.

Investigations

- Full history and examination including BMI
- Full endocrine profile (FSH, LH, Prolactin, thyroid function tests, 17-OH progesterone)

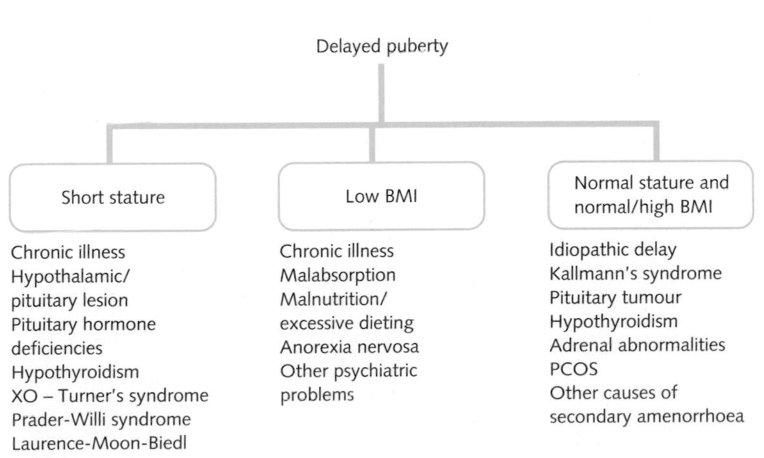

Fig. 16.7 Aetiology for delayed puberty.

- Chromosome analysis
- Bone age studies
- Imaging: CT or MRI of the head.

Management

Management of delayed puberty is aimed at treating the underlying cause:

- congenital conditions (abnormal chromosomes and syndromes) will need paediatric and genetic input
- chronic illness will need supervising by relevant specialist input (renal, malabsorption)
- anorexia nervosa may require psychiatric input
- tumours are likely to require surgical removal
- removal of gonads in conditions that predispose to gonadal malignancy (XY gonadal dysgenesis, Androgen insensitivity syndrome)
- correction of hypothyroidism
- management of PCOS (see under hirsutism and virilism)
- steroid replacement with CAH.

HIRSUTISM AND VIRILISM

Hirsutism – excess facial and body hair growth – can be either genetic (idiopathic) or due to increased androgen levels or sometimes both.

Virilism occurs secondary to high circulating levels of androgens and is diagnosed when clitoral hypertrophy, breast atrophy, deepening of the voice and male-pattern balding occur either alone or together.

Approximately 10% of healthy normal women can be said to have some degree of hirsutism without signs of virilism. However, virilism rarely occurs in the absence of hirsutism (except in the newborn). Virilism is never idiopathic whereas hirsutism can be. Rapid-onset hirsutism and virilism is suggestive of an androgen-producing tumour. The causes of hirsutism and virilism are shown in Figure 16.8.

Aetiology

Hirsutism and virilism occur due to excess circulating endogenous or exogenous androgens. Endogenous production by the ovary is the most common source.

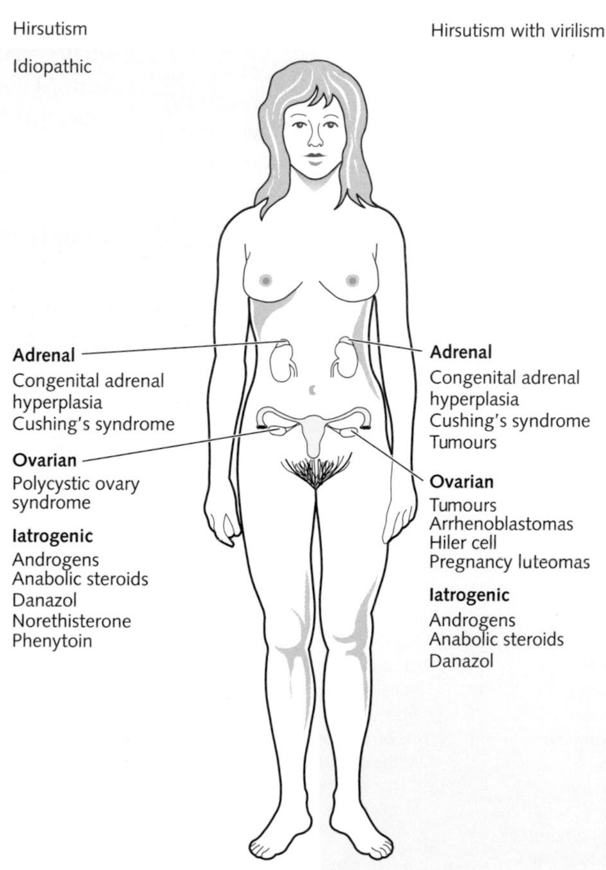

Fig. 16.8 Causes of hirsutism and virilism.

Ovarian androgens

PCOS is the most common cause of hirsutism (90%) and occurs in about 20% of women. Raised levels of circulating LH and sex steroids are characteristic of this syndrome and occur through different pathways (Figure 16.9). Pituitary production of LH is raised in PCOS causing increased ovarian androgen production. This leads to a reduced production of SHBG by the liver and, as SHBG binds to circulating androgens, free testosterone levels increase. Androgens are converted to oestrogens in adipose tissue, raising oestradiol levels, which further stimulate pituitary production of LH. Obesity not only increases insulin levels, which stimulates further ovarian androgen production, but also reduces SHBG levels and increases the peripheral conversion of androgens to oestrogens.

Androgen-secreting tumours of the ovary are rare and include arrhenoblastomas and hilar cell tumours. Pregnancy luteomas are a rare source of excess ovarian androgen secretion. They develop due to an exaggerated response by the ovarian stroma to hCG.

Adrenal androgens

CAH is the term used to describe a group of rare disorders caused by defects in hydroxylation of cortisol precursors, most commonly 21-hydroxylase deficiency. The net effect is increased circulating levels of cortisol precursors and androgens. Excessive stimulation of the adrenal cortex produces raised cortisol levels and is often associated with excess androgen production (Cushing's syndrome). Adenomas and adenocarcinoma of the adrenal gland produce high levels of androgens but are rare.

Exogenous androgens

Androgens and anabolic steroids will cause hirsutism and virilism, depending on the amount and length of time taken. Certain drugs prescribed for medical disorders have androgenic properties and, if taken in high enough doses and for long periods of time, can cause hirsutism (norethisterone, phenytoin) and virilism (danazol).

HINTS AND TIPS

- Although the most common cause of hirsutism in women is PCOS, it is vital to exclude an androgen-secreting tumour.
- The psychological effects of precocious and delayed puberty can be profound and should not be neglected.

History

The timing of onset and the speed of progression of symptoms need to be elicited from the history. For instance, women with PCOS typically have mild symptoms that have been present since menarche, whereas androgen-secreting tumours of the ovary characteristically produce high levels of androgens, which cause severe symptomatology over a short period of time. A detailed menstrual history is important because oligomenorrhoea (infrequent periods) is associated with PCOS and amenorrhoea is often associated with virilism. A family history of hirsutism is often present with idiopathic hirsutism and the menstrual history is usually normal.

PCOS typically presents with oligomenorrhoea and hirsutism from the time of menarche. There might be a history of subfertility secondary to chronic anovulation or a history of glucose intolerance. Although acne and seborrhoea occur relatively commonly, the androgen levels are not usually high enough to produce symptoms of virilism.

CAH usually presents in infancy with ambiguous genitalia but milder cases might not present until puberty and might have a history similar to women with severe PCOS.

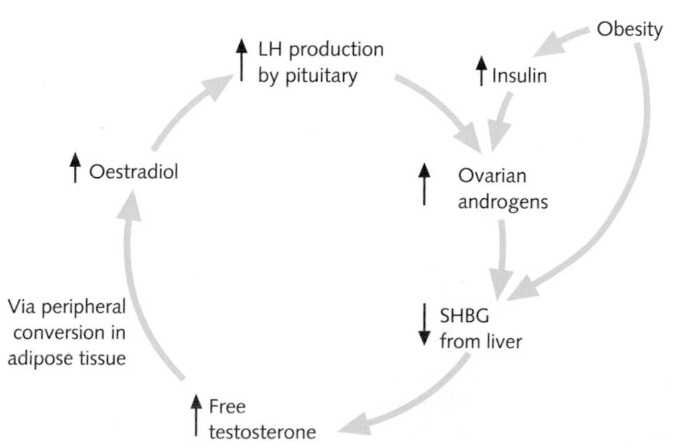

Fig. 16.9 Mechanism of increased androgen production in polycystic ovary syndrome.

Cushing's syndrome (excess cortisol) presents commonly with a gradual change in appearance associated with a host of other symptoms, including central obesity, muscle wasting and weakness, hypertension and purple striae.

A careful drug history is imperative as not only do many of the hormonal therapies used in gynaecology have androgenic properties but there is an increase in the use of anabolic steroids even among women.

Examination

- Hirsutism can be objectively scored using scoring systems, but simple descriptive assessments are more practical. Signs of virilism should be looked for.
- Women with PCOS are often obese, although not always so. Acanthosis nigricans (pigmented raised patches found on the neck and skin flexures) is sometimes present in women with PCOS associated with insulin resistance.
- Severe CAH will have been diagnosed during childhood due to ambiguous external genitalia or salt-losing conditions. Women with milder, late-onset forms of CAH have little to distinguish them from those with PCOS, that is, obese, hirsutism/virilism with menstrual disorder.
- Women with Cushing's syndrome will have the typical appearance of central obesity, peripheral muscle wasting, hypertension and striae.
- Androgen-producing tumours cause little in the way of systemic upset apart from marked signs of virilism. They are usually too small to cause palpably enlarged ovaries.
- Women with idiopathic hirsutism usually have no abnormal findings on examination.

Investigations

Investigation is determined by the degree of symptoms (Fig. 16.10). Having excluded a history of exogenous androgens, if hirsutism is the only presenting complaint then PCOS is the likely cause accounting for 90% of cases. Diagnosis is made from the history, biochemical tests and ultrasound imaging of the ovaries. A rapid onset of symptoms, especially where virilism is present, would suggest high circulating levels of androgens secondary to more serious pathology. Testosterone levels more than twice the upper limit of normal suggest an ovarian or adrenal androgen-secreting tumour, which could be identified by imaging test such as ultrasound or CT scanning. Small tumours might be missed so a high level of suspicion is needed. Investigations for CAH and Cushing's syndrome should be performed if symptoms and clinical signs suggest these diseases. Idiopathic hirsutism is a diagnosis made by excluding other pathology.

Complications

- The main complication of hirsutism is psychosocial.
- Some signs of virilism, such as deepening of the voice and cliteromegaly might be irreversible.
- Complications associated with PCOS include obesity, insulin resistance and glucose intolerance.
- Chronic anovulation affects fertility and can cause endometrial hyperplasia and adenocarcinoma as a result of the unopposed effect of oestrogens.

Treatment

Idiopathic hirsutism can be treated cosmetically using bleaching or electrolysis. Encouraging weight loss is important in PCOS.

Medical treatment of hirsutism in women with PCOS is most effective using a combination of ethinyloestradiol with an anti-androgen such as cyproterone acetate (Dianette). Although improvement can take many months, the progestogenic effect of cyproterone acetate will protect the endometrium from the effects of unopposed oestrogen. Recent data suggest that PCOS might be driven by insulin resistance – as such, good results have been obtained by the use of the oral hypoglycaemic agent metformin.

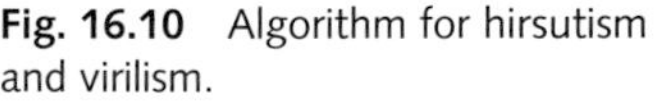
Fig. 16.10 Algorithm for hirsutism and virilism.

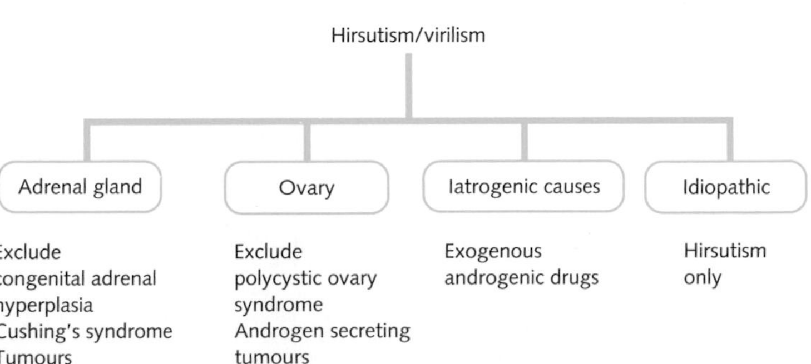

Androgen-secreting ovarian and adrenal tumours should be surgically removed with preservation of the ovary in younger women.

Glucocorticoid and often mineralocorticoid replacement is the mainstay of treatment in CAH. Hirsutism and virilism should improve with therapy but it is sometimes necessary to perform surgical reconstructive procedures to the external genitalia.

Treating the cause of excess cortisol production in Cushing's syndrome should result in normal circulating levels of adrenal androgens.

Women with gynaecological conditions requiring treatment with drugs that have androgenic properties should be forewarned of the potential virilizing side effects and the lowest therapeutic dose advocated. Phenytoin should not be stopped suddenly because this could precipitate status epilepticus.

Further reading

Bain, C., Burton, K., Mcgavigan, J., 2011. Gynaecology Illustrated, sixth ed. Churchill Livingstone, London.

Llewellyn-Jones, D., 2010. Fundamentals of Obstetrics & Gynaecology, ninth ed. Mosby, London.

Shaw, R.W., Soutter, W.P., Stanton, S.L., 1997. Gynaecology, third ed. Churchill Livingstone, London.

RCOG, 2007. Polycystic Ovary Syndrome, Long-Term Consequences (Green-top 33). Available online at: www.rcog.org.uk/guidelines.

Menopause 17

Objectives

By the end of this chapter, you should be able to:

- Understand what the menopause is, when it occurs and what its symptoms are
- Understand how to diagnose the menopause and how to investigate it
- Outline what treatments are available and their risks.

DEFINITIONS

'Menopause' is derived from the Greek *Men* (month) and *Pausis* (Cessation) and refers specifically to last menstrual period. This diagnosis can only be made retrospectively after 1 year of absent cycles. Women may experience symptoms and irregular periods before their last period when they are said to be 'perimenopasal'. This period of time is also referred to as the 'climacteric'.

The menopause generally occurs between the ages of 45 and 55 with the average age being 51 years. A premature menopause (<45 years of age) can occur for a number of reasons, e.g. surgery, chemo/radiotherapy or, indeed, naturally. A small percentage of women (1%) will experience premature ovarian failure below the age of 40 years.

PATHOPHYSIOLOGY

In order to understand the physiology of the menopause it is necessary to briefly review the physiology of the menstrual cycle.

At around 20 weeks of gestation the developing female fetus can have up to 7 million oocytes within the ovaries; this number will eventually fall to around 2 million at birth with approximately 50% of these being atretic. The ovaries are then quiescent until puberty when from a woman's first period (menarche) onwards, each month, her ovaries will recruit a cohort of oocytes. These oocytes then secrete oestrogen and progesterone and the whole process results in one oocyte becoming a dominant follicle and releasing an egg ready for fertilization.

After 40 years of age as a result of successive cycles in a woman's fertile period, only a few thousand oocytes remain. The depletion of the remaining oocytes coupled with their increased resistance to pituitary hormones (FSH and LH) will then lead to the cessation of menstruation – the hallmark of the menopause. In the perimenopausal patient anovulatory cycles become more common and oestrogen secretion can continue without the progesterone opposition required to protect the endometrium. These patients are at risk of endometrial hyperplasia and, rarely, endometrial cancer. Figure 17.1 summarizes the hormonal changes after the menopause.

CLINICAL FEATURES

Several symptoms are associated with the menopause, which can even begin before the last menstrual period and can cause a great deal of distress to patients (Fig. 17.2).

Making a diagnosis

In most cases, menopause can be diagnosed by history-taking and examination. As this is an important point in a woman's life it should be dealt with sensitively.

History

When taking a history, key features include:

- any vasomotor symptoms and mood disturbances
- date of the last menstrual period (LMP)
- pattern of menses in the past few years.

During the climacteric periods may become irregular and heavier, resulting in some intermenstrual bleeding. Urinary symptoms such as dysuria, frequency, incontinence should prompt further investigation (see below).

A sexual history should be taken, including dyspareunia and contraception. It is still possible to get pregnant during the climacteric and patients should continue using contraception beyond the menopause.

Fig. 17.1 Hormonal changes with the menopause.

	Menopause
FSH	↑↑
LH	↑↑
Oestrogen	↓↓
Progesterone	↓↓

Other important points include a cervical smear history and family history of conditions such as osteoporosis or cardiovascular disease so primary prevention can be initiated if required.

HINTS AND TIPS

Remember that all of the above symptoms can be due to other pathology, so the diagnosis should not be based on one symptom alone.

Examination

Important points include height, weight, blood pressure measurement, abdominal palpation and pelvic examination. A breast examination and cervical smear should be performed if clinically indicated.

Investigations

Serum FSH levels will confirm the diagnosis of menopause (see Fig 17.1). All other investigations should be tailored to the patient's symptoms (Fig. 17.3).

Treatment

As with many conditions lifestyle changes are beneficial; regular aerobic exercise can reduce bone loss and improve muscle tone. A reduction or cessation in alcohol consumption and smoking are also beneficial.

Hormone replacement therapy

There are many preparations available, both hormonal and non-hormonal which can be administered by a number of routes.

Oestrogen-based hormone replacement therapy (HRT) preparations were the first to be used to alleviate menopausal symptoms, but some women developed endometrial hyperplasia (a precursor for endometrial cancer). Progesterone was, therefore, added to

Immediate

- **Hot flushes and night sweats** (vasomotor symptoms) thought to be due oestrogen deficiency leading to thermodysregulation. More common in Caucasian and Afro-Caribbean than Japanese and Chinese women.
- **Mood disturbances** can include mood swings, insomnia, anxiety, fatigue, loss of libido and poor concentration. Symptoms can lead to perimenopausal depression compounded by oestrogen deficiency-driven reduction in serotonin secretion.

Intermediate

- **Atrophy of vaginal tissues** leading to dyspareunia and vaginal bleeding.
- **Atrophy of the urethra** leading to dysuria, urinary frequency and urge incontinence

Long Term

- **Osteoporosis** more common in women and in menopause oestrogen deficiency-driven imbalance in favour of bone resorption rather than formation predisposes to osteoporosis.
- Other contributory factors include family history, smoking, nulliparity, drugs, and a sedentary lifestyle.
- Diagnosis is confirmed by a bone scan in patients with bone mineral density 2.5 standard deviations below mean.
- Significant cost burden to health services from osteoporosis and related patient morbidity and mortality.
- **Cardiovascular disease** in postmenopausal women markedly increased compared to premenopausal women. Usual gender bias (men more susceptible than women) no longer apparent by age 70. Thought to be due to oestrogen deficiency having a direct effect on lipid levels (HDL:LDL ratio) and myocardial perfusion.

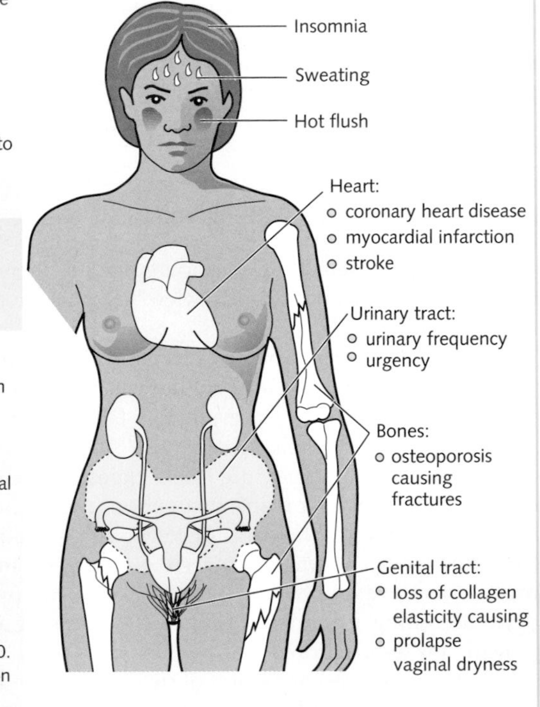

Fig. 17.2 Hormonal changes after the menopause.

Fig. 17.3 Investigating menopausal symptoms.

Urinary symptoms (dysuria, frequency, urgency)
Urine Dipstick +/− Urine microscopy, culture and sensitivities +/− Urodynamic Testing
Intermenstrual/post coital bleeding
Cervical Smear +/−Colposcopy
Low impact fractures/family history of osteoporosis
X-Ray Dual energy X-ray absorptiometry (DEXA) scan

preparations to protect the endometrium. In patients who have had a hysterectomy, progesterone is not required as there is no endometrium to protect.

There are many different types of oestrogen and prior to the menopause the main circulating oestrogen is oestradiol, produced by the granulosa cells of the developing follicle. Following the menopause oestrone is produced by peripheral tissues. The aim of HRT is readdress this and, therefore, most preparations contain oestradiol. Figure 17.4 shows the available routes of administration for HRT preparations as well as their potential advantages and disadvantages.

When prescribing HRT the lowest effective dose should be used. Oral preparations can be given as sequential preparations where patients will experience a monthly withdrawal bleed or continuous preparations where there will be no monthly bleed. In general cyclical preparations should not be continued for more than 5 years and in those patients experiencing symptoms after a period of 1 year's amenorrhoea with an intact uterus, continuous combined HRT should be commenced.

Side effects

Side effects described are nausea, fluid retention, hirsutism, leg cramps and breast discomfort. Modifying the preparation, as well as reducing the dose, can be beneficial. The progestogen component must be altered particularly carefully as there is a risk of not adequately protecting the endometrium. The Mirena® IUS can be beneficial as it secretes the progestogen locally with low systemic levels.

Contraindications

Figure 17.5 displays the contraindications to HRT use.

Risks

Over the past 20 years the use of HRT has come under intense scrutiny due to some studies showing an increased risk of cardiovascular disease, breast cancer and stroke in patients taking combined forms of HRT. In breast cancer it is thought that the risk increases with the duration of use, but this increased risk is not seen in those patients taking HRT for an early menopause. Evidence around cardiovascular risk is somewhat conflicting,

Fig. 17.5 Contraindications to hormone replacement therapy.

- Endometrial carcinoma
- Breast carcinoma
- Undiagnosed vaginal bleeding
- Undiagnosed breast lumps
- Severe active liver disease
- Pregnancy (always rule out before starting therapy)
- Personal history of venous thromboembolism – ORAL therapy is contraindicated but if benefits of treatment outweigh risks then TRANSDERMAL preparations can be used

Fig. 17.4 Route of administration for hormone replacement therapy.

	Advantages	Disadvantages
Oral	Cheap Effective	First pass metabolism Variable plasma levels Higher doses required
Transdermal (Patch/Gel)	Avoids first-pass metabolism Reduce risk of VTE Continuous administration	Cost Skin reactions
Vaginal	Good for urogenital symptoms Minimal systemic absorption Licensed for 3 months use without progesterone opposition (in the UK)	Unlikely to treat other symptoms
Mirena®IUS	Licensed for 4 yrs to provide the progesterone arm of HRT Contraceptive	Only provides progesterone for endometrial protection. Patients will still need oestrogen

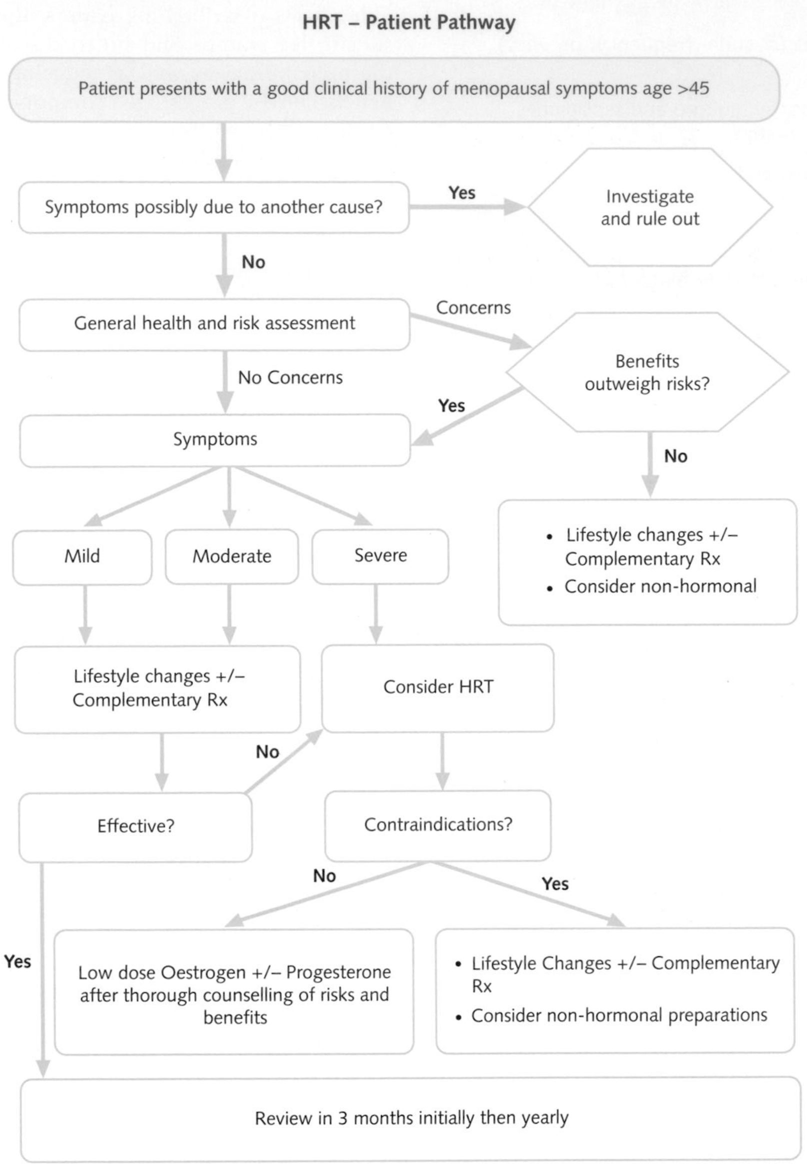

Fig. 17.6 Hormone replacement therapy – patient pathway. Adapted from Panay 2011, with permission. (Adapted from Panay N (2011) Menopause. In Oxford Desk Reference: Obstetrics and Gynaecology. Oxford University Press.)

although there appears to be a protective effect in the younger age group of patients taking HRT (50–59) and a detrimental effect in older patients (70–79 years).

Non-hormonal pharmacological agents

If hormonal agents are not tolerated or contraindicated for vasomotor symptoms, consider:

- clonidine – a centrally active alpha-2 agonist.
- selective serotonin reuptake inhibitors (SSRIs) and selective noradrenaline reuptake inhibitors (SNRIs).

CONTRACEPTION

Women in the climacteric remain at risk of pregnancy. Women should continue contraception for 1 year after their last menstrual period if they are >50 years old and for 2 years if they are <50 years old.

OSTEOPOROSIS

Although it is not a first-line treatment for osteoporosis prophylaxis in older age groups (due to the risk profile), HRT is still recommended for women under the age of 50 undergoing menopause for bone protection. Once they reach the age of 51, HRT should be reviewed and other methods to prevent osteoporosis considered.

Other pharmacological agents include bisphosphonates, and Selective oEstrogen Receptor Modulators (SERMs). Calcium and vitamin D supplementation, cessation of smoking and regular weight-bearing exercises are also important.

PREMATURE MENOPAUSE (PREMATURE OVARIAN FAILURE)

Premature ovarian failure occurs in 1% of women. It is diagnosed in patients under the age of 40 with secondary amenorrhoea, with a high FSH on two separate occasions. Causes include chemo or radiotherapy or viral infections such as mumps. Diagnosis is based on FSH and LH levels, whilst treatment is primarily HRT and dietary advice to prevent osteoporosis. Women affected by premature ovarian failure must be counselled on the need for IVF, together with the possibility of developing other autoimmune disorders such as thyroid disorders.

Once again, although it is not a first-line treatment for osteoporosis prophylaxis in older age groups (due to the risk profile), HRT is still recommended.

Reference

Panay, N., 2011. Menopause. In: Arulkumaran, S., Regan, L., Papageorghiou, A.T., et al. (Eds.), Oxford Desk Reference Obstetrics & Gynaecology. Oxford University Press, Oxford.

Further reading

Beresford, S., Weiss, N., Voigt, L., et al., 1997. Risk of endometrial cancer in relation to use of oestrogen combined with cyclic progestogen therapy in postmenopausal women. Lancet 349, 458–461.

British Menopause Society. Available online at: www.thebms.org.uk.

RCOG, 2011. Venous Thromboembolism and Hormone Replacement Therapy. Green-top Guideline No. 19. Royal College of Obstetricians and Gynaecologists, London. Available online at: www.rcog.org.uk.

Subfertility 18

Objectives

By the end of this chapter, you should be able to:

- Understand what subfertility is and how common it is
- Understand how to take a history from a couple and the necessary examinations/investigations
- Understand the causes of subfertility
- Understand the approaches to treatment and management.

INTRODUCTION

Around 84% of couples trying to conceive will do so successfully within 1 year. This figure rises to 92% by 2 years. Infertility is defined as the failure to conceive after regular unprotected sexual intercourse for 2 years, in the absence of known reproductive pathology. Subfertility is often sub-classified as being either primary or secondary. Primary subfertility refers to couples who have never had a previous pregnancy whereas secondary subfertility refers to those that have had a previous pregnancy.

Couples who are having difficulty conceiving after 1 year should be investigated for any possible underlying causes. In some couples, i.e. those with a history of menstrual irregularities, pelvic infection or where the female is aged >35 years, investigations may be needed earlier.

Female fertility decreases with age and as more women defer pregnancy, the problem is becoming more prevalent. The cause for subfertility can lie in either the male partner, female partner or both (Fig. 18.1).

Couples seeking advice and help with subfertility are often very anxious as they may fear not being able to have children, so an empathetic approach is very important.

To understand the causes and management of subfertility, first consider what is necessary for conception, i.e. an XX woman and an XY male must have penetrative intercourse resulting in male ejaculation. The sperm must pass through the cervical mucus, the uterine cavity and into the fallopian tube. The egg must have been picked up by the fimbrial end of the fallopian tube and transported down to meet the sperm so that fertilization occurs within the tube, and the fertilized embryo must implant within the endometrium. Conception generally occurs in the 4 days around ovulation, sperm can survive for around 3 days and an egg can be fertilized for up to 1 day after it is released.

TAKING THE HISTORY

A detailed history is very important when assessing a couple with subfertility.

History of the couple

When taking a history from the couple, find out the duration of subfertility and whether the frequency of intercourse is adequate. Current guidelines recommend intercourse every 2–3 days. Any coital problems should be identified, especially female vaginismus, dyspareunia or male erectile/ejaculatory dysfunction.

History from the woman

Causes of subfertility in the female are shown in Figure 18.2 and it is useful to keep these in mind when taking a history.

Past obstetric history

Ask about any previous pregnancies, their outcomes and mode of delivery. This includes a history of a previous ectopic pregnancy as this may indicate a tubal problem.

Past gynaecological history

A menstrual history should be taken to assess the following:

- Menorrhagia (heavy periods) may be due to fibroids which can contribute to subfertility
- Dysmenorrhoea (painful periods), might suggest:
  - Endometriosis, which can cause tubal problems, either due to adhesions or by interfering with the ciliary action of the tubal lining, or

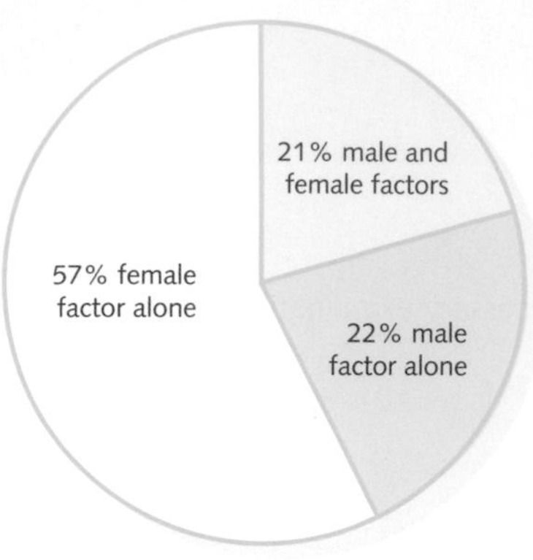

Fig. 18.1 Pie chart of causes of subfertility.

Fig. 18.2 Causes of female infertility.

Problem	Cause
Ovulatory dysfunction	Chronic systemic illness Eating disorders Polycystic ovarian syndrome Hyperprolactinaemia Hypo/hyperthyroidism Cannabis use NSAIDs
Tubal factor	Pelvic inflammatory disease Previous tubal surgery Previous ectopic pregnancy Endometriosis
Uterine problem	Fibroid Uterine septae Congenital anomaly Ashermann's syndrome
Coital dysfunction	Vaginismus Dyspareunia

  - Ashermann's syndrome – the presence of intrauterine adhesions that form after curettage or termination of pregnancy.
- Dyspareunia is an important symptom, suggesting pelvic inflammatory disease (PID) or endometriosis
- Oligo- or amenorrhoea (few or absent periods) may point to anovulation
- Any previous pelvic infections should be noted as they may have caused tubal damage, in addition, any previous intrauterine contraceptive device (IUCD) use, tubal surgery or ectopic pregnancy should be identified.

HINTS AND TIPS

One episode of pelvic inflammatory disease (PID) gives a 10% chance of tubal blockage; three episodes of PID give a 50% chance of tubal blockage.

Past medical history

Chronic medical conditions (e.g. renal disease, hypo- and hyperthyroidism) and eating disorders – especially anorexia nervosa – decrease the number of ovulatory cycles, reducing the chance of conception.

Drug history

A drug history is essential (both prescription or otherwise). Regular use of non-steroidal anti-inflammatory drugs and cannabis reduces the number of ovulatory cycles. This is an opportunity to review any medications not recommended for use in pregnancy, considering alternatives if appropriate. All women trying to conceive should take folic acid supplements.

Social history

Smoking reduces fertility so smoking cessation should be encouraged. Alcohol consumption should be limited to 1–2 units once or twice a week. Regular exercise should be encouraged and those with a body mass index (BMI) >29 should be advised to lose weight. Those with a BMI of <19 who have oligo/amenorrhoea should be advised that moderate weight gain may increase conception rates.

History from the man

Past surgical history

Relevant operations include:

- inguinal hernia repairs, which may lead to obstruction of the vas deferens in its inguinal portion
- undescended testes – this affects semen quality (regardless of timing of orchidopexy)
- testicular torsion reduces fertility
- bladder neck surgery, including transurethral resection of the prostate (TURP) can cause retrograde ejaculation.

Past medical history

- Cystic fibrosis (CF) – patients with CF may have agenesis of the vas deferens and therefore an obstruction.

- Epididymo-orchitis, most commonly caused by sexually transmitted infections such as chlamydia can also result in epididymal obstruction.
- Post pubertal mumps orchitis can cause significant testicular atrophy resulting in very poor-quality sperm.
- Chronic medical conditions (e.g. renal disease, diabetes) impair spermatogenesis.

Drug history

Several drugs are known to decrease sperm number and/or function:

- Anabolic steroids, cannabis, cocaine, sulfasalazine (taken for inflammatory bowel disease), colchicine (used to treat gout), nitrofurantoin and tetracyclines (antibiotics)
- α-blockers (used for treatment of benign prostatic hypertrophy) and some antidepressants are known to interfere with ejaculation
- β-blockers may cause impotence.

Social history

- Smoking can impair the quality of the sperm
- Excessive alcohol intake reduces semen quality
- Occupational history is important. Sperm count might be affected in men whose jobs result in raised testicular temperature such as prolonged driving
- Heavy metals, solvents and agricultural chemicals are all associated with oligospermia.

HINTS AND TIPS

Consultation with the subfertile couple should be carried out with compassion and dignity. The inability to conceive may result in psychological, social, ethnic and religious pressures that may not always be apparent but may have profound consequences for the individuals.

EXAMINATION

Examination of the woman

General

- The presence or absence of secondary sexual characteristics should be noted.
- The BMI should be calculated (weight (kg)/height (m^2)).
- Hirsutism and acanthosis nigricans may indicate PCOS.
- Other syndromes linked to infertility have other typical facies (e.g. hyper/hypothyroidism, Cushing's syndrome, Turner's syndrome).

Abdominal examination

Initial inspection may reveal scars from previous surgery which could raise the possibility of adhesions or indicate previous treatment (e.g. laparoscopy for endometriosis/PID). Palpation may reveal the presence of a mass which may be due to a large fibroid uterus or ovarian cyst and lower abdominal tenderness may be due to endometriosis or PID.

Vaginal examination

- Vaginal discharge may be physiological or a sign of PID and if there is doubt, triple swabs should be taken.
- The cervix should be visualized and concerns followed up with a colposcopy. Previous cervical surgery may have caused stenosis.
- The uterus is palpated; a non-mobile uterus may be due to adhesions from endometriosis or PID; an enlarged uterus is likely to be due to fibroids.
- The practice of female genital mutilation is widespread in some parts of the world and may cause dyspareunia and even apareunia.
- Occasionally an intact hymen is discovered.

Examination of the man

- Calculate the BMI as obesity is known to decrease testosterone levels.
- Look for secondary sexual characteristics – inadequate virilization could be due to abnormal karyotype.
- Scars from inguinal hernia repair might point to an obstructive problem.
- Consider the impact of clothing; tight underwear raises the scrotal temperature and can impair sperm function.
- Measure testicular size using an orchidometer, and palpate to check the presence of the vas deferens on both sides.

INVESTIGATION

Target investigations for subfertility to a specific cause (if indicated from the history). In some cases not all investigations are necessary. Investigations which may be required include:

Blood tests

The following should be checked in women:

- Mid-luteal phase progesterone: the level rises after ovulation. The test should be performed a week before the next period is due, e.g. day 21 of a 28-day cycle, or day 28 of a 35-day cycle.
- Rubella immunity: this is not an investigation of subfertility but must be checked in any woman who is intending to conceive so that she can be vaccinated if not immune to prevent infection in pregnancy.

Pelvic ultrasound

Performed to look for:

- congenital or structural abnormalities of the uterus
- fibroids
- bulky ovaries with multiple peripheral follicles in PCOS
- Hydrosalpinx.

Microbiology

Screen for Chlamydia in both women (endocervical swab/urine) and men (urethral swab). Infection is asymptomatic in up to 70% of women so there might not be any clues in the history. Treatment itself may not improve fertility but failure to identify and treat prior to hysterosalpingogram or laparoscopy and dye (see below) can exacerbate the infection, which may worsen tubal disease

Testing tubal patency

Testing for tubal patency is a very important part of a work up in subfertility and is performed in the first half of the cycle to ensure the patient isn't already pregnant. The method used will depend upon patient's history:

- A hysterosalpingogram (HSG) is generally used in patients with no comorbidities (PID, previous ectopic, endometriosis). Radio-opaque dye is introduced through the cervix into the uterus and an X-ray is taken to look for passage of the dye. Blockage inside or outside the tubes can prevent the dye flowing; however, tubal spasm in response to the dye can also prevent flow (see Fig. 18.3).
- Hysterosalpingo contrast sonography (HyCoSy) is an alternative. It is performed by ultrasound and involves the passage of fluid through the cervix into the uterus and tubes monitored using Doppler.
- Where there is suspicion of pathology a laparoscopy and dye is performed under general anaesthetic. It enables direct visualization of the pelvis in order to diagnose endometriosis or PID and the resulting adhesions. Methylene blue dye is introduced through the cervix and its progress through the uterus and out of the fallopian tubes can be directly visualized. Lack of 'fill and spill' of dye indicates tubal occlusion.
- Infection screening should be done before any investigations of tubal patency to prevent ascending infection. Where it has not been done antibiotic cover should be prescribed. A semen analysis (see below) is mandatory prior to laparoscopy as an abnormal semen analysis may be the cause of subfertility and make the operation unnecessary.

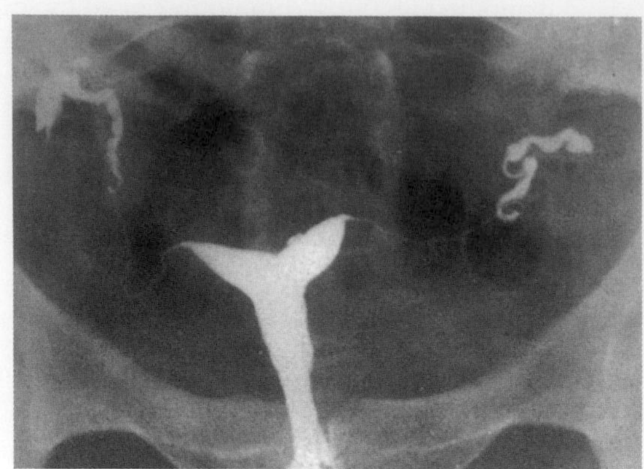

Fig. 18.3 Hysterosalpingogram. From Letterie 2011, with permission.

Semen analysis

Here, the patient is asked to provide a specimen after 3 days' abstinence and after a period of good health (a systemic illness within the previous 72 days can reduce the quality of sperm produced).

The sample should be examined within 1 hour of production. The sperm are counted and evaluated for motility, progression and morphology, and the volume of the specimen is recorded (Fig. 18.4 gives the normal parameters). The presence of more than 106 white blood cells suggests epididymo-orchitis. Ideally, at least two samples at least 12 weeks apart should be examined (to sample different populations of sperm).

Fig. 18.4 Normal parameters of semen analysis.

Volume	1.5–5 mls
Count	>20 million/ml
Progression	>50%
Normal forms	>30%

HINTS AND TIPS

Definitions:

- Azoospermia: no sperm in ejaculate
- Oligozoospermia: < 15 million/mL
- Asthenozoospermia: < 32% motile sperm
- Teratozoospermia: < 4% normal forms
- Oligo-terato-asthenospermia (OAT) is the most common diagnosis in male infertility.

Further investigations

These might be prompted by specific points in the history or examination, and include:

- prolactin, LH and FSH levels done if the woman has irregular cycles. Prolactin may also be required if the patient has galactorrhoea
- thyroid function tests done only if the patient has signs/symptoms of thyroid disease
- karyotyping: if secondary sexual characteristics are absent
- testosterone: if the man appears hypoandrogenic (non-hirsute, small soft testes) or if the woman is overly hirsute
- antisperm antibodies: should only be performed in tertiary centres. Both women and men might have antibodies to sperm. In men they occur on the sperm surface, in the seminal plasma and in the blood serum, whereas in women they are found in blood and in cervical mucus. They affect sperm motility and function, but their presence is not a significant predictor of infertility – they are found in 5–10% of infertile men, but also in 2% of fertile men
- hysteroscopy: should only be performed if the ultrasound suggests abnormality (e.g. intrauterine adhesions, endometrial polyps or fibroids). Polyps and submucosal fibroids are associated with subfertility, but the exact causal relationship is unclear.

TREATMENT

Where identified, treatment for subfertility can be aimed at the specific cause. Many couples, however, suffer unexplained subfertility, but can still be helped by the methods described below.

Anovulation

Anovulation can be due to failure of the hypothalamo-pituitary-ovarian (HPO) axis (GnRH deficiency), dysfunction of the HPO axis (polycystic ovary syndrome (PCOS)) or ovarian failure. Most commonly it is due to PCOS. It is confirmed by measuring serum progesterone levels during the luteal phase of the cycle. If the woman is not ovulating due to PCOS:

- optimize general health (correct thyroid disease, diabetes, etc.)
- consider BMI (ovulation is less likely at the extremes of weight)
- consider clomiphene (see below) to induce ovulation
- if BMI >25 and not responding to clomiphene alone consider adding metformin
- consider ovarian drilling – performed laparoscopically with a series holes drilled into the ovaries.

Clomiphene is an antioestrogen that occupies oestrogen receptors in the hypothalamus, thereby increasing GnRH release, which leads to increased release of LH and FSH. This induces follicular development and ovulation. It is given on days 2–6 of the cycle. Ovulation should be confirmed by a raised progesterone level. If ovulation does not occur the dose can be increased the next cycle month.

The patient must be warned of the risk of multiple pregnancy. Often ultrasound is used to assess the ovaries during the cycle and couples may be advised to use barrier contraception if multiple follicles are seen to prevent multiple pregnancy. In addition the patient should be warned of the possible association between ovulation induction and ovarian cancer.

HINTS AND TIPS

Couples who are subfertile may not understand why they are warned about the risk of multiple pregnancy with ovarian stimulation. They may actually view multiple pregnancy as an advantage. It is important to explain that multiple pregnancies have a higher overall complication rate including miscarriage, three times the rate of cerebral palsy and five times the perinatal mortality rate.

Uterine, tubal and pelvic problems

- Submucous fibroids, polyps and uterine septae, all distort the uterine cavity. They can impair fertility and may cause miscarriage. Often they will be removed prior to in vitro fertilization (IVF) to maximize the chances of success.
- Hydrosalpinges reduce the implantation rate and can be removed or drained for this reason prior to IVF.
- Surgical treatment of even mild endometriosis (i.e. diathermy or laser at time of laparoscopy) has been shown to improve fertility in the short term.
- Tubal surgery – proximal tubal blockage can be treated hysteroscopically using new cannulation techniques. Distal damage may be treated by

laparoscopic salpingostomy. Tubal patency, however, does not guarantee function and these patients are at risk of an ectopic pregnancy.

Male factor infertility

If the semen analysis is persistently abnormal despite advice regarding loose underwear and reduction of alcohol and nicotine intake, assisted fertility can be considered. Up to six cycles of intrauterine insemination (IUI) may be tried before IVF or intracytoplasmic sperm injection (ICSI), because it is less invasive.

Intrauterine insemination

IUI is a technique which is suitable for patients with mild male factor infertility, unexplained infertility or mild endometriosis. The male partner provides a semen sample. Fast-moving sperm are selected and introduced into the uterine cavity. In the female partner the cycle ovulation can be stimulated or unstimulated.

In vitro fertilization

In vitro (in glass) fertilization involves inducing ovulation followed by harvesting the oocytes and fertilizing them in a laboratory using sperm from the partner or donor. The subsequent embryo is then transferred back to the patient with the hope of an ongoing pregnancy.

IVF has advanced hugely over the past few years with variations on techniques and protocols. It generally involves several steps:

- Down-regulation of the woman's own hormones using GnRH agonists. They initially stimulate LH and FSH but then cause down-regulation, leading to reduction in oestrogen production and 'menopausal' side effects. These drugs are given by nasal spray or subcutaneous injection
- Induction of multiple follicular development using gonadotrophins such as human menopausal gonadotrophin (hMG), which contains FSH and LH and is prepared from the urine of menopausal women, hCG, which is obtained from the urine of pregnant women and has a similar action to LH, or recombinant FSH, an expensive but pure form of FSH
- Egg collection: performed transvaginally using ultrasound, under sedation (Fig. 18.5)
- Sperm preparation
- In vitro fertilization of the oocytes with sperm
- Transfer of the healthy embryos (maximum of two) back into the uterine cavity (Fig. 18.6).

HINTS AND TIPS

Pre-implantation genetic diagnosis (PGD) is a technique whereby couples affected by a hereditary disorder can screen embryos to see which may be affected. Cells from each embryo are removed and analysed so that only unaffected embryos are transferred to the patient.

Intracytoplasmic sperm injection

Intracytoplasmic sperm injection (ICSI) is an advanced form of IVF where one sperm is directly injected into the egg (Fig. 18.7). This technique has revolutionized treatment for couples where the partner's sperm count is very low or showing increased abnormal forms. If there are

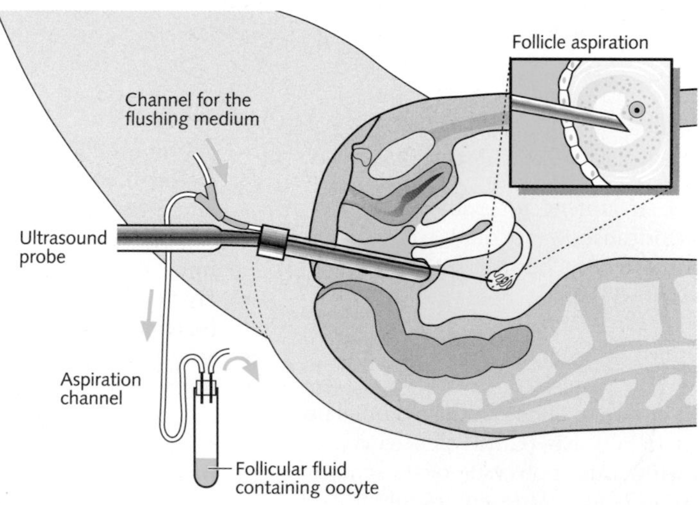

Fig. 18.5 Egg collection.

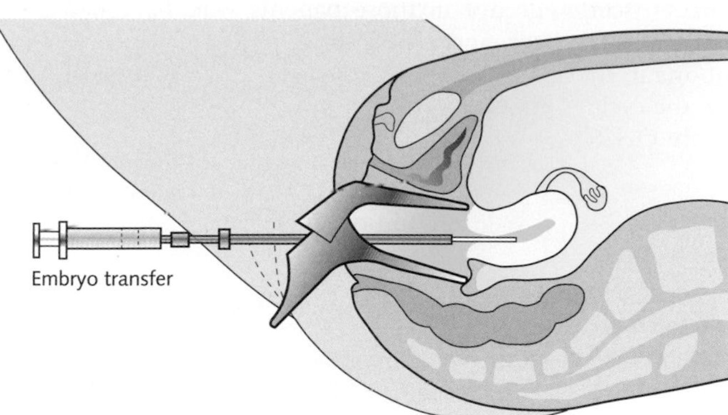

Fig. 18.6 Embryo transfer.

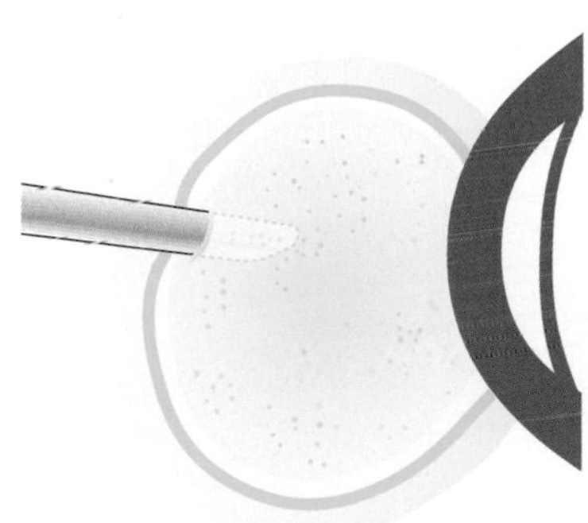

Fig. 18.7 Sperm injection into an egg.

no sperm in the semen at all (due to obstruction or to congenital absence of the vas) sperm can sometimes be extracted from the vas, the epididymis, or even from a testicular biopsy. It has recently been suggested that spermatids (i.e. immature spermatozoa) could be used, but at present this has not been licensed by the Human Fertilisation and Embryology Authority (HFEA).

HINTS AND TIPS

The Human Fertilisation and Embryology Authority (HFEA) was established in 1991 and regulates all centres in the UK that offer assisted conception. Their website www.HFEA.gov.uk is an excellent source of advice and information for couples.

Surgical options for male subfertility

If the sperm count is suboptimal because of epididymal blockage, surgery can be performed to restore patency. If a varicocoele is present this can be repaired. This has not been proven conclusively to improve spermatogenesis but it is known that the incidence of varicocoele in the male partner of couples with subfertility is 40% compared with 15% in the general population.

RISKS OF ASSISTED REPRODUCTIVE TECHNIQUES

- IVF has a well-known association with multiple pregnancy and studies have shown children born through IVF have a slightly lower birth weight compared to spontaneous conceptions.
- ICSI has been shown to have an increased risk of children being born with congenital malformations especially affecting the urogenital system.
- Ovarian hyperstimulation syndrome (OHSS) which is discussed below.

Ovarian hyperstimulation syndrome

Ovulation induction can lead to OHSS, which is a systemic disease with potentially very serious consequences. It occurs as a consequence of high levels of oestrogen and increased vascular permeability. This can lead to accumulation of fluid in the 'third space' (abdomen, chest, etc.) and leads to intravascular fluid depletion.

In its mild form the patient suffers only mild abdominal discomfort. In worse cases, however, nausea and vomiting develop, there is pronounced, painful abdominal distension, and fluid shifts resulting in ascites and pleural effusions. Hepatorenal failure and adult respiratory distress syndrome (ARDS) can ensue and the patient is at greatly increased risk of thromboembolism. Treatment is hospitalization and careful fluid balance. Thromboprophylaxis is very important and some patients may require therapeutic drainage of accumulated fluid by an ascitic or chest drain.

As with many conditions prevention is better than cure and careful ultrasound monitoring of patients undergoing ovulation induction is very important. In some cases it may be necessary to abandon the cycle if too many follicles have developed to prevent OHSS occurring.

Prognosis

The age of the female partner has been shown to be the most important prognostic factor in IVF. Women aged between 23 and 35 years have a 20% chance of live birth per IVF cycle compared with 6% for those aged 40 years or more. Older women may choose to use donor eggs, which can increase success rates. IVF is also more effective in those patients who have had a previous pregnancy.

Reference

Letterie, G.S., 2011. Management of congenital uterine abnormalities. Reprod. Biomed. Online 23, 40–52. http://dx.doi.org/10.1016/j.rbmo.2011.02.008, Epub 2011 Feb 17.

Further reading

NICE, 2004. Clinical Guideline 11. National Institute for Health and Care Excellence, London.

RCOG, 2006. Ovarian Hyperstimulation Syndrome. Green-top Guideline No. 5. Royal College of Obstetricians and Gynaecologists, London.

Contraception, sterilization and unwanted pregnancy

Objectives

By the end of this chapter, you should be able to:

- Describe contraceptive failure rates
- Discuss the contraindications to using the combined contraceptive pill
- Name the non-contraceptive benefits of the combined contraceptive pill
- List the progestogen-only methods of contraception and describe their mechanism of action
- Explain the options for emergency contraception and how long after intercourse they can be used
- Describe the methods used for sterilization.

INTRODUCTION

The ideal contraceptive is one that is 100% effective, with no side effects, is readily reversible and does not need medical supervision: this does not exist. Hence, it is important that the doctor assesses the patient's requirements at the particular time in her life that she requests contraception, and reviews the advantages and disadvantages so that the patient can make an informed choice (see *Crash Course in Endocrinology*).

Informed choice regarding the method of contraception used by each individual patient is important. It is essential to take a sexual history in a sensitive, non-judgemental way and to check for any medical contraindications that may be relevant.

Consideration must be given to a woman's risk of sexually transmitted infections (STI), her future fertility needs and, in some cases, her medical history. The effectiveness of a particular method can be measured by the number of unwanted pregnancies that occur during 100 women years of exposure; this is known as the Pearl Index. Figure 19.1 shows effectiveness in terms of percentage.

NATURAL FAMILY PLANNING METHODS

Rhythm method

The rhythm method involves predicting the fertile and infertile times of the menstrual cycle, by using several fertility indicators:

- A menstrual calendar
- Charting the basal body temperature, which rises 0.2–0.4 °C when progesterone is released from the corpus luteum
- Recognizing changes in cervical mucus
- An ovulation predictor kit, e.g. Persona®.

Advantages

This method has no side effects and does not involve hormones. It might be useful if other methods are unacceptable to the couple, such as with certain religious groups or because of unwanted side effects.

Disadvantages

The method relies on a regular menstrual cycle, lengthy instruction and commitment. The couple may wish to avoid sex or use a condom at fertile times of the cycle.

Coitus interruptus

Advantages

Still widely practised, this method is free and without side effects.

Disadvantages

The failure rate is high due to variable ejaculatory control and the fact that pre-ejaculatory fluid contains some sperm. There is no protection against STIs.

BARRIER METHODS

These methods include the male condom and, for women, the diaphragm, the cervical cap and the female condom. Their effectiveness increases with concomitant use of a spermicide such as nonoxynol-9, which alters sperm membrane permeability resulting in sperm death (use of spermicides alone as contraception is not recommended).

Fig. 19.1 Methods of contraception and their relative effectiveness.

Method	Effectiveness
Sterilization Female	lifetime failure rate 1 in 200
Sterilization Male	lifetime failure rate 1 in 2000
Combined oral contraceptive pill	<1 in 100 pregnancies in 1 year
Progesterone-only pill	1 in 100 pregnancies in 1 year
Depot injection	<1 in 100 pregnancies in 1 year
IUCD	1-2 in 100 pregnancies in 1 year
Mirena IUS (has lowest failure rate in IUCD)	5 per 1000 pregnancies in 5 years
Condom:male	2 in 100 pregnancies in 1 year
Diaphragm	4-8 in 100 pregnancies in 1 year

In 2001, a World Health Organization (WHO) report stated that nonoxynol-9 offered no protection against sexually transmitted infections and is even shown to increase the risk of HIV infection when used frequently by women at high risk of infection.

Advantages

When used properly, these are effective, free from side effects and widely available. They offer protection against STIs, in particular the male condom, which protects against HIV.

Disadvantages

They must be applied before penetration (which can interrupt sex) and can reduce the level of sensation. The diaphragm and the cap have to be fitted and checked regularly by a trained professional. In all these methods, effectiveness is dependent on correct use and sustained motivation.

HORMONAL CONTRACEPTION

Combined oral contraceptive pill

Since their introduction in 1961, various combinations of different oestrogens and progestogens have been used to prevent pregnancy. Combined oral contraceptive pills (COCP) have the following modes of action:

- Inhibiting ovulation by:
  - inhibiting follicular stimulating hormone (FSH) release
  - preventing follicular ripening
- Preventing the luteinizing hormone (LH) surge
- Thinning the endometrium
- Thickening the cervical mucus to prevent sperm reaching the egg.

Contraindications

Figure 19.2 lists the contraindications to the COCP.

Advantages

This method is reliable if taken correctly, convenient and not intercourse related. Its use reduces dysmenorrhoea, menorrhagia and premenstrual syndrome (PMS) symptoms. It also controls functional ovarian cysts and is associated with a reduced incidence of carcinoma of the ovary and endometrium.

Disadvantages

The main risks of the COCP are thromboembolism and cardiovascular complications. These are exacerbated by:

- age
- obesity
- cigarette smoking

Fig. 19.2 Contraindications to the combined oral contraceptive pill.

Degree of contraindication	Description
Absolute	Pregnancy Arterial or venous thrombosis Liver disease Undiagnosed vaginal bleeding History of oestrogen-dependent tumour Recent hydatidiform mole
Relative	Family history of thrombosis (consider investigations for thrombophilia) Hypertension Migraine Varicose veins

- diabetes
- hypertension
- familial hyperlipidaemia.

Other more minor side effects include weight gain, decreased libido, breast discomfort, mood disturbance and breakthrough bleeding. The effectiveness of the COCP is limited by some antibiotics, hepatic-enzyme-inducing drugs and by vomiting and diarrhoea. Use is associated with an increase in cervical intraepithelial neoplasia and carcinoma of the cervix. This may be because of the increased risk of exposure to STIs with a non-barrier method of contraception. The effect on breast cancer is uncertain.

The COCP should be discontinued 4 weeks before major surgery because of the risk of venous thromboembolism. Heparin prophylaxis may still be necessary depending on other risk factors such as immobility or BMI over 30. Alternative contraception should be advised.

Progesterone-only pill

Although slightly less effective than the COCP, the progesterone-only pill (POP) is used in women in whom oestrogens are contra-indicated or who cannot tolerate the side effects. This includes women aged over 35 who smoke and those who are breast-feeding.

The mode of action differs from the COCP in that ovulation is suppressed in only 50–60% of cycles, but with similar changes in cervical mucus and in the endometrium, as well as reduced tubal motility.

Advantages

Without oestrogen, few serious side effects occur.

Disadvantages

Efficacy is reduced if the time of pill-taking is delayed by more than 3 hours. The main problem is a change in menstrual pattern, with spotting or breakthrough bleeding that does not settle despite continued use. There is a small increase in the risk of ectopic pregnancy.

Injectable progestogens (Depo-provera)

Intramuscular injections of medroxyprogesterone acetate given every 3 months ensure that high-dose progestogen is gradually released into the circulation and inhibits ovulation; it is almost as effective as the COCP.

Advantages

This method of contraception is highly effective and is not intercourse related. It also does not require daily motivation.

Disadvantages

- Because it is injected, it cannot be removed and any side effects must be tolerated for 3 months.
- Most women become amenorrhoeic but heavy, unpredictable bleeding patterns can sometimes occur.
- Being a slow-release depot preparation, there might be a delay in return to fertility of 12 to 18 months.
- Prolonged use is associated with an increased risk of osteoporosis.
- Other side effects include headache, spotty skin, mood changes and breast tenderness.

Progestin implant (Implanon)

This is an inert flexible tube, 2–3 cm in length that is inserted subdermally, usually under the skin of the upper arm under local anaesthetic. It releases the man-made hormone progestin.

Advantages

Its effects last for 3 years but the device can be taken out any time. It has the advantage over the depo preparation of a quicker return to normal fertility and regular menses once discontinued. It is not intercourse-related.

Disadvantages

Periods can be irregular and some women gain weight. Training is needed for insertion using a local anaesthetic and tenderness, bruising and swelling may occur.

INTRAUTERINE CONTRACEPTIVE DEVICES AND MIRENA INTRAUTERINE SYSTEM

Insertion of one of a variety of synthetic devices into the uterine cavity (Fig. 19.3) is likely to ensure that blastocyst implantation is prevented. There is also some foreign body reaction to the intrauterine contraceptive device (IUCD) in the endometrium, resulting in altered cell numbers and fluid compositions, which may affect gamete viability. There may also be changes in the cervical mucus which reduce sperm penetration. The latter effects are particularly applicable to the progestogen-containing MIRENA intrauterine system (IUS), which also acts to thin the endometrium.

Contraindications

Figure 19.4 lists the contraindications to IUCD/IUS use.

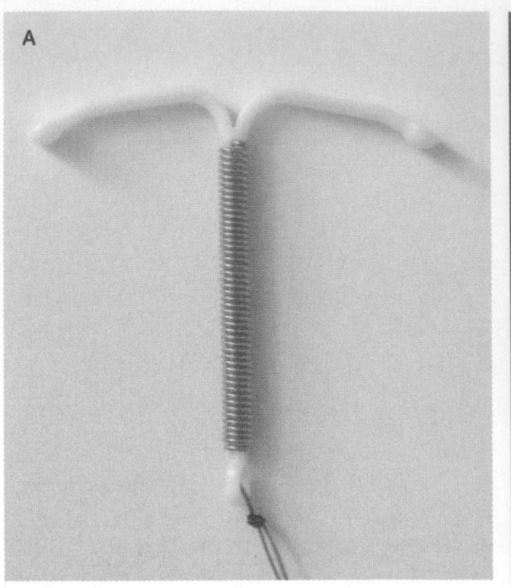

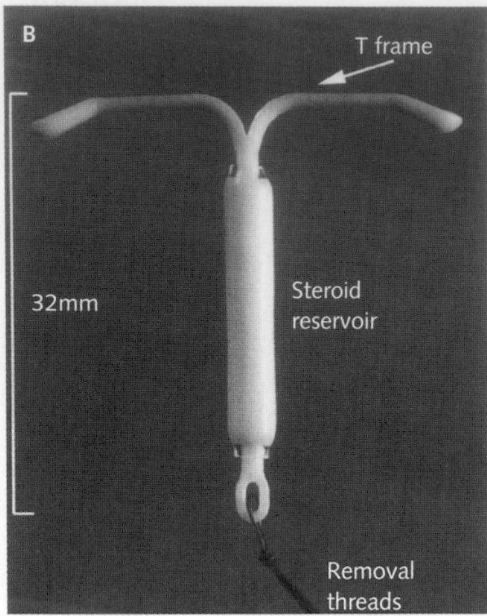

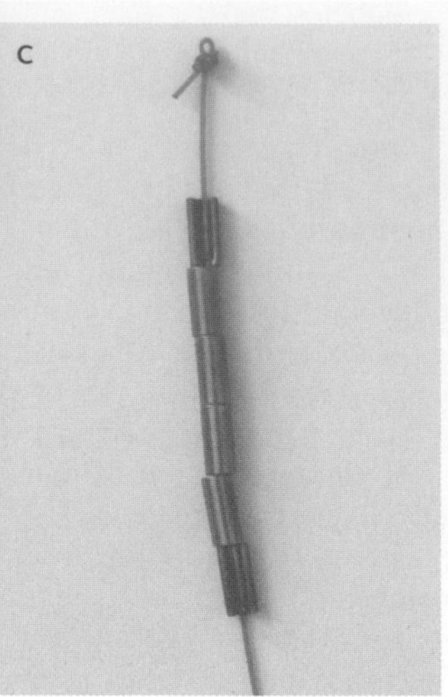

Fig. 19.3 Types of intrauterine contraceptive device: (A) Copper T. (B) Mirena IUS. (C) Gynefix.

Advantages

Once inserted by a trained operator, the IUCD/IUS is effective immediately. It can remain in place for 3 to 5 years and its effect on preventing conception is almost immediately reversible when removed. The MIRENA IUS has the extra advantages related to local secretion of progestogen, which acts on the endometrium; this results in amenorrhoea in up to 85% of patients at 6 months. Hence this type of system has various gynaecological indications, such as treating menorrhagia and dysmenorrhoea. It should also be considered as an alternative to sterilization since it has at least a similar success rate. The IUCD should not be used in women with menorrhagia as it can increase menstrual blood loss.

Disadvantages

- Infection
- Uterine perforation
- Expulsion of IUCD/IUS
- Menorrhagia (except with MIRENA) and/or abdominal pain
- Ectopic pregnancy.

Fig. 19.4 Contraindications to the intrauterine contraceptive device.

- Pregnancy
- Undiagnosed uterine bleeding
- Active and/or past history of PID
- Previous ectopic pregnancy
- Previous tubal surgery

Introduction of infection at the time of insertion of the IUCD/IUS is one of the main risk factors for using this form of contraception. For this reason, it is advisable to exclude chlamydia infection and/or give prophylactic antibiotics. The possibility of developing pelvic inflammatory disease (PID) means that an IUCD/IUS is less commonly used in nulliparous women, especially if they have multiple partners.

Other disadvantages that the patient should be told about include risk of uterine perforation at the time of coil insertion or possibly at a later date. The woman should be taught to check that she can feel the threads of the coil to ensure that it has not fallen out. If either of these situations arises, attempts to locate the IUCD/IUS should be made by X-ray, ultrasound and possibly laparoscopy.

The most common reasons for a patient requesting removal of the IUCD are menorrhagia and abdominal pain; these symptoms are much less common with a Mirena® than with other IUCDs. If a pregnancy does occur with a coil in situ, the risk of an ectopic pregnancy is higher than with other forms of contraception.

FEMALE STERILIZATION

Sterilization is a permanent way of preventing pregnancy, involving having an operation. The more commonly used techniques include the application of Falope rings or Filshie clips to each tube laparoscopically as a day-case procedure. At laparotomy, a modified Pomeroy tubal ligation is usually performed, for example at caesarean section. Hysteroscopic techniques inserting microcoils into the Fallopian tubes are not yet in common use (e.g. Essure).

Counselling

Sterilization should be regarded as an irreversible procedure and therefore the patient must be sure that she has completed her family and that she has considered all other methods of contraception. There is a higher risk of regret if the patient makes the request at the time of termination of a pregnancy or caesarean section. This is particularly the case in a younger woman, under the age of 30; the MIRENA IUS, therefore, should be considered since it has a similar rate of success but is reversible and avoids the need for surgery.

Sterilization has a lifetime failure rate of about 1 in 200; this might be due to failure to exclude pregnancy preoperatively or incorrect application of a clip. If a pregnancy does occur, the risk of an ectopic pregnancy is higher than other forms of contraception.

MALE STERILIZATION

Compared to female sterilization, a vasectomy is a relatively easy operation, avoiding the risks of a general anaesthetic. The vas deferens is ligated via bilateral incisions in the scrotum under local anaesthesia. Another method of contraception must be used until two azoospermic samples have been obtained 3 and 4 months after the procedure. The failure rate is much lower than for the female operation (1:2000 after azoospermia confirmed). It may be associated with chronic testicular pain. Nearly 75% of men who undergo vasectomy will develop antisperm antibodies.

CONTRACEPTION AND BREAST-FEEDING

Breast-feeding can act as a very effective contraceptive when a woman is fully breast-feeding a baby under 6 months of age. However, in the UK, where contraception is free and readily available, it should not be relied upon. Depending on the woman's medical history, the POP or an IUCD/IUS may be appropriate.

POSTCOITAL CONTRACEPTION (EMERGENCY CONTRACEPTION)

Since 1999, Levonelle has superceded the Yuzpe method as the choice for emergency contraception and is currently available over the counter in the UK. Within 72 hours of unprotected intercourse or with a failed method of contraception, levonorgestrel, a synthetic progestogen, 1.5 mg, is taken as a single dose.

It interferes with ovulation and prevents fertilization. There is little evidence to suggest that it inhibits implantation. If it is taken before the preovulation oestrogen surge, ovulation can be inhibited. Vomiting occurs in approximately 1% of patients and necessitates repeat treatment if it occurs within 2 hours of ingestion. The failure rate is approximately 1%, being more effective when taken as close as possible to the episode of unprotected intercourse. Counselling is essential so that the patient understands the implications of the failure rate.

Another method of emergency contraception is to insert an IUCD within 5 days of unprotected intercourse (see above for more details). It can be removed after the patient's next period or left in situ to provide ongoing contraception. The patient ensures she is followed up, both to check that she has a period and also to decide on future long-term contraception.

A relatively new method, Ulipristal acetate, is a selective progesterone receptor modulator, which has been licensed for emergency contraception in the UK since October 2009. It inhibits ovulation and causes alteration in the endometrium which may also impair implantation. It is given as a single oral dose (30 mg) as soon as possible within 5 days (120 hours) of the earliest episode of unprotected sexual intercourse.

Postcoital or emergency contraception is not for routine use:

- High-dose oral progestogen contraceptive Levonelle – 1 dose within 72 hours
- Insert an intrauterine contraceptive device within 5 days
- Ulipristal acetate 1 dose within 120 hours.

TERMINATION OF PREGNANCY

Since the Abortion Act of 1967 (amended in 1991 to reduce the upper limit of gestation from 28 weeks to 24 weeks), termination of pregnancy has been legal in England, Scotland and Wales. Two registered medical practitioners must agree on one of five circumstances relevant to the individual patient; this is most commonly clause C, which states that continuing the pregnancy involves greater risk to the woman's physical or mental health than termination.

Surgical methods

Up to 12 weeks of pregnancy, vacuum aspiration is the most commonly used method. Preoperative prostaglandin to ripen the cervix is often used, especially in nulliparous women, followed by cervical dilatation and evacuation of the uterus using a plastic cannula.

After 12 weeks, dilatation and evacuation can be used; the uterine contents must be crushed prior to curettage. It is essential to ascertain the patient's blood group for anti-D administration, if she is Rhesus negative.

Medical methods

In the first trimester, medical termination is offered with up to 63 days of amenorrhoea. Mifepristone, an anti-progesterone is given orally 36–48 hours before vaginal insertion of a prostaglandin E1 analogue pessary; complete abortion occurs in 95% of patients.

In the second trimester, mifepristone is followed again by synthetic prostaglandin pessaries, placed in the posterior fornix every 3–4 hours. At any gestation, incomplete abortion may occur and surgical evacuation must be performed.

Counselling

Alternatives to abortion should be discussed with the woman, including support if she continues the pregnancy or adoption. If she decides to proceed with the termination, the appropriate method must be agreed. This may depend on ultrasound confirmation of the patient's last menstrual period. Future contraception should be arranged. Screening and/or prophylaxis should be offered for chlamydia infection. The offer of psychological counselling may be appropriate.

Complications

These are generally more common with the surgical methods:

- Infection: screen for chlamydia preoperatively and/or give prophylactic antibiotics including cover for anaerobic infection
- Trauma: to cervix or uterus including perforation (cervical incompetence only usually occurs with repeated procedures)
- Haemorrhage: might be secondary to the above or the result of incomplete evacuation
- Retained products of conception and re-doing the procedure.

Further reading

Faculty of Family Planning and Reproductive Health Care. Available online at: www.ffprhc.org.uk.

Guillebaud, J., 2007. Contraception Today, fifth ed. Informa Healthcare, London.

Guillebaud, J., 2012. Contraception: Your Questions Answered, sixth ed. Churchill Livingstone, Edinburgh.

NICE, 2005. Long-Acting Reversible Contraception. National Institute for Health and Care Excellence, London.

RCOG, 2010. Venous Thromboembolism and Hormonal Contraception. Green-top Guideline No. 40. Royal College of Obstetricians and Gynaecologists, London.

Early pregnancy complications 20

Objectives

By the end of this chapter, you should be able to:

- Understand the important points in the history for a patient presenting with bleeding and/or pain in early pregnancy
- Perform an examination on a patient presenting with bleeding and/or pain in early pregnancy
- Undertake appropriate investigations on a patient presenting with bleeding and/or pain in early pregnancy in order to establish a diagnosis
- You will understand the definition of recurrent miscarriage and how to investigate this condition
- You will understand the biochemical management of a suspected ectopic pregnancy and how to treat if confirmed
- The genetic differences between a partial and complete molar pregnancy will be discussed.

BLEEDING AND/OR PAIN IN EARLY PREGNANCY

Early pregnancy is defined as being the first trimester of pregnancy, up to and including the twelfth week of pregnancy. The history, examination and investigations are predominantly aimed at distinguishing an ectopic pregnancy from a miscarriage. However, other aetiology such as a torted ovarian cyst or appendicitis must also be considered. Women with bleeding or pain in early pregnancy will be anxious so sensitive explanations are important, especially when the diagnosis is uncertain and further investigations are necessary. Note that the definitions in Figure 20.1 refer to miscarriage. The term 'miscarriage' is used in preference to 'abortion', which many women will equate with a termination.

HISTORY

Last menstrual period

The first day of the last menstrual period (LMP) will allow you to calculate the gestation. This becomes important when interpreting early pregnancy scans. While an empty uterus on a scan at 7 weeks might indicate an ectopic pregnancy, a small gestation sac with no fetal pole is common at 5 weeks. However, it is important to establish whether the woman is sure of her dates and whether her cycle is regular; if not, the estimated gestation may be wrong. If she conceived while taking the pill then the last period cannot be relied upon to predict the gestation as it was a hormonally induced withdrawal bleed.

Last cervical smear

Bleeding could be the result of a local cause which could be benign such as cervical ectropian or sinister, such as cervical carcinoma. Ensure that the woman was up to date with her smear tests and they were normal prior to pregnancy.

Presenting complaint

Bleeding

Some women might not realize that there is a problem with their pregnancy until they have a scan (see Fig. 20.1). Miscarriage does not always start with heavy bleeding, and the loss seen with ectopic pregnancy is variable, so the amount of bleeding cannot be used to predict the problem unless the woman has seen products of conception mixed with the bleeding, in which case she is having an inevitable miscarriage. Products may be described as 'pieces of tissue'. Heavy blood flow will form clots that can be described as being 'like liver'– it is worth asking the woman the size of the clots in relation to coins ('Were they 5p-sized or 50p-sized?'). You can often quantify the blood flow by asking how many pads she has needed to change in a day.

The woman might connect the onset of bleeding to an event such as intercourse or exercise. It is possible for the cervix, which is more friable in pregnancy, to bleed postcoitally but actual miscarriage is not provoked by intercourse. It is important to emphasize this point as many women will blame themselves for the miscarriage.

Fig. 20.1 Types of miscarriage.

Type of miscarriage	Description
Threatened	Bleeding occurring before 24 weeks, where the cervix is closed on examination
Inevitable	Bleeding occurring before 24 weeks, where the cervix is open on examination
Missed/delayed/silent	Scan shows a non-viable fetus or an empty intrauterine gestation sac. The cervix is closed on examination. Patient might not have had any bleeding
Complete	Scan shows that there are no products of conception left in the uterus in a case where the patient has had bleeding. The cervix will be closed on examination
Incomplete	Scan shows that there are products of conception left inside the uterus in a case where the patient has bleeding. The cervix will be open on examination

Pain

Miscarriage typically causes cramping, central, lower abdominal pain. The patient might describe it as 'like period pains' or 'like contractions'. It might have started suddenly or could have been preceded by days or weeks of spotting.

The pain of a tubal ectopic pregnancy may be worse on one side than the other, and centred around the iliac fossa. There might have been dyspareunia on that side over the previous few days and, as a result of blood irritating the bowel, the woman might have had some diarrhoea. If an ectopic pregnancy ruptures it causes pain all over the abdomen and referred shoulder-tip pain because of blood irritating the inferior surface of the diaphragm.

Fig. 20.2 Conditions predisposing to ectopic pregnancy.

Factor	Reason
Pelvic inflammatory disease	Tubal damage and pelvic scarring
Tubal surgery, e.g. previous ectopic or sterilization	Tubal damage
Peritonitis or pelvic surgery in past, e.g. appendicitis	Pelvic scarring
Endometriosis	Tubal damage and pelvic scarring
IUCD in situ IVF pregnancy	Abnormal implantation Abnormal implantation

Past obstetric history

A history of miscarriage or ectopic pregnancy increases the risk of these problems happening again.

Past medical history

This should focus on any conditions that predispose to ectopic pregnancy (see Fig. 20.2). Also, remember that a woman who has a non-viable or an ectopic pregnancy might need an operation, so attention should be paid to conditions that may affect fitness for anaesthetic.

EXAMINATION

Observations

The woman might be experiencing significant pain if the uterus is expelling clots or products, or if an ectopic pregnancy has ruptured. Her pulse and blood pressure should be measured.

Miscarriage is unlikely to cause shock due to hypovolaemia but, rarely, cervical shock is seen, in which there is a vagal response to the dilatation caused by products of conception distending the cervical canal. In this case pulse and blood pressure would both be low.

Haemorrhage from a ruptured ectopic pregnancy can be massive; the pulse will be weak and tachycardic and blood pressure will be low. The patient will look pale, sweaty and unwell and might collapse.

Abdominal examination

With miscarriage, the abdomen will be soft. If more than 12 weeks, or if the uterus is fibroid, it might be palpable above the symphysis pubis. With ectopic pregnancy the uterus will not be palpable abdominally.

Before it ruptures there will be tenderness on the affected side, and there might be some guarding and rebound. Once ruptured, the entire abdomen will be tense and tender with guarding and rebound.

Remember to consider an ectopic pregnancy in any woman of reproductive age who presents to casualty with shock and collapse. A pregnancy test must be done on all such women.

Cusco's speculum examination

The cervix should be visualized and swabs taken from the endocervix and vagina. An ectropion or, rarely, a cervical carcinoma, might be visible. It might be possible to see if the os is open or closed but this is best determined by palpation.

An ectropion is not pathological – it is simply an extension of endocervical columnar epithelium, which bleeds easily, onto the ectocervix and is common in pregnancy due to the influence of oestrogen. Bleeding from an ectropion is usually light but can be heavier if provoked by intercourse or in the presence of infection, so cervical swabs should be taken. No treatment is necessary unless infection is proven.

Vaginal examination

When performing a vaginal examination, check whether the os is open or closed. In early pregnancy, if the woman has had a labour in the past, the external os may be open ('multip's os'), but the internal os should be closed, so this question refers to the internal os. If it is open there will be no resistance, and the cervix will admit a finger. An open os indicates an inevitable miscarriage; a closed os might be seen with miscarriage (see Fig. 20.3) or with ectopic pregnancy. The uterine size in weeks should be estimated. The adnexa should be examined – an ectopic pregnancy may cause fullness and tenderness on the affected side. Cervical excitation is present with an ectopic pregnancy.

Cervical excitation pain is sudden severe pain that occurs when the cervix is moved at the time of vaginal examination. This is different from the discomfort that many women feel at the time of examination.

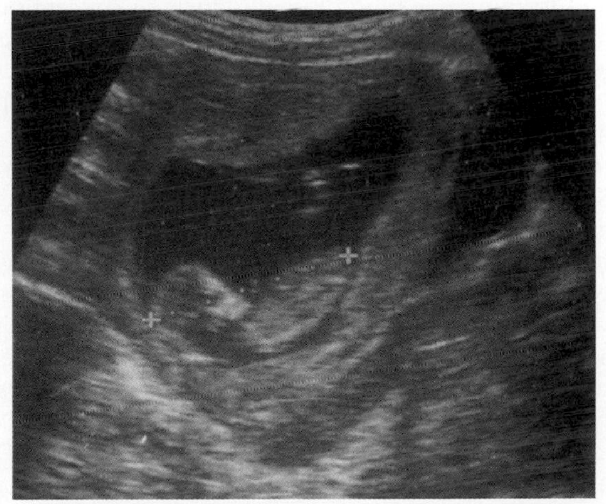

Fig. 20.3 Transvaginal scan showing intrauterine pregnancy, 7-week-sized fetus.

INVESTIGATION

Blood tests

- Full blood count: the woman is unlikely to be anaemic due to the bleeding of a threatened miscarriage but there might be pre-existing anaemia, which will be important from an anaesthetic point of view. An ectopic, if ruptured, may result in severe anaemia. Electrophoresis, if appropriate, must also be requested.
- Blood group: women who are Rhesus negative will require anti-D after an operation for ectopic pregnancy, after an evacuation of the retained products of conception (ERPC) at any gestation or after an episode of bleeding after 12 weeks.
- The serum β-hCG level can be helpful in diagnosing an asymptomatic ectopic pregnancy. An intrauterine pregnancy should be seen on a transvaginal scan with levels of above 1500.

Ultrasound scan

Transvaginal scans give the best view in early pregnancy (Fig. 20.4). The uterus is examined, looking for a gestation sac and fetal pole, and then for a fetal heartbeat. If the uterus is empty, raising the possibility of ectopic pregnancy, the adnexa are scanned, looking for a mass. Sometimes a live ectopic is seen, where the ectopic gestation sac contains a fetus with a heartbeat. Free fluid, due to bleeding from the ectopic pregnancy, might be seen in the pouch of Douglas. With a miscarriage, retained products of conception may be seen.

Once a fetal heartbeat is seen on ultrasound scan there is a 90% chance of the pregnancy continuing and the woman can be reassured. Fetal heart activity can be seen from around 6 weeks' gestation.

MISCARRIAGE

Miscarriage is the most common complication of pregnancy and will be experienced by 1 in 4 women at some point in their lives. It is defined as the spontaneous loss of a pregnancy before 24 weeks.

Fig. 20.4 Common questions asked by women who have suffered a miscarriage.

Why has this happened?
She should be reassured that she has done nothing wrong and is not to blame, but told that in most cases we do not find the cause for early miscarriage. Flying, working, having smear tests, using mobile phones and VDUs and making love when pregnant do not cause miscarriage.

Will it happen again?
Many women who have had a miscarriage will go on to have a healthy term pregnancy. Realising how common early miscarriage is may reassure her.

When can I start trying to get pregnant again?
Physically there is no reason why she cannot conceive with her next cycle, and this has no adverse effects on a resulting pregnancy, but mentally it may be better to have a few months to recover from the miscarriage. Couples can be advised to use condoms if they wish to wait for this time, as condoms are an instantly reversible form of contraception.

When will my next period come?
The next period may be early or late, but should be expected in roughly one month (or sooner or later depending on her usual cycle length). If she does not use contraception after the miscarriage and the next period is late she should seek a pregnancy test.

Aetiology

It is often difficult to identify the cause of a miscarriage but factors that have contributed can be noted. These include:

- fetal abnormality: 50% of miscarried fetuses are genetically (e.g. trisomy, monosomy) or structurally (e.g. neural tube defect) abnormal. Multiple pregnancies are more likely to be affected in these ways
- infection: *Toxoplasma* species, the rubella virus, tuberculosis, *Listeria* species, malaria, *Salmonella* species and cytomegalovirus are just a few of the potential causes. Bacterial vaginosis, where there is a change in the natural flora of the vagina, has been linked to second trimester miscarriage
- maternal age: the miscarriage rate begins to increase when the mother reaches the age of 35. The risks of miscarriage in relation to mother's age are:
  - under 35: 6.5%
  - 5–40: 15%
  - over 40: 23%.
- abnormal uterine cavity: the presence of an intrauterine contraceptive device (IUCD or 'coil'), submucous fibroids, a congenital septum or adhesions (Ashermann's syndrome)
- maternal illness, including Wilson's disease, poorly controlled diabetes, thyroid or renal disease
- intervention: e.g. amniocentesis, chorionic villus sampling.

Antiphospholipid antibodies and cervical weakness ('incompetence') can result in second trimester loss (see the section 'Recurrent miscarriage', below). Investigation of the cause of miscarriage is usually delayed until the woman has had three consecutive miscarriages. This affects 1% of couples (see the section 'Recurrent miscarriage', below).

Management of miscarriage

Once the fetus has died, the uterus will expel the products of conception. This process can take some weeks if left to happen spontaneously. Because of the fear of infection of retained products women have traditionally been advised to have a surgical evacuation to empty the uterus (a procedure that many women still think of as a 'D&C'). Studies comparing the operative route with expectant management have now confirmed no difference in infection rates. Evacuation of retained products of conception (ERPC) is a minor operation that can be performed as a day case; the cervix is dilated to allow suction or sharp curettage. The pregnant uterus is easily perforated, so curettage must be gentle. Syntocinon can be given intravenously during the procedure to encourage uterine contraction and to minimize blood loss. Products of conception are sent for histology after maternal consent is obtained.

If the patient is offered the choice of expectant management she should be booked for follow-up appointment and scan to confirm that the uterus is empty. She should be counselled with regards to the bleeding and pain she will experience. They, and women who have had an ERPC, should be warned of the possibility of endometritis and told of the symptoms and signs to watch out for. These are: fever, feeling unwell, lower abdominal pain and a change in vaginal bleeding, which can become offensive smelling and suddenly heavy.

If the woman is Rhesus negative she needs anti-D after an ERPC or miscarriage after 12 weeks.

Unless investigation for recurrent miscarriage is needed, no follow-up in hospital is necessary. Before going home the woman should be given a contact

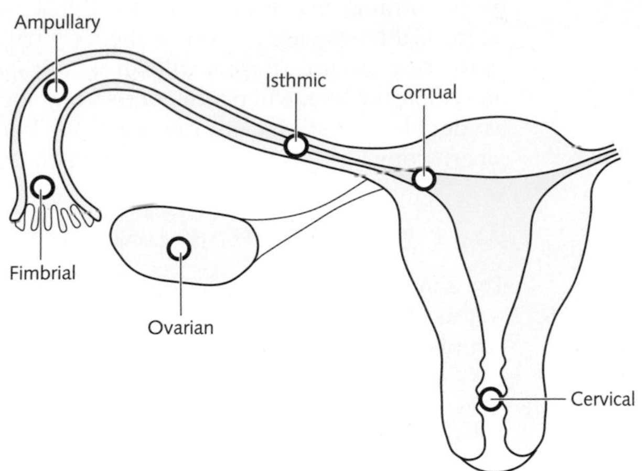

Fig. 20.5 Implantation sites of ectopic pregnancy.

number for a local support group that can help her answer the questions that will arise after the miscarriage (Fig. 20.5). If she is not going to try to get pregnant again in the near future, methods of contraception should be discussed.

RECURRENT MISCARRIAGE

A woman who has had three or more consecutive first trimester miscarriages should have the same history taken and undergo the same examination as above.

Extra investigations should also be considered:

- Karyotyping of both partners and of products of conception where appropriate
- An ultrasound scan (USS) to assess the uterine cavity and the ovaries. This has been shown to be as useful and more acceptable to patients as hysterosalpingography. It is also, unlike the hysterosalpingogram (HSG), without the risk of infection
- A high vaginal swab (HVS) to screen for bacterial vaginosis
- Antiphospholipid antibodies assay on two occasions at least 6 weeks apart. The test is performed twice to avoid the false negatives that occur due to fluctuations in antibody levels, and the false positives caused by a temporary rise in levels at times of viral illness. If the two results are different, the test is repeated. The diagnosis is made after two positive results
- Cervical weakness is best diagnosed by careful history taking, where there will be a story of painless cervical dilatation or spontaneous rupture of membranes in the second trimester. Transvaginal scan of the cervical canal can aid diagnosis, showing an open internal os and short canal.

ECTOPIC PREGNANCY

This is a pregnancy that has implanted outside the uterine cavity (see Fig. 20.6 for likely sites). The incidence of ectopic pregnancy is increasing due to the rising number of cases of pelvic inflammatory disease (PID), asymptomatic chlamydial infection and as the number of IVF pregnancies increase. Currently in the UK the incidence is around 1 per 100 term deliveries; 10–15% of ectopics occur after IVF.

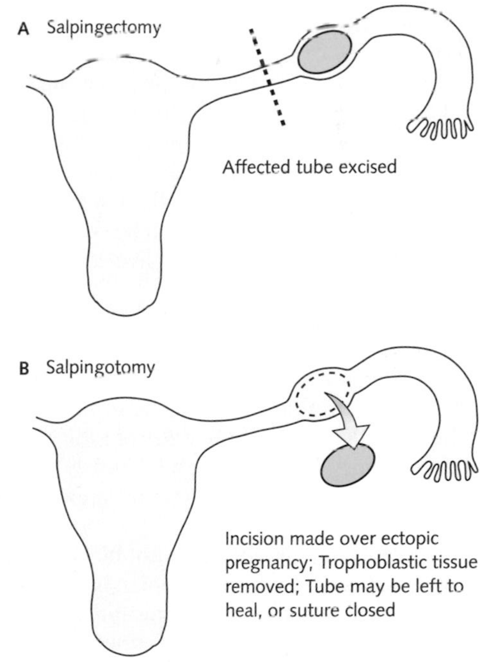

Fig. 20.6 Surgical options for treatment of tubal ectopic pregnancy.

Aetiology of ectopic pregnancy

Ectopic pregnancy is caused by conditions that damage the uterine tubes or their ciliary lining, thus hindering the passage of the fertilized egg towards the uterine cavity, and anything that distorts the cavity itself or predisposes to abnormal implantation. These include:

- PID
- tubal surgery, e.g. sterilization, reversal of sterilization, previous ectopic pregnancy
- peritonitis or pelvic surgery in the past (e.g. appendicitis)
- IUCD ('coil') in situ
- IVF
- endometriosis
- progesterone-only ('mini') pill – this does not cause ectopic pregnancy but if a woman conceives when using it the pregnancy is more likely to be ectopic than if she is using no contraception at all. The progesterone reduces tubal motility.

Clinical evaluation of ectopic pregnancy

In a few cases the patient will require immediate resuscitation and, as soon as possible, laparotomy. Those who have an acute abdomen, but who are haemodynamically stable can have a laparoscopy to confirm the diagnosis. Treatment can then be performed laparoscopically or at laparotomy, depending on the surgeon's skill and the patient's haemodynamic status.

If, as in most cases, the presentation is subacute – it is not necessary to head straight for the operating theatre. An ultrasound scan can be arranged; this may not identify the ectopic pregnancy, but will demonstrate the fact that the uterus is empty. If there has been bleeding from the ectopic, the scan will show free fluid in the pelvis. In some cases a mass in the adnexae can be visualized and, uncommonly, this might contain a live ectopic, with a fetal heartbeat present.

The appearance of an empty uterus on scan in the presence of a positive pregnancy test should always raise the strong suspicion of ectopic pregnancy, which can be confirmed at laparoscopy. However, in some cases there might be uncertainty about the dates of LMP, meaning that the pregnancy could still be a very early gestation, which might account for the 'empty' appearance of the uterus.

In other cases the history might not be clear cut and there could be suspicion that the woman has had a complete miscarriage, which also gives the appearance of an empty uterus on scan, and, as β-hCG does not return to a non-pregnant level immediately, can cause confusion. In these cases, if the patient is stable and there is doubt about the diagnosis it is reasonable to delay laparoscopy by performing two blood tests for β-hCG 48 hours apart. If the pregnancy is viable the level will double. In the case of miscarriage it will fall significantly. With an ectopic the level will plateau or rise, but not as much as double – the patient can then be booked for laparoscopy.

Treatment of tubal pregnancy

The aim is to eliminate the ectopic pregnancy in such a way as to minimize the risk of future pregnancies being ectopic. Various methods are used.

Surgical management

These techniques can all be performed at laparotomy, through a low transverse incision, or at laparoscopy. The skill of the operator will dictate the choice (Fig. 20.7).

Salpingectomy, complete or partial

Here, the affected fallopian tube, or part of it, is removed. This might be the only option if the ectopic has ruptured because the tubal anatomy will have been destroyed. In the event that an ectopic has occurred following IVF where the tubes are scarred, the patient and surgeon might decide that it would be wise to remove both tubes at operation so that future IVF attempts do not lead to further tubal pregnancies.

Salpingotomy

An incision is made in the fallopian tube over the ectopic, which is removed, and the tube is usually allowed to heal by secondary intention.

Medical treatment

The use of the cytotoxic drug methotrexate to treat ectopic pregnancy is increasing. It can be given as intramuscular injections or by injection directly into the ectopic pregnancy either at laparoscopy or transvaginally under ultrasound control.

Asymptomatic patients are carefully selected for medical management – it is only suitable if the pregnancy is small and the tube is intact. The sac is measured on ultrasound scan as less than 3 cm in size with no cardiac activity, and the β-hCG level should be less than 3000 iu/L.

Follow-up of ectopic pregnancy

Patients treated with methotrexate or by conservative surgery (i.e. salpingotomy) must have serial serum β-hCG levels performed to ensure the resolution

- Complete mole: a pregnancy within the uterus consisting of a multivesicular mass of trophoblastic tissue with hydropic change (looking like a bunch of grapes on ultrasound), and no evidence of a fetus, formed by mono or dispermic fertilization of an oocyte which has deleted all maternal genetic material, i.e. all genes are paternal (see below)

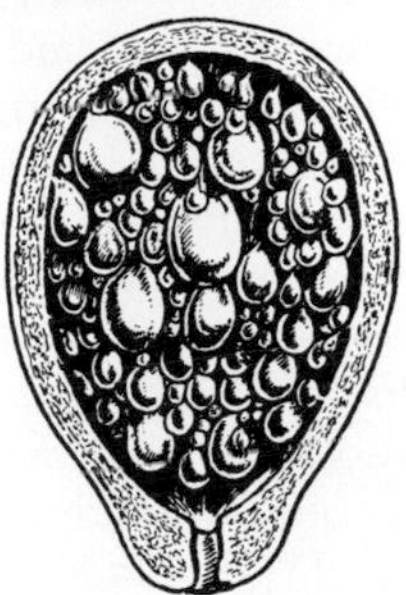

- Partial mole: a pregnancy within the uterus consisting of some trophoblastic proliferation and some hydropic change, where a fetus (usually non-viable) may also be seen. Formed by dispermic fertilization of an oocyte resulting in triploidy i.e. maternal and paternal genes
- Choriocarcinoma: a tumour of trophoblastic cells which secrete hCG occurring when molar pregnancies do not regress after surgical evacuation or, more rarely, after a non-molar pregnancy

Fig. 20.7 Trophoblastic disease comprises of a group of conditions which includes molar pregnancy (complete and partial) and the malignant choriocarcinoma. From McKay Hart & Norman 2000, with permission.

or removal of all trophoblastic tissue. Around 5% of patients treated medically will require further treatment with either methotrexate or a surgical procedure.

Prognosis after ectopic pregnancy

The chance of a repeat ectopic pregnancy is dependent on the health of the remaining tubal tissue. If management was conservative the affected tube will have been scarred by the ectopic pregnancy. Rates of ectopic implantation in future pregnancies are around 11% after medical treatment, 12% after 'conservative' surgery and 9% after salpingectomy. The chance of conception after salpingectomy is obviously lower, so the risks must be weighed up when deciding on management.

Other sites of ectopic pregnancy

These have high rates of maternal mortality and morbidity. Cervical, interstitial and intramural pregnancies are best treated with methotrexate. The haemorrhage that can ensue from rupture or from attempted surgical treatment can be severe, necessitating hysterectomy and sometimes proving fatal. Cornual pregnancy is treated surgically, to remove the rudimentary horn in which the pregnancy has implanted and the tube on the affected side. Ovarian pregnancy can be treated surgically, performing wedge resection of the ovary, or medically. Abdominal pregnancy, if the fetus survives, should be delivered as soon as the fetus is viable.

Heterotopic pregnancy

The extremely rare combination of intra- and extrauterine pregnancy is becoming more common with the increase in IVF pregnancies where at least two embryos are replaced. Treatment is usually surgical, with the procedure being performed laparoscopically, but avoiding instrumentation of the uterus. There is an increased risk of miscarriage for the intrauterine pregnancy, being around 25%.

TROPHOBLASTIC DISEASE

This term covers partial and complete molar pregnancies and the choriocarcinoma that can follow them.

Definitions

See Figure 20.8.

Incidence of molar pregnancy

In the UK, complete mole occurs around 1 per 1000 normal pregnancies. Partial mole is more common, but the exact incidence is harder to calculate as many go unreported. Three per cent of molar pregnancies do not regress spontaneously and therefore require chemotherapy – this is more common with complete moles than partial moles.

Some ethnic groups are more prone to molar pregnancy – it is more common in the Far East – but the

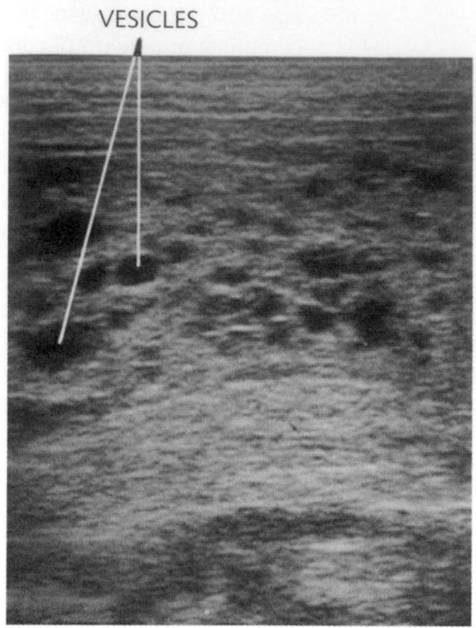

Fig. 20.8 Molar pregnancy. From Chudleigh 2004, with permission.

incidence there is decreasing prompting the suspicion that there is a nutritional element.

Women at the extremes of reproductive age are more likely to experience trophoblastic disease.

Diagnosis and clinical evaluation of molar pregnancy

There is likely to be bleeding early in the pregnancy investigated by ultrasound scan which reveals molar pregnancy with a characteristic 'bunches of grapes' appearance (Fig. 20.9). Alternatively, it could be diagnosed first by the histopathologist after the study of retained products of conception. The trophoblastic tissue secretes hCG, so serum levels are very high and might lead to exaggerated symptoms of pregnancy (e.g. severe hyperemesis, vaginal bleeding). The uterus may also appear large for dates on palpation.

Management of molar pregnancy

Molar pregnancies are treated with surgical evacuation in the same way as miscarriage. The products of conception are sent for histology. The patient must then be followed up with fortnightly serum samples for β-hCG to ensure that levels are falling, as this will confirm that the trophoblastic tissue is regressing. This follow-up is coordinated by the nearest specialist centre (Sheffield, Dundee or Charing Cross). Once the levels are normal, urine samples are tested every month for β-hCG in case of reactivation of trophoblast tissue.

If hCG levels return to normal within 8 weeks, follow-up is limited to 6 months. All other cases are followed for 2 years. Women are advised not to use hormonal contraceptives and not to become pregnant until levels have been normal for 6 months. In future pregnancies serum β-hCG will be measured at 6 and 10 weeks postpartum because of the possibility of choriocarcinoma occurring.

If hCG levels rise, plateau or are still abnormal 6 months after surgical evacuation, chemotherapy is started. Most are given methotrexate and folinic acid, although some with adverse prognostic factors might need different combinations of other chemotherapies.

The current survival rate of patients requiring chemotherapy is 94%. Metastases from choriocarcinoma are seen in the lung, liver and brain.

Reference

Chudleigh, P., 2004. Obstetric Ultrasound, third ed. Churchill Livingstone, London.

McKay Hart, M.D., Norman, J., Callander, R., 2000. Gynaecology Illustrated, fifth ed. Churchill Livingstone, London.

Further reading

Gonick, L., Wheelis, M., 2005. The Cartoon Guide to Genetics. Harper Collins, New York.

Hanretty, K.P., 2010. Obstetrics Illustrated, seventh ed. Churchill Livingstone, London.

McKay Hart, D., Norman, J., 2000. Gynaecology Illustrated, fifth ed. Churchill Livingstone, London.

Nelson-Piercy, C., 2010. Handbook of Obstetric Medicine, fourth ed. Informa Healthcare, New York.

Reid, R., Roberts, F., MacDuff, E., 2011. Pathology Illustrated, seventh ed. Churchill Livingstone, Elsevier.

Smith, N.C., Smith, A.P.M., 2006. Obstetric Ultrasound Made Easy, 2nd ed. Churchill Livingstone, London.

RCOG, 2004. Why Mothers Die, Report on Confidential Enquiries into Maternal Deaths in the United Kingdom, 2000–2002. Royal College of Obstetricians and Gynaecologists, London.

Health Education Development. Available online at: www.swot.org.uk.

RCOG. Available online at: www.rcog.org.uk/guidelines.

Hydatidiform Mole and Choriocarcinoma UK Information and Support Sevice. Available online at: www.hmole-chorio.org.uk.

Update Software Ltd. Available online at: www.update-software.com/cochrane.

Antepartum haemorrhage

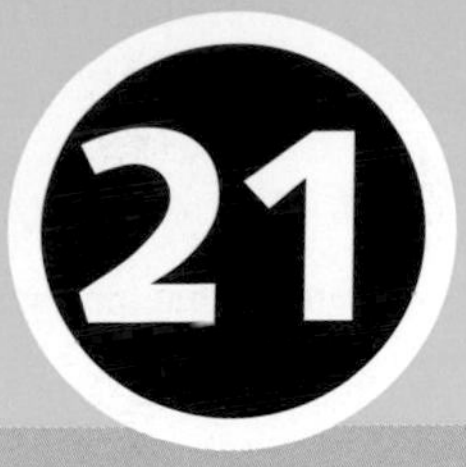

Objectives

By the end of this chapter, you should be able to:

- List the common causes of antepartum haemorrhage
- Distinguish between placenta praevia and placental abruption
- Describe the investigations appropriate for the patient who presents with an antepartum haemorrhage
- Understand the place for conservative management in antepartum haemorrhage
- List the main complications of placenta praevia.

DEFINITION

Antepartum haemorrhage (APH) is defined as any bleeding from the genital tract that occurs after 24 + 0 weeks gestation and before the birth of the infant.

HINTS AND TIPS

Antepartum haemorrhage (APH) is an important cause of increased maternal and perinatal morbidity and mortality. Up to 20% of very preterm infants are born in association with APH.

INCIDENCE

The incidence of APH is 3–5%.

AETIOLOGY

A summary is shown in Figure 21.1. Placenta praevia combined with placental abruption account for about 50% of the causes of an APH. In both cases, the bleeding comes from maternal vessels that are exposed as the placenta separates from the decidua, i.e. it is not fetal blood. Fetal hypoxia can occur as a secondary process.

HINTS AND TIPS

With any bleeding in pregnancy, don't forget ABC – assess the patient including the estimated blood loss and resuscitate.

HISTORY

When taking a history, it is important to elicit certain points including:

- amount of bleeding
- association with abdominal pain and/or contractions
- association with mucoid discharge.

The presence or absence of constant abdominal pain is particularly important to differentiate between placenta praevia and a placental abruption. With the latter, there may also be uterine contractions as the myometrium is infiltrated with blood that makes the uterus irritable.

There may be an obvious trigger event, for example, recent sexual intercourse can cause bleeding from a cervical ectropion. The date of the patient's last smear test is relevant to exclude a cervical cause for the bleeding. The patient should be asked about fetal movements.

HINTS AND TIPS

The presence of abdominal pain typically distinguishes placental abruption from placenta praevia.

EXAMINATION

The aim is to assess maternal and fetal well-being. This includes the following:

Maternal well-being:

- Pulse/blood pressure/respiratory rate
- Pallor
- Abdominal palpation for uterine tenderness/contractions

Fig. 21.1 Aetiology of antepartum haemorrhage.

Source of haemorrhage	Type of haemorrhage
Uterine source	Placenta praevia Placental abruption Vasa praevia Circumvallate placenta
Lower genital tract source	Cervical ectropion Cervical polyp Cervical carcinoma Cervicitis Vaginitis Vulval varicosities
Unknown origin (approx. 50%)	
Note bloody mucoid vaginal loss may be the "show" or cervical mucus plug associated with the onset of labour	

- Speculum examination for cervical abnormalities
- Digitial examination in the presence of contractions to assess cervical change, only if placenta praevia has been excluded.

Fetal well-being:

- Abdominal palpation for lie/presentation/engagement
- Auscultation of fetal heart to determine viability.

INVESTIGATIONS

Figure 21.2 lists the investigations appropriate for the patient with an APH.

Blood tests

Blood should be cross-matched if the bleeding is significant and ongoing, e.g. major placenta praevia. Blood group must be checked – anti-D immunoglobulin should be given if the patient is rhesus negative, in order to prevent haemolytic disease of the newborn in a future pregnancy. A Kleihauer test examines the maternal blood film for the presence of fetal blood cells, suggesting feto-maternal haemorrhage. This can be seen with placental abruption.

Fig. 21.2 Investigations for a patient with an antepartum haemorrhage.

- Haemoglobin
- Group and save/cross-match
- Rhesus status
- Coagulation profile
- Kleihauer test
- Renal function tests
- Liver function tests
- Cardiotocograph
- Ultrasound scan

Fetal monitoring

A cardiotocograph (CTG) should be done to confirm fetal well-being after 26 + 0 weeks gestation. It may also show uterine irritability or established contractions.

Ultrasound scan

The placental site is checked at the routine 20 week anomaly scan. If it is found to be low-lying at this stage, then repeat scan should be arranged for approx 36 weeks to make the diagnosis of placenta praevia. In the majority of patients, as the lower segment begins to form and the upper segment enlarges upwards, so the placenta appears to move up away from the cervical os. A transvaginal scan is safe and may improve accuracy over the transabdominal mode, particularly with a posterior placenta.

An abruption is usually diagnosed on clinical grounds. A small retroplacental clot may not be seen on ultrasound scan, but this does not exclude the diagnosis. A large retroplacental clot that can be seen on scan is likely to be obvious clinically.

PLACENTA PRAEVIA

Definition

The placenta is wholly or partially attached to the lower uterine segment. The degree of attachment has traditionally been divided into four grades (Fig. 21.3), but should now be classified as either minor – which encompasses grades I and II – or major – covering grades III and IV.

Incidence

Placenta praevia occurs in 0.4–0.8% of pregnancies; this figure has altered with routine use of ultrasound scanning. The incidence is increased with the following risk factors:

- Previous caesarean section including previous placenta praevia
- Advanced maternal age
- Multiparity
- Multiple pregnancy
- Presence of a succenturiate placental lobe
- Smoking.

Fig. 21.3 Grading of placenta praevia determined by ultrasound scan.

Grade	Description	Degree of placenta praevia
I	Encroaches the lower segment	Minor
II	Reaches the internal os	Minor
III	Overlies the internal os in part	Major
IV	Centrally placed in the lower segment	Major

It is associated with a maternal mortality rate of about 0.03% in the developed world. However, both maternal and fetal morbidity are substantially higher in developing countries due to complications such as haemorrhage and prematurity.

Particularly with increasing numbers of caesarean sections, there is an increased incidence of placenta accreta. This is a condition found in up to 15% of those with placenta praevia, in which the placenta is morbidly adherent to the uterine decidua and may even penetrate through the myometrium to invade surrounding organs. MRI scan is thought to be helpful to aid diagnosis of this complication.

History

Painless vaginal bleeding

Bleeding from a placenta praevia is usually unprovoked and occurs in the third trimester, in the absence of labour.

Examination

General observations including maternal pulse and blood pressure must be performed. On abdominal palpation, the uterus is soft and non-tender. The low-lying placenta may displace the presenting part from the pelvis so that a cephalic presentation is not engaged, or there is a malpresentation.

With a minor degree of bleeding, a speculum can be passed to exclude a lower genital tract cause for the APH. A digital examination should be avoided because it may provoke massive bleeding.

Diagnosis

As described above, the placental site is localized as part of the routine 20-week ultrasound scan. If a low-lying placenta is noted then a follow-up scan in the third trimester is usually performed to make the diagnosis of placenta praevia.

Investigations

These are outlined in Figure 21.2. Blood should be sent for haemoglobin, and group and save. Anti D is indicated if the patient is rhesus negative. If the bleeding is heavy, cross-matching blood for transfusion is indicated and a baseline clotting screen. Renal function tests are important if the urine output is poor secondary to hypovolaemia. A cardiotocograph should be performed to check fetal well-being. An ultrasound scan should be performed if the placental location is unknown (Fig. 21.2). An MRI scan may be indicated if there is a high index of suspicion about placenta accreta, as outlined above.

Management

Management depends first on assessing the severity of the bleeding and resuscitation of the patient. Immediate delivery by caesarean section may be appropriate if there is either maternal or fetal compromise.

Expectant management depends on the severity of bleeding, the gestation of the pregnancy and the placental site. If the placenta remains at or over the cervical os, massive bleeding is likely to occur if the patient goes into labour and the cervix starts to dilate. Therefore, in-patient management is appropriate in the third trimester with immediate recourse to caesarean section if necessary. Steroids to improve fetal lung maturity should be considered following liaison with the paediatricians. Caesarean section is usually advised if the placenta is encroaching within 2 cm of the internal cervical os. If the head of the fetus becomes engaged (i.e. it passes below the leading edge of the placenta) then vaginal delivery may be possible.

Complications

Placenta praevia is associated with an increased risk of postpartum haemorrhage (PPH) (see Chapter 33). The lower uterine segment where the placenta is sited is less efficient at retraction following delivery of the placenta compared to the upper segment. Thus occlusion of the venous sinuses is less effective resulting in heavier blood loss. This may be further complicated by the presence of placenta accreta. Therefore, preparations should be in place for potential PPH. This includes cross-matching blood and both consultant obstetrician and anaesthetist input. The patient should be given adequate counselling regarding the possible need for medical and surgical measures to control bleeding including hysterectomy.

Future pregnancy

Placenta praevia has a recurrence rate of 4–8% with an increased risk of placenta accreta in each pregnancy.

PLACENTAL ABRUPTION

Definition

The placental attachment to the uterus is disrupted by haemorrhage as blood dissects under the placenta, possibly extending into the amniotic sac or the uterine muscle.

Incidence

Placental abruption occurs in about 1% of pregnancies in the UK. In the majority of cases the cause is unknown, but it is associated with:

- previous abruption
- advanced maternal age
- multiparity
- maternal hypertension or pre-eclampsia
- abdominal trauma, e.g. assault, road traffic accident
- cigarette smoking
- cocaine use
- lower socioeconomic group
- external cephalic version.

History

Vaginal bleeding associated with abdominal pain

The patient can present at any stage of pregnancy with a history of bleeding and constant abdominal pain, which is usually unprovoked. There may be associated uterine contractions.

As maternal blood escapes from the placental sinuses, it tracks down between the membranes and the uterus and escapes via the cervix; this is known as a revealed haemorrhage. Sometimes, the blood remains sealed within the uterine cavity such that the degree of shock is out of proportion to the vaginal loss; this is known as a concealed haemorrhage (Fig. 21.4).

Depending on the patient's previous antenatal history, she should be asked about symptoms of pre-eclampsia, including headache, blurred vision, nausea and epigastric pain (see Chapter 22).

Examination

The general maternal condition, including pulse and blood pressure, should be assessed. On abdominal palpation the uterus is typically tender. As bleeding extends into the uterine muscle, a tonic contraction can occur, making the uterus feel hard. Fetal parts are difficult to palpate. If the placental site is known (i.e. if placenta praevia has been excluded) a digital examination is appropriate in the presence of uterine contractions to diagnose the onset of labour.

Maternal hypertension and proteinuria must be excluded due to the association between abruption and pre-eclampsia. If present, liver tenderness, hyperreflexia and clonus should be excluded (see Chapter 22).

Investigations

These are outlined in Figure 21.2. Blood should be sent for haemoglobin, and group and save. Anti D is indicated if the patient is rhesus negative. If the bleeding is heavy or if the patient is shocked, cross-matching units of blood for transfusion is indicated and a baseline clotting screen. A Kleihauer test should be requested to diagnose feto-maternal haemorrhage, which occurs in an abruption.

Renal function tests are necessary if the urine output is poor or in conjunction with liver function tests if pre-eclampsia is suspected. Urinalysis should be done to exclude proteinuria; if present, a protein-creatinine ratio or a 24-hour urine protein level may be helpful to determine the degree of renal involvement (see Chapter 22).

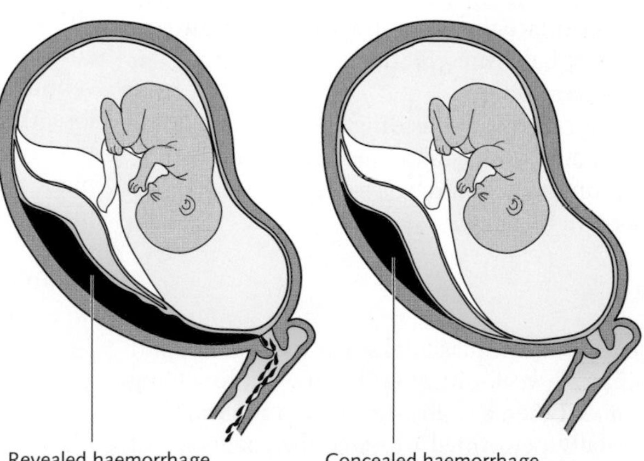

Fig. 21.4 Types of placental abruption.

A cardiotocograph (CTG) should be done to check fetal well-being. A sinusoidal pattern can be seen with feto-maternal haemorrhage. The CTG will also monitor uterine activity, either contractions or a uterus that might simply be irritable with irregular activity.

An ultrasound scan is of limited value since only a large retroplacental haemorrhage will be seen. The diagnosis of abruption is usually made on clinical grounds.

Management

As for placenta praevia, management of a placental abruption must start with assessment of the severity of the symptoms and prompt resuscitation. Immediate delivery of the fetus may be necessary as a life-saving procedure for the mother, regardless of gestation.

In a situation where the patient is clinically well and the fetus is not compromised, expectant management might allow the symptoms to resolve. Again, steroids should be considered to aid fetal lung maturity.

Complications

Accurate assessment of blood loss is necessary to assess the risks of developing disseminated intravascular coagulation and renal failure. Post-partum haemorrhage occurs in 25% of cases, which rarely leads to Sheehan's syndrome (pituitary necrosis secondary to hypovolaemic shock – see Chapter 33).

Future pregnancy

The risk of recurrence is about 8%.

VASA PRAEVIA

This is a rare cause of antepartum haemorrhage, 1 in 2000–6000 pregnancies. There is a velamentous insertion of the cord and the vessels lie on the membranes that cover the internal cervical os, in front of the presenting part. When the membranes rupture, either spontaneously or iatrogenically, the vessels can be torn and vaginal bleeding occurs. Unlike placenta praevia and placental abruption, this blood is fetal blood and the fetus must be delivered urgently before it exsanguinates.

If the diagnosis is unclear, a Kleihauer test can be performed on the vaginal blood loss to test for the presence of fetal red blood cells. However, this may delay delivery inappropriately and should only be considered if the CTG is normal.

CIRCUMVALLATE PLACENTA

This type of placenta develops secondary to outward proliferation of the chorionic villi into the decidua, beneath the ring of attachment of the amnion and chorion. This does not interfere with placental function, but it is associated with antepartum and intrapartum haemorrhage.

UNEXPLAINED ANTEPARTUM HAEMORRHAGE

In up to 50% of cases of APH, no specific cause is found. A history should be taken as described above including date of last smear test. The cervix should be visualized with a speculum examination and referral to colposcopy considered if any abnormality is seen.

However, overall, perinatal mortality with any type of APH is double that of a normal pregnancy, suggesting that placental function might be compromised. Therefore, with recurrent APH, it is appropriate to perform serial ultrasound scans to monitor fetal growth and to consider delivery at term, by inducing labour.

Further reading

Chamberlain, G., Steer, P., 2001. Turnbull's Obstetrics, third ed. Churchill Livingstone, Edinburgh.

Enkin, M.W., Keirse, M.J.N.C., Neilson, J., et al., 2000. A Guide to Effective Care in Pregnancy and Childbirth, third ed. Oxford University Press, Oxford.

RCOG, 2011. Antepartum Haemorrhage. Green-top Guideline 63. Royal College of Obstetricians and Gynaecologists, London. Available online at: www.rcog.org.uk.

RCOG, 2011. Placenta Praevia, Placenta praevia Accrete and Vasa Praevia: Diagnosis and Management. Green-top Guideline 27. Royal College of Obstetricians and Gynaecologists, London. Available online at: www.rcog.org.uk.

Hypertension in pregnancy

Objectives

By the end of this chapter, you should be able to:

- Understand the possible causes of hypertension in pregnancy
- Understand how to investigate, diagnose and treat hypertension in pregnancy
- Understand pre-eclampsia and its impact on pregnancy.

INTRODUCTION

Management of hypertensive disorders in pregnancy forms a large part of antenatal care. Hypertensive disorders fall into three main categories, and accurate diagnosis with prompt treatment is essential to ensure a good outcome for both mother and fetus. The three categories are as follows:

- Pre-existing or chronic hypertension: patients may have a known history of hypertension or, indeed, be found to be hypertensive at booking or < 20 weeks. Early treatment and monitoring is important
- Gestational or pregnancy induced hypertension (PIH), which is hypertension presenting after 20 weeks of the pregnancy with no proteinuria
- Proteinuric hypertension, also known as pre eclampsia (PET) is hypertension presenting after 20 weeks with significant proteinuria.

When assessing pregnant patients, the history and examination are aimed at differentiating between the three groups.

HISTORY TAKING

Presenting complaint

Interestingly, hypertensive patients may be asymptomatic and the hypertension may only be picked up as part of the routine antenatal check. Therefore, the importance of accurate blood pressure measurement cannot be underestimated.

Symptoms of pre-eclampsia are shown in Figure 22.1. However, it is important to ask specifically about:

1. headache
2. visual disturbance (typically in the form of flashing lights)
3. right upper quadrant or epigastric pain (due to oedema of the liver capsule)
4. vomiting
5. swelling of the face, hands or feet.

Past gynaecological history

A history of high blood pressure when taking the oral contraceptive pill indicates a susceptibility to high blood pressure in pregnancy.

Past obstetric history

Hypertensive episodes in previous pregnancies should be enquired about and their exact nature. Pre-eclampsia does not always recur with every pregnancy; it is more common in primigravida or in the first pregnancy with a new partner.

Past medical history

Those with a history of pre-existing hypertension are very unlikely to have normal blood pressure in pregnancy and may even have evidence of end organ damage if it has previously been poorly managed. Conditions that predispose to hypertension include diabetes, renal and cardiac disease.

Family history

Pre-eclampsia is familial, with the strongest association being a sister affected in her pregnancy. The more severe the pre-eclampsia and the earlier it occurs in pregnancy the more likely it is to be familial.

Drug history

Patients with pre-existing hypertension might already be on medication. This might need to be changed to avoid the use of drugs contraindicated in pregnancy.

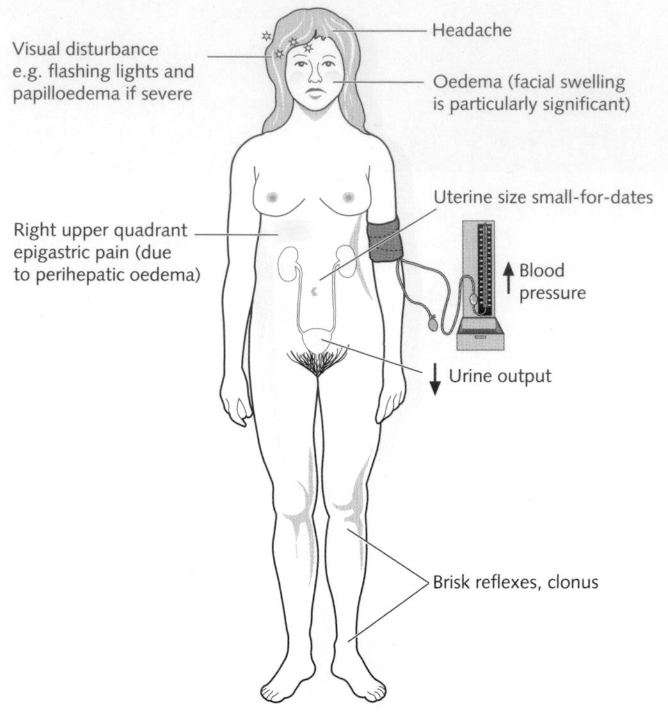

Fig. 22.1 Signs and symptoms of pre-eclampsia.

EXAMINATION

Examination begins with a general inspection. Any facial oedema should be noted and if it is not obvious to the physician, the patient or her partner may be asked to confirm its presence. If it has not been done already, the patient's blood pressure should be taken.

> **HINTS AND TIPS**
>
> Blood pressure should be measured with the patient sitting or lying at 45°. The arm should be at the same level as the heart, and when auscultating, one should observe the point at which the sounds disappear rather than muffle as the cut-off for the diastolic. It is essential that the correct size of cuff is used; if a small cuff is used for an obese woman, the blood pressure will be artificially (and worryingly) high and vice versa for large cuffs in small women.

Abdominal palpation should then be performed to elicit liver tenderness followed by palpation of the uterus to ascertain if the uterine size is appropriate for the gestational age. A small-for-dates fetus may be as a result of pre-eclampsia.

Reflexes should be assessed and the presence of any clonus noted. Brisk reflexes and clonus are seen in pre-eclampsia. Fundoscopy should be performed to look for papilloedema, which can occur in pre-eclampsia, or retinopathy, which may be seen in severe pre-existing hypertension.

INVESTIGATIONS

Investigating hypertension in pregnancy is aimed at establishing which of the three categories the patient falls into. The key points are discussed below.

Urinalysis

> **HINTS AND TIPS**
>
> When seeing a pregnant woman with raised blood pressure, one of your first questions must be 'Is there any proteinuria?' The presence of proteinuria should always raise the suspicion of pre-eclampsia.

As you will be able to see from the definitions above, the presence of proteinuria is very important when differentiating between PIH and PET. Therefore, in all cases, the urine should be tested using a urinary 'dipstix' to provide a rapid bedside assessment.

The presence of protein may be due to PET, but may also be the result of contamination with blood, liquor (if the membranes have ruptured), vaginal discharge or be caused by a urinary tract infection (UTI). A UTI should be suspected if the proteinuria is associated with the presence of nitrites, leucocytes and/or blood. However, PET must still be suspected until a UTI is excluded by sending a midstream sample (MSU) for microbiology testing.

Proteinuria assessed as ≥2+ on urinary dipstix should be quantified by sending samples to the laboratory for:

- protein-creatinine ratio (PCR), or
- 24 hour urine collection.

These will help to distinguish between contaminants giving a false positive and true proteinuria. A PCR >30 or a level of more than 0.3 g of protein in 24 hours should be regarded as significant.

Blood tests

In patients with pre-existing hypertension, baseline investigations (FBC, U&E and LFTs) should be performed at booking as they will be an important reference point later in the pregnancy if the hypertension gets worse or the patient develops pre-eclampsia. During pregnancy, hypertension is investigated using a standard set of blood tests, which are displayed in Figure 22.2 along with the changes that may occur.

Ultrasound

PET may cause intrauterine growth restriction, oligohydramnios and abnormal Dopplers secondary to placental insufficiency. Essential hypertension, if poorly controlled, may also affect fetal growth. Therefore, in these cases an ultrasound scan for fetal growth, liquor volume and Dopplers should be requested.

For patients with pre-existing hypertension, some units offer ultrasound assessment of uterine artery Dopplers at around 22 weeks in an attempt to predict those who may go on to develop pre-eclampsia.

TREATMENT

Pre-existing/essential hypertension

Those with pre-existing hypertension should be ideally seen pre-pregnancy and have their blood pressure optimized. In addition, any potentially teratogenic medications should be changed.

HINTS AND TIPS

In a young person who is being diagnosed with hypertension for the first time it is important to exclude an underlying disease such as coarctation of the aorta, renal artery stenosis, Conn's syndrome, Cushing's syndrome or a phaeochromocytoma.

The aim of treatment in this group is to maintain blood pressure readings below 150/100 mmHg. Those with evidence of end organ damage (renal or retinal) may need even tighter control, below 140/90 mmHg. The risks of uncontrolled hypertension in this group are cerebral haemorrhage and other end organ damage.

Low-dose aspirin (75 mg daily) from 12 weeks' gestation until delivery has been shown to be beneficial in this group for reducing the risk of developing PET.

Pregnancy induced hypertension

PIH presents after 20 weeks of pregnancy in patients with no history of hypertension and in the absence of proteinuria. The risks of uncontrolled blood pressure are those described above and, therefore, monitoring is very important:

- Mild hypertension, i.e. <140/99 mmHg does not always require treatment, blood pressure and urine should be checked weekly.
- Moderate hypertension (between 150/100 mmHg and 159/109 mmHg) should be treated (Fig. 22.3) and monitored twice weekly.
- Severe hypertension >160/110 mmHg requires inpatient treatment and close monitoring.

Both pre-existing hypertensives and those with PIH are at increased risk of developing pre-eclampsia so continued monitoring is very important. Early delivery before 37 weeks of gestation is not usually indicated unless the blood pressure is very difficult to control or there are signs of fetal compromise. In those who require delivery before 37 weeks a course of steroids should be administered to aid fetal lung maturity.

Pre-eclampsia

Pre-eclampsia is defined as new hypertension developing after 20 weeks with significant proteinuria. It is a multi-system disorder which, if left untreated, can be fatal for both mother and fetus. Risk factors for PET are shown in Figure 22.4 and, once identified at booking, consideration should be given to prescribing aspirin 75 mg daily from 12 weeks' gestation until delivery in order to reduce the risk.

Fig. 22.2 Blood tests in the patient with hypertension.

	Chronic HTN	PIH	PET
Full blood count	Normal	Normal	↓ Platelets ↑ Haematocrit
Urea & electrolytes	Normal*	Normal	↑ Creatinine
Liver function tests	Normal	Normal	↑ ALT/AST
Serum urate	Normal	Normal	↑
△Clotting screen	Normal	Normal	Can be deranged
△Lactate dehydrogenase	Measured if concerns regarding haemolysis◇		

**Chronic hypertensives may have an element of pre-existing renal impairment and therefore baseline renal function tests should be sent at booking to compare with later tests in pregnancy*

△done only if indicated by clinical picture or low platelets

◇HELLP syndrome ***H****aemolysis* ***E****levated* ***L****iver enzymes and* ***L****ow* ***P****latelets is a severe variant of PET which is named after its features.*

The aetiology of PET is still not fully understood, but it is felt that failure of the normal trophoblastic invasion of myometrial spiral arteries leads to a high resistance circulation and utero-placental under perfusion. This process then results in the release of antiangiogenic factors into maternal circulation causing vasoconstriction (hence hypertension) and endothelial damage causing proteinuria.

Treatment

The process of PET can only be ended by delivery of the placenta. Therefore, when treating PET in pregnancy there is a fine balance between continuing pregnancy (with an aim to allow more time for fetal maturity) and risk to the mother.

Fig. 22.3 Anti-hypertensives.

Labetalol
α and β-Blocker – regarded as first line treatment. Has direct cardiac effects and also lower peripheral vascular resistance. Should be avoided in asthmatics.
Nifedipine
Calcium channel blocker which causes arterial vasodilatation. Can cause headaches.
Methyldopa
α agonist which prevents vasoconstriction. It has been used for many years with a good safety profile. Should be stopped within two days of delivery and changed to another agent due to the risk of postnatal depression.
Hydralazine
Intravenous drug which causes vasodilatation. Can cause rapid hypotension so is often given after a bolus of colloid.

Again, the severity of hypertension will influence whether or not anti-hypertensives are commenced:

- Mild PET 140/90 – 149/99 mmHg does not always require anti-hypertensives.
- Moderate PET 150/100 – 159/109 mmHg requires treatment (see Fig. 22.3).
- Severe PET >160/110 mmHg requires urgent treatment and if not responsive to first-line treatments may require intravenous anti-hypertensives.

In severe cases where there is a real risk of eclampsia (seizures), intravenous magnesium sulphate (MgSO4) has been shown to be beneficial as prophylaxis. It is usually used if the mean arterial pressure (MAP; Fig. 22.5)

Fig. 22.4 Risk factors for pre-eclampsia.

High risk
- Previous PET
- Chronic kidney disease
- Diabetes (Type I and Type II)
- Systemic Lupus Erythematosus, Antiphospholipid syndrome

Moderate risk
- Primips
- Age >40 yrs
- BMI >35 kg/m^2
- Family Hx of PET
- Twins

Fig. 22.5 Calculation of mean arterial pressure.

Mean Arterial Pressure (MAP) can be estimated by using the following formula:

$$MAP = \frac{(2x \text{ Diastolic BP}) + \text{Systolic BP}}{3}$$

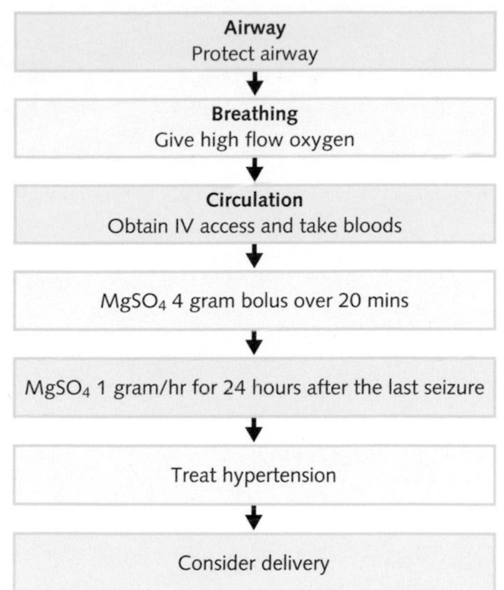

Fig. 22.6 Management of eclampsia.

remains above 125 mmHg despite initial treatment and there are other features:

- Headaches
- Visual disturbance
- Epigastric pain
- Brisk reflexes or clonus (>3 beats)
- Deranged blood tests such as low platelets, high ALT or high creatinine.

Using $MgSO_4$ generally means the clinical picture necessitates delivering the baby once the mother is stable and/or steroids have been given (if required).

Severe PET also requires a fluid restriction to prevent fluid overload and this is accepted as 1 ml/kg/h. Generally, 85 ml/h is used unless the patient is very under- or overweight. Strict input/output measurement is essential.

Eclampsia

Eclampsia is defined as the occurrence of seizures in pregnancy on a background of PET. Eclampsia affects 1 in 2000 pregnancies with around 40% of seizures occurring postnatally (usually within 48 h of delivery). Seizures presenting for the first time in pregnancy should always be assumed to be eclamptic seizures until proven otherwise. The differential diagnosis includes:

- epilepsy
- meningitis
- cerebral thrombosis
- intracerebral bleed
- intracerebral tumour.

Management

The management of eclampsia is detailed in Figure 22.6. As always, the initial management of eclampsia should always follow the ABC approach. Again, stabilization of the mother is paramount and should be ensured before any consideration is given to the fetus.

Further reading

Levine, R.D., Lam, C., Qian, C., et al., 2006. Soluble endoglin and other circulating antiangiogenic factors in preeclampsia. N. Engl. J. Med. 355, 992–1005.

NICE, 2010. Guidelines – Hypertension in Pregnancy. National Institute for Health and Care Excellence, London.

Medical disorders in pregnancy 23

Objectives

By the end of this chapter, you should be able to:

- Understand the common medical problems encountered in pregnancy
- Understand their impact on pregnancy to both the mother and fetus
- Understand how to diagnose, investigate and treat them.

INTRODUCTION

Medical disorders in pregnancy can have a significant effect upon the outcome for both the mother and fetus. Early optimization of certain conditions (ideally pre-pregnancy) can help to minimize the adverse effects and ensure a good outcome for both. The aim of this chapter is to highlight common medical problems that complicate pregnancy and discuss their management.

ANAEMIA

The term anaemia comes from the Greek – *anaimia* meaning lack of blood. Anaemia is a very common problem to encounter in pregnancy. The normal physiological changes in pregnancy result in an increased plasma expansion and since haemoglobin (Hb) levels are expressed as a concentration, it therefore follows that an increase in circulating volume results in a decrease in the concentration of Hb. Despite an increase in gastrointestinal absorption during pregnancy, iron requirements increase almost threefold.

As part of booking investigations all patients should have a full blood count (FBC) performed and repeated at 28 weeks. Treatment should be advised with Hb levels:

- <11 g/dl at booking
- <10.5 g/dl at 28 weeks.

Some individuals may have pre-existing anaemia, which is most commonly due to iron deficiency. Iron deficiency can be caused by lack of dietary iron, heavy periods, gastrointestinal bleeding or, indeed, as a result of a recent pregnancy and it is these individuals that need thorough treatment. It is also important to note whether or not the patient has a haemoglobinopathy, which can be responsible for their anaemia. In these patients, measurement of serum ferritin levels is vital to prevent iron overload.

Folate deficiency can also be responsible for anaemia and, therefore, estimation of serum haematinics may need to be performed to allow correction of the depleted factor.

Iron supplements are known to cause constipation which often leads to patients discontinuing therapy. Vitamin C has been shown to increase its absorption from the gut and patients should be advised to take orange juice or a similar vitamin-C-containing juice. Tannins found in tea and coffee reduce absorption so should be avoided.

During pregnancy patients who complain about fatigue, dizziness or collapsing should be investigated for anaemia in addition to the routine screening that occurs at booking and 28 weeks.

HINTS AND TIPS

Correction of anaemia is essential as it has been linked with low birth weight and pre-term delivery. In addition patients with adequate Hb levels are less likely to need a blood transfusion following delivery.

ASTHMA

Asthma is frequently encountered in antenatal clinics and affects up to 7% of females of a child-bearing age. The course of asthma in pregnancy varies but those with the most severe asthma should be closely monitored.

New diagnoses of asthma in pregnancy, although not common, should be considered in patients complaining of cough, shortness of breath, wheezing or chest tightness. Classically these symptoms will be worse at night or associated with certain triggers like dust, exercise or pollen.

For known asthma sufferers, a detailed enquiry should include:

- current treatments
- peak flow record
- previous hospital admissions (especially those requiring admission to intensive care).

The peak expiratory flow rate (PEFR) trend will form an important part of monitoring in pregnancy and, therefore, its importance should not be underestimated.

Some patients may discontinue their therapy due to fears over the effect they may have on the fetus. They can be reassured and encouraged to continue, to prevent any deterioration in their condition. The cessation of smoking and avoidance of trigger factors should also be emphasized.

DIABETES

Management of diabetes in pregnancy forms a major part of antenatal care, so much so that most units have specialist joint multidisciplinary obstetric diabetic clinics to optimize care. Patients can either have pre-existing diabetes or develop gestational diabetes which, left untreated, can have severe ramifications for both mother and fetus.

Glucose metabolism is altered during pregnancy such that pregnancy itself is a state of impaired glucose tolerance, especially as it advances towards term. A major contribution to this is made by hormones secreted by the placenta:

- Glucagon
- Cortisol
- Human placental lactogen.

These effects are to some extent offset by increased insulin secretion. However, those who have an insufficient response will develop gestational diabetes. For the same reason, patients with pre-existing Type 1 diabetes will require an increase in the amount of insulin they administer. Those with Type 2 diabetes may need conversion to insulin from oral hypoglycaemics as pregnancy progresses.

Pre-existing diabetes

Care of patients with pre-existing diabetes, either Type 1 or Type 2, should ideally start pre-conception, including:

- optimizing glycaemic control by monitoring glucose pre and postprandial
- educating the patient about diabetes in pregnancy and the risks (Fig. 23.1)
- Educating the patient about the risks of hypoglycaemia
- prescribing folic acid at the higher dose of 5 mg daily (pre-conception until 12 weeks)
- screening for nephropathy and retinopathy.

Fig. 23.1 Risks of diabetes in pregnancy.

Miscarriage
Congenital anomalies in particular cardiac
Fetal macrosomia and/or polyhydramnios
Induction of Labour
Caesarean Section
Birth Trauma
Shoulder Dystocia
Stillbirth
Neonatal Hypoglycaemia
Obesity/Diabetes in the baby (later in life).

Patients suffering with nephropathy and/or retinopathy may warrant specialist review prior to pregnancy to identify their risks, including review of hypertension and any medication.

Dietary advice regarding a low sugar, low fat and high fibre intake as well as the benefits of exercise and weight loss if their body mass index is >27 kg/m^2 should be discussed.

Ultrasound scans

Patients with pre-existing diabetes have a higher rate of miscarriage and, therefore, may request an early ultrasound scan. In addition there is an increased risk of congenital anomalies so nuchal translucency and a detailed anomaly scan including detailed assessment of the fetal heart should be arranged. Poor glycaemic control can lead to fetal macrosomia and increased liquor volume (see Chapter 26), therefore diabetic patients are advised to have serial growth scans in the 3rd trimester.

Antenatal care

Both diabetic retinopathy and diabetic nephropathy can worsen during pregnancy. Patients should have their eyes checked at booking and at 28 weeks, as well as regular blood pressure checks and assessment of proteinuria. Aspirin 75 mg daily is advised because of the increased risk of development of pre-eclampsia.

In the event of complications such as pre-eclampsia, the patient may require early delivery and may be offered steroids for fetal lung maturation. This commonly requires admission and an insulin sliding scale since administration of steroids will cause a worsening in glycaemic control.

Delivery and postnatal care

In the absence of complications, the timing of delivery needs to be carefully planned with the risks of prematurity and induction of labour against the risk of stillbirth (the rate of which is increased in diabetic mothers, as is the rate of caesarean section). Glucose control with a sliding scale is usually needed in labour. In addition macrosomic babies have an increased risk of shoulder dystocia so senior assistance must be available.

Immediately following delivery the fetus will be at risk of hypoglycaemia as it is no longer in a hyperglycaemic environment, although fetal insulin levels will still be high. Close monitoring and early feeds are important. Also, once the placenta has been delivered, maternal requirements of insulin will fall and the doses of insulin should return to pre-pregnancy levels or slightly less than pre-pregnancy levels if breast-feeding.

Gestational diabetes

Gestational diabetes is described as a condition leading to impaired glucose metabolism first recognized in pregnancy. This will, therefore, include those patients who had unknown pre-existing diabetes, who will be found to have a high blood sugar level at booking.

Diagnosis

In the UK, the gold standard for diagnosis is widely accepted as the 75 g oral glucose tolerance test (OGTT). The World Health Organization (WHO) define frank diabetes as a fasting glucose level of >7 mmol/l or a 2-hour level of >11.1 mmol/l. Gestational diabetes is defined as a fasting glucose level of >7 mmol/l or a 2-hour level >7.8 mmol/l (Fig. 23.2).

HINTS AND TIPS

When undergoing an oral glucose tolerance test (OGTT) the patient is asked to starve the night before the test and will then have a venous blood glucose level measured. Following this they will be asked to drink a glucose load (75 g) and have a second glucose level taken 2 hours later.

Screening for gestational diabetes is offered to 'at-risk' groups. Risk factors for gestational diabetes are shown in Figure 23.2 and patients with one or more risk factors should be offered an OGTT at around 26–28 weeks. Patients who have had gestational diabetes in a previous pregnancy will be offered an earlier OGTT (usually 16–18 weeks) followed by another at 28 weeks if negative.

Fig. 23.2 Risk factors for gestational diabetes.

BMI above 30 kg/m2
Previous macrosomic baby weighing ≥4.5 kg
Previous gestational diabetes.
First-degree relative with diabetes.
Country of family origin
- South Asian
- Black Caribbean
- Middle Eastern

Antenatal care

Risks of gestational diabetes to both the mother and fetus are similar to pregnancies in patients with pre-existing diabetes (Fig. 23.1) with the exception of miscarriage and congenital anomalies, as this period has passed. Patients should be seen in joint obstetric diabetic clinics and advised to self monitor with regular pre- and post-prandial capillary blood glucose levels. They may respond to changes in diet (consider referral to a dietician) and exercise alone. If these measures are insufficient, oral hypoglycaemic agents +/- insulin may be required. They should have serial growth scans to look for macrosomia +/- polyhydramnios.

Delivery and postnatal care

The planning of delivery is not always as rigid as in those with pre-existing diabetes as the risk to the fetus may be less. Each case should be assessed individually taking into account any complications that may have developed.

Postnatally patients can discontinue their hypoglycaemic agents and should have an OGTT taken at 6 weeks. The fetus will still be at risk of hypoglycaemia in the immediate period post delivery and, therefore, early feeds and close monitoring is advised. Patients with GDM should also be advised regarding weight loss and maintenance of a healthy diet with exercise and told of the high possibility of recurrence in future pregnancies.

EPILEPSY

Epilepsy affects around 1 in 200 women of child bearing age. Similar to diabetes, the management of epilepsy should, ideally, begin pre-conceptually with the counselling of patients about the risks to the mother and fetus. It is very important that epileptic women who are of a child bearing age and **who do not want to conceive** be offered effective contraception.

Anti-epileptic drugs and the complications

Pre-conception counselling should include the recommendation that all epileptic women take folic acid 5 mg daily. Anti-epileptic drugs (AEDs) are known to be teratogenic and patients are often concerned about the fetus, opting to discontinue therapy. The patient

Fig. 23.3 Fetal and neonatal complications of anti-epileptic drug use in pregnancy.

Orofacial clefts
Neural tube defects
Congenital heart disease
Haemorrhagic disease of the newborn.

should be carefully counselled against doing so and warned about the risk of status epilepticus and sudden unexpected death in epilepsy (SUDEP).

The aim of treatment of epilepsy in pregnancy is to maintain a seizure free status with monotherapy at the lowest possible AED dose. The approximate risk for one AED appears to be around 6%, which is double the background rate. In addition, data on sodium valproate appears to show an increased risk of fetal malformations. Figure 23.3 lists the known complications of AED use in pregnancy. Therefore, patients should undergo a detailed ultrasound scan with particular attention to:

- cardiac function
- neural tube status
- skeletal condition
- orofacial structures.

The course of epilepsy is variable; from an improvement in seizure frequency to a deterioration. Levels of AEDs can decrease during pregnancy due to increased hepatic metabolism and renal clearance. Seizures may, therefore, be difficult to control and dose changes may be required. Patients on hepatic enzyme inducing drugs should be given vitamin K 10 mg orally and the neonate should receive 1 mg of vitamin K IM soon after birth.

Delivery and postnatal care

There is an increase in the risk of seizures around the time of delivery and the following 24 hours. This risk is sufficient enough to recommend that patients deliver in hospital.

Breast-feeding is generally regarded as safe and should be encouraged. Postnatal education about safety measures should be given to all epileptic mothers such as the avoidance of excessive tiredness, changing the baby on the floor to prevent falls if a seizure occurs and also bathing the baby with another adult present, again in case of seizures.

THYROID DISEASE

Thyroid disorders again are commonly encountered in antenatal clinics. Preconception counselling and close monitoring reduces the impact on both mother and fetus.

Hypothyroidism

Hypothyroidism affects around 1% of pregnancies and is more common in those patients with a family history. Symptoms in pregnancy are similar to the non-pregnant patient:

- Lethargy
- Tiredness
- Weight gain
- Dry skin
- Hair loss.

These may be confused with normal pregnancy symptoms (cold intolerance, slow pulse rate and slow relaxing tendon reflexes are said to be discriminatory features in pregnancy). A goitre may also be present and should be carefully assessed when examining the patient.

In cases of known hypothyroidism preconceptual optimization of thyroid hormone levels with replacement therapy is very important as hypothyroidism itself can lead to subfertility. Up until 12 weeks the fetus is entirely dependent upon maternal thyroid hormones and, therefore, if left untreated there is an association with miscarriage, reduced intelligence, neuro-developmental delay and brain damage.

Most cases of hypothyroidism encountered in pregnancy are due to either autoimmune (Hashimoto's/atrophic) thyroiditis or treated Graves' disease, but it can also be due to drugs or following treatment for hyperthyroidism.

In patients who are adequately treated, it is usual to continue the current dose of thyroxine and check levels in each trimester. Those who require modifications of their dosing will need more frequent thyroid function tests (TFTs). When interpreting TFTs, it is important to use pregnancy adjusted values (Fig. 23.4). The importance of compliance with medication to minimize the impact on the fetus should be emphasized to all patients.

Hyperthyroidism

Hyperthyroidism, although less common than hypothyroidism, still affects around 1 in 800 pregnancies. Approximately 50% of those suffering with the disease will have a family history of thyroid disease.

Symptoms of hyperthyroidism are the same as in the non-pregnant population and again can mimic normal

Fig. 23.4 Pregnancy specific thyroid hormone values.

	Non Pregnant	First Trimester	Second Trimester	Third Trimester
TSH	0 – 4	0 – 1.6	0.1 – 1.8	0.7 – 7.3
Free T_4	11 – 23	11 – 22	11 – 19	7 – 15
Free T_3	4 – 9	4 – 8	4 – 7	3 – 5

pregnancy symptoms. These include sweating, palpitations, heat intolerance and vomiting. When examining the patient, look for the following signs:

- Tachycardia
- Tremor
- Eye signs (exopthalmos)
- Goitre
- Palmar erythema.

The presence of the first three signs are said to help distinguish hyperthyroidism from normal pregnancy symptoms.

Ninety-five per cent of hyperthyroidism encountered in pregnancy is due to Graves' disease, a condition where thyroid receptor antibodies stimulate thyroid hormone production. It can also be due to:

- drugs
- multi-nodular goitre
- thyroiditis.

Again if untreated patients may have difficulty conceiving so pre-conceptual counselling and optimization is vital as untreated hyperthyroidism is associated with miscarriage, preterm labour and growth restriction.

Patients with hyperthyroidism should have their TFTs measured in each trimester and assessed using pregnancy specific values (Fig. 23.4). Anti-thyroid drugs such as propylthiouracil (PTU) and carbimazole should be continued. β-blockers may be required to improve symptoms of sweating, tachycardia and palpitations, and rarely surgery may be required, especially if obstructive symptoms from the goitre are present.

One per cent of fetuses or neonates can suffer from neonatal thyrotoxicosis due to transplacental passage of thyroid antibodies. The condition should also be considered in fetuses or neonates of patients who are now hypothyroid as a result of thyroid treatment for Graves' disease. Fetuses will exhibit signs of tachycardia, growth restriction and possibly a goitre, whilst neonates may present with jaundice, failure to gain weight, irritability or in severe cases heart failure.

GASTROINTESTINAL DISORDERS

Obstetric cholestasis

Obstetric cholestasis (OC) is a condition in pregnancy which presents with characteristic itching of the palms and soles of the feet. Classically there is no rash but excoriations from excessive scratching may be present.

OC affects around 0.5% of pregnancies in the UK and is more common in certain ethnic groups (1.2–1.5% Indian or Pakistani origin and up to 5% in Chileans). The cause is not clearly understood but a susceptibility to the cholestatic effects of oestrogen and progesterone is thought to be key. Given that a family history of the condition is often found (35%) genetic factors are thought to play a role.

Diagnosis

OC is a diagnosis of exclusion, made in patients complaining of the classical symptoms of itchy palms and soles in the absence of a rash, and abnormal liver function tests (LFTs). Alanine transaminase (ALT) levels and bile acids are usually raised. In some cases there may be dark stools, pale urine, anorexia and steatorrhoea. All other causes of deranged LFTS should be excluded. Occasionally patients may present with classical symptoms, but have normal LFTs. These patients should have LFTs repeated every 1–2 weeks.

Treatment

Treatment of the condition is usually with chlorphenamine (Piriton®), aqueous creams and ursodeoxycholic acid (UCDA) for symptom control. UCDA is unlicensed in pregnancy but no adverse effects have been reported. It works by altering the bile acid pool balance by reducing the number of hydrophobic bile acids which are thought to be hepatotoxic.

Antenatal care

Once diagnosed, patients need to be monitored with weekly LFTs until delivery. Bile acid levels of >40 mmol/l are associated with pregnancy complications:

- Stillbirth
- Preterm delivery
- Passage of meconium
- Fetal anoxia.

Fetal surveillance with cardiotocograph (CTG) monitoring (although lacking evidence) is often offered to ease anxiety. Discussion about induction of labour after 37 + 6 weeks should take place, although this is associated with an increased rate of caesarean section. Those patients with severe derangements of their bile acids and LFTs have a greater indication for intervention. Vitamin K supplementation should be provided for those with abnormal clotting.

Postnatal care

Once delivered it is important to ensure LFTs have normalized (after at least 10 days). Patients should be warned of the likelihood of recurrence in a future pregnancy and advised to avoid oestrogen containing contraceptive pills as these may trigger cholestasis.

ACUTE FATTY LIVER OF PREGNANCY

Acute fatty liver of pregnancy (AFLP) is a rare (1 in 20 000) potentially fatal condition, which needs prompt recognition and management. Although the aetiology is poorly understood a disorder of mitochondrial fatty acid oxidation may play a role. Risk factors include:

- primips
- those carrying male fetuses
- multiple pregnancy.

The condition may be the same spectrum as pre-eclampsia and it may be difficult to distinguish from HELLP syndrome. It is a reversible condition which affects both the liver and kidneys.

Patients may present with nausea, vomiting, anorexia, malaise, abdominal pain or polyuria. Jaundice, ascites, encephalopathy and mild proteinuric hypertension may also be present. The haematological and biochemical derangements are shown in Figure 23.5.

Confirmation of the diagnosis with imaging is not always possible as changes may not be seen on ultrasound, CT or MRI. Liver biopsy may be considered, but in practice is not usually done due to the coagulopathy.

Patients diagnosed with AFLP need multidisciplinary input and urgent delivery. Supportive measures with fluids, correction of hypoglycaemia and correction of coagulopathy are important and patients may need intensive care and dialysis. In severe cases, liver transplant may be necessary.

THROMBOEMBOLISM

Until the last confidential report into maternal deaths (see Chapter 35), venous thromboembolism (VTE) was the leading direct cause of maternal death. It remains an important cause and all clinicians must be alert to the signs, symptoms, investigations and treatment.

The normal physiological adaptations to pregnancy mean that it is a prothrombotic state, increasing the risks of VTE. These include:

- increase in certain clotting factors
- increase in fibrinogen levels
- decrease in fibrinolytic activity
- decrease in protein S and antithrombin (endogenous anticoagulants)
- increased venous stasis in lower limbs (left > right).

Fig. 23.5 Acute fatty liver of pregnancy blood test results.

↑ Alanine Transaminase (ALT)
↑ Alkaline Phosphatase (ALP)
↑ Bilirubin
↑ White Cell Count
Hypoglycaemia (severe)
↑ Uric acid
Coagulopathy

Fig. 23.6 Risk factors for venous thrombo-embolism in pregnancy.

Thrombophilia (Factor V Leiden, Protein C deficiency, antiphospholipid syndrome)
Age >35
BMI>30
Parity >3
Smoker
Immobility (Surgery, disability)
Gross Varicose Veins
Multiple pregnancy
Medical comorbidities
Systemic Infection

Risk factors

Risk factors for VTE are given in Figure 23.6 and consideration should be given to prophylactic anticoagulation once a risk assessment has been made.

Thromboprophylaxis

Given the increased risk of VTE in pregnancy, the Royal College of Obstetricians and Gynaecologists (RCOG) recommend that all patients undergo a risk assessment in early pregnancy to identify those at high risk who might benefit from prophylactic anticoagulation.

Obstetric patients admitted to hospital should undergo a risk assessment and be offered prophylactic LMWH, especially if they are going to be immobile for a period of time. Most patients should be offered graduated compression stockings.

A key point to remember is that the risk of VTE is not abolished once the fetus is delivered, but remains high until 6 weeks post delivery. Therefore, any prophylactic measures should continue up until this point. In fact the puerperium is regarded as a particularly high-risk period. Delivery by caesarean section poses a significant risk of VTE and all patients (except those who have an uncomplicated elective operation with no risk factors) are offered 7 days of LMWH.

Symptoms and signs

Deep vein thrombosis (DVT) may present with pain, swelling and redness of the calf. Pulmonary emboli (PE) can present with shortness of breath, chest pain (pleuritic), collapse, cough or haemoptysis.

Patients found to be tachypnoeic, tachycardic, dyspnoeic or hypoxic (reduced saturations on pulse oximetry or low pO_2 on arterial blood gas ABG) need to have a PE ruled out. **In all cases a high index of suspicion is advised and when suspected, treatment must be initiated until the diagnosis is ruled out.**

Investigations

Investigation of a DVT usually starts with a clinical examination followed by venous Dopplers. It is important to bear in mind that the thrombosis may be located higher than the calf (propensity for ileofemoral DVT in pregnancy compared with popliteofemoral) and, therefore, imaging should include this area.

PE investigations usually begin again with a thorough examination followed by an ECG, ABG, FBC, chest X-ray (CXR). On the ABG the patient may be hypoxic and hypercapnic, the ECG may reveal a sinus tachycardia and the CXR is important to rule out other potential causes of the symptoms, such as infection or pneumothorax.

If the CXR is normal, the patient may proceed to a ventilation/perfusion scan. This may identify an area of under-perfusion indicating a PE. If the CXR is abnormal, a computed tomographic pulmonary angiogram (CTPA) may be indicated. This is very sensitive at diagnosing a PE but involves high doses of radiation.

Treatment

With a confirmed DVT or PE, patients require anticoagulation with therapeutic doses of low-molecular-weight heparin (LMWH). Warfarin is generally avoided as it crosses the placenta and is known to be teratogenic, as well as carrying the risk of fetal intracranial bleeding. In the puerperium patients can be converted to warfarin even if they are breast-feeding as it is regarded as safe.

CEREBRAL VEIN THROMBOSIS

A cerebral vein thrombosis is an uncommon yet fatal problem encountered by obstetricians. It is more common in the puerperium and presents with headaches, seizures, vomiting, photophobia, reduced consciousness or even focal neurology. It is usually diagnosed with a magnetic resonance imaging (MRI) venous angiogram and treatment is usually with hydration and anticoagulation.

HUMAN IMMUNODEFICIENCY VIRUS

Human immunodeficiency virus (HIV) is a chronic condition caused by infection with the human immunodeficiency virus via:

- sexual intercourse
- injecting drug use
- blood transfusion
- mother to fetus or neonate vertically during pregnancy or breast-feeding.

Infection with the virus leads to immunosupression and individuals become susceptible to infections and certain malignancies. However, advances in modern medicine and the production of anti-retroviral drugs (**H**ighly **A**ctive **A**nti-**R**etroviral **T**reatment HAART) have led to a significant decline in the morbidity and mortality from the illness.

Screening

In the UK all women are advised to have screening for HIV infection as part of their booking investigations. Identification of HIV infected individuals then allows appropriate care to improve maternal health and reduce the risk of transmission to the fetus from approximately 25% to less than 1%.

Additional interventions for HIV positive women include screening for hepatitis C, offering vaccinations against hepatitis B and screening for genital infection in the 1st trimester and at 28 weeks.

Testing for the patient's partner and any other children should be offered.

HINTS AND TIPS

A major barrier to compliance with testing and treatment is the fear of stigmatization and patients should be reassured regarding confidentiality.

Antenatal care

Care for patients with HIV should be given by a multidisciplinary team composed of HIV specialists, obstetricians, specialist midwives and paediatricians. The use of HAART has been shown to dramatically reduce the risk of vertical transmission; therefore, if a patient falls pregnant whilst taking HAART, she should continue to do so. Patients who are not on HAART but require it (following assessment) should commence treatment as soon as possible. Patients who are not on HAART (i.e. that do not require treatment after assessment) should commence HAART regardless from 20 weeks onwards until delivery.

HINTS AND TIPS

Patients on certain HAART should be screened for gestational diabetes due to their association with impaired glucose tolerance.

Delivery and postnatal care

The mode of delivery is usually confirmed at 36 weeks of gestation. Patients will have their viral load measured and if <50 copies/ml will be offered a vaginal delivery. When the patient is in labour, however, to reduce the risk of transmission, one should avoid performing invasive procedures such as fetal blood sampling or attaching a fetal scalp electrode.

Patients who have a high viral load will be offered a planned caesarean section with zidovudine cover (an antiretroviral 4 hours prior and continued until cord clamping).

In resource rich countries the avoidance of breast-feeding is recommended (to prevent transmission) and formula milk used as an alternative. It is, however, not always possible in developing countries.

Once delivered all neonates are treated with antiretrovirals as soon as possible (ideally within 4 hours). The neonate will be tested at regular intervals and, if not breast-fed, a negative test at 18 months ensures the child is not affected.

HINTS AND TIPS

Three steps known to reduce rates of vertical transmission of HIV:
- Avoidance of breast-feeding
- Anti-retroviral medication (HAART)
- Elective caesarean section.

PSYCHIATRIC ILLNESS

Identifying psychiatric illnesses in pregnancy is a vital part of assessing risk. Early specialist referral and multidisciplinary management are very important.

Depression

Symptoms of depression are thought to affect around 1 in 3 women at some stage in their pregnancy and it can be associated with suicide. Symptoms of low mood, anxiety, loss of appetite, insomnia, low self-esteem, lack of energy, failure to find enjoyment and suicidal ideation should be actively enquired about.

Risk factors for depression are shown in Figure 23.7. Any patient with a history of depression or who is currently suffering with depression should be referred for specialist counselling, usually in the form of a perinatal mental health team. Both pharmacological and non-pharmacological (cognitive behavioural therapy CBT) treatments may be required.

Fig. 23.7 Risk factors for depression during and after pregnancy.

- History of postnatal depression
- History of depression unrelated to pregnancy
- IVF pregnancy
- History of abuse
- Multiple pregnancy
- Drug misuse
- Poor social support
- Low socioeconomic status
- Low educational achievement
- Poor pregnancy outcome, e.g. illness in pregnancy, premature or difficult delivery, neonatal illness or death, diagnosis of congenital anomaly antenatally or neonatally

Patients with a history of depression outside or during pregnancy are at risk of postnatal depression (PND). PND can present as more mild 'baby blues', which are usually short lasting (24–72 hours) and begin around the fifth day after delivery. Tearfulness, labile mood and irritability are possible symptoms. In more severe cases, especially with signs of neglect and suicidal ideation, prompt specialist intervention is important.

Puerperal psychosis

Puerperal psychosis is a serious disorder which affects around 1 in 500 births. It usually starts abruptly around 2 weeks postnatally and presents with mania, delusions and hallucinations (both auditory and visual). Patients appear agitated and may exhibit disinhibited behaviour.

Puerperal psychosis is more common in patients who have a previous psychiatric history. Treatment invariably involves admission to hospital for both the safety of the mother and baby, ideally to a specialist mother and baby unit to prevent separation. Antipsychotic medications such as haloperidol may be required. Organic causes of the symptoms (infection, drug withdrawals, etc.) must be excluded.

Schizophrenia

Schizophrenia affects around 1 in 100 women of child-bearing age and again needs specialist management in pregnancy. As well as caring for the mother's health, an assessment must be conducted to identify any potential difficulties the patient may have in caring for the child and what risks an acute episode may pose.

Hallucinations, delusions or an abnormal affect may be encountered and should prompt specialist help. Antipsychotic medications may be indicated during the pregnancy, although the evidence regarding their safety is not clear. In practice the lowest dose is used with a reduction in the dose towards term to prevent toxicity in the neonate. Breast-feeding on antipsychotics is not advised.

Bipolar disorder

Bipolar disorder (BD) is a condition characterized by episodes of acute illness mixed with periods of relative normality. Many of the drugs used to treat BD are teratogenic and, therefore, careful assessment must be made to balance the risk of harm from a relapse in pregnancy against the risk of damage to the fetus. Lithium use is associated with cardiac defects. Again, management by specialist perinatal mental health teams is advised and particular attention needs to be paid to the puerperium when acute episodes are common.

SUBSTANCE ABUSE

Substance abuse in pregnancy poses a risk to the health of the mother and the fetus. This risk is both direct, i.e. from the abused substance itself and indirect, i.e. from risk allied to drug use like the transmission of infection from injecting drug use.

Booking assessments should be used as an opportunity to screen for substance abuse. Early cessation will help to minimize risk and enable implementation of other care such as screening for infection. This particular group may represent a challenge as their attendance for antenatal care may be poor.

Cocaine abuse is associated with growth restriction, placental abruption, stillbirth and neonatal death. Opiates are associated with growth restriction, preterm labour and neonate dependence. Again, referral to drug and alcohol treatment services is important.

Referral to drug and alcohol treatment services is important and patients should be offered a detoxification program where appropriate.

Smoking cessation advice should be offered at every visit and when accepted, appropriate referral made. Smoking is associated with growth restriction, placental abruption, cot death and childhood asthma, and, therefore, educating patients about the risks posed by both active and passive smoking is very important.

Alcohol abuse is known to cause fetal anomalies and fetal alcohol syndrome. Safe amounts of alcohol intake are the subject of much continuing debate and most people would recommend no alcohol at all, especially in the first trimester. Patients who wish to continue drinking alcohol should not exceed 1–2 units once or twice a week and binge drinking should be strongly discouraged.

Further reading

Anaemia, n.d. Collins English Dictionary - Complete & Unabridged, 10th ed.

De Swiet, M., 2002. Medical Disorders in Obstetric Practice, fourth ed. Blackwell Publishing, London.

Dhanjal, M., 2011. Thyroid and parathyroid disease in Oxford Desk Reference Obstetrics & Gynaecology. Oxford University Press, Oxford.

Murphy, V., Namazy, J., Powell, H., et al., 2011. A meta-analysis of adverse perinatal outcomes in women with asthma. BJOG. 118, 1314–1323. http://dx.doi.org/10.1111/j.1471-0528.2011.03055.x.

Myles, J., 2011. Substance Abuse in Pregnancy in Oxford Desk Reference Obstetrics & Gynaecology. Oxford University Press, Oxford.

Nelson-Piercy, C., 2010. Handbook of Obstetric Medicine, fourth ed. Informa Healthcare, New York.

NICE, 2008. Guidelines – Antenatal Care. National Institute for Health and Care Excellence, London.

NICE, 2008. Guidelines - CG63 Diabetes in Pregnancy: Full Guideline. National Institute for Health and Care, London.

RCOG, 2007. The Acute Management of Thrombosis and Embolism During Pregnancy and the Puerperium, Green-top Guideline No. 37b. Royal College of Obstetricians and Gynaecologists, London.

RCOG, 2009. Reducing the Risk of Thrombosis and Embolism during Pregnancy and the Puerperium, Green-top Guideline No. 37a. Royal College of Obstetricians and Gynaecologists, London.

RCOG, 2010. Management of HIV in Pregnancy, Green-top Guideline No. 39. Royal College of Obstetricians and Gynaecologists, London.

RCOG, 2011. Obstetric Cholestasis, Green-top Guideline No. 43. Royal College of Obstetricians and Gynaecologists, London.

Williamson, C., 2011. Obstetric Cholestasis in Oxford Desk Reference Obstetrics & Gynaecology. Oxford University Press, Oxford.

Multiple pregnancy

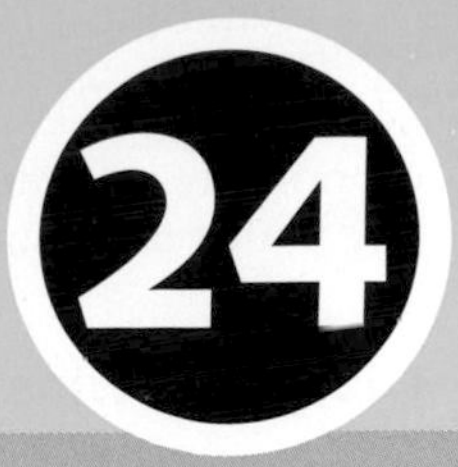

Objectives

By the end of this chapter, you should be able to:

- Understand the difference between zygosity and chorionicity
- List the methods of diagnosing chorionicity
- Plan the antenatal care of a woman with a multiple pregnancy
- Describe the intrapartum management of a twin pregnancy
- Consider the potential advantages and disadvantages of selective fetal reduction.

A multiple pregnancy is one in which two or more fetuses are present, i.e. it is not a singleton pregnancy. Such pregnancies are important to the obstetrician because they represent a high-risk pregnancy. The risk of all pregnancy complications is greater than in a singleton pregnancy; in particular preterm labour (see Chapter 29) and intrauterine growth restriction (IUGR). Perinatal mortality for a multiple pregnancy is about six times greater than that of a singleton.

HINTS AND TIPS

- A multiple pregnancy is a high-risk pregnancy.
- Perinatal mortality rate is increased six times compared with a single fetus, mainly due to the risk of preterm delivery.

INCIDENCE

The most common type of multiple pregnancy is a twin pregnancy, with an incidence of 1 in 80 pregnancies. The incidence of spontaneous triplets is 1 in 80^2 or 1 in 6400. The incidence of any multiple pregnancy increases with:

- increasing maternal age
- increasing parity
- ethnic variation, e.g. more common in Africa compared with Far East
- improved nutrition
- assisted conception.

The latter accounts for a significant rise over the last two decades, especially in Western countries.

DIAGNOSIS

Nowadays, multiple pregnancies are normally diagnosed by routine dating ultrasound scan at 11–14 weeks gestation. Other clinical situations in which the diagnosis should be suspected are if patient presents with hyperemesis gravidarum or if clinical examination reveals either a large-for-dates uterus or multiple fetal parts in later pregnancy.

AETIOLOGY

Twins

The majority of twins (75%) are dizygotic, that is they arise from the fertilization of two ova by two sperm. Monozygotic twins (25%) arise following the fertilization of a single ovum by a single sperm, which then completely divides, so that each twin has the same genetic make-up.

However, the clinically important issue is the chorionicity of the pregnancy. This relates to the placentation. If the placentae are separate, with separate amnions and chorions (dichorionic diamniotic twins), the blood supply to each fetus during the pregnancy is independent.

Conversely, if there are blood vessel anastomoses between the placentae (monochorionic diamniotic twins or monochorionic monoamniotic twins), then there is a risk of uneven distribution of blood. This may result in discordant growth, with one twin showing signs of growth restriction and the other getting larger (see below Twin to twin transfusion). Thus diagnosing chorionicity determines the level of surveillance necessary in that particular pregnancy.

Dizygotic twins

Two ova from the same or different ovaries are released simultaneously and fertilized by two separate sperm. Each fetus has its own chorion, amnion and placenta — dichorionic diamniotic placentation. The placentae can appear fused if implantation occurs close together. These twins can be of the same or different sexes and will have different genetic constitutions, i.e. they have no more similarities than any siblings.

The incidence of dizygotic twins varies widely between different populations, probably for multifactorial reasons such as genetic and nutritional factors. It also increases with increasing maternal age and increasing parity.

Monozygotic twins

A single ovum is fertilized by a single sperm and the zygote divides into two. This may occur at different stages of embryonic development, giving rise to different structural arrangements of the membranes (Fig. 24.1).

A third of monozygotic twins establish at the eight-cell stage, so that two separate blastocysts form and implant. These twins will thus have dichorionic diamniotic placentation. About two-thirds of monozygotic twins have monochorionic diamniotic placentation: that is a single blastocyst implants, developing a single chorion; the inner cell mass divides into two so that each embryo has its own amnion.

The least common type of monozygotic twins occurs by later splitting of the inner cell mass, before the appearance of the primitive streak, to produce a single amniotic cavity — monochorionic monoamniotic twins. Splitting even later than this results in conjoint twins.

The incidence of monozygotic twins is constant around the world, at about 4 per 1000 births.

Triplets

Pregnancies of higher-order multiples (i.e. three or more fetuses) are less commonly formed by separate ova. In the case of a triplet pregnancy, there are usually two ova, one of which splits as described above to form a monochorionic pair of twins.

With triplets or more, it is appropriate to counsel the parents about selective fetal reduction (see below). The chorionicity of the pregnancy must be known in order to select the appropriate fetus. The procedure cannot be performed on a monochorionic twin because it shares placental circulation with its co-twin and, therefore, the drugs would affect both fetuses.

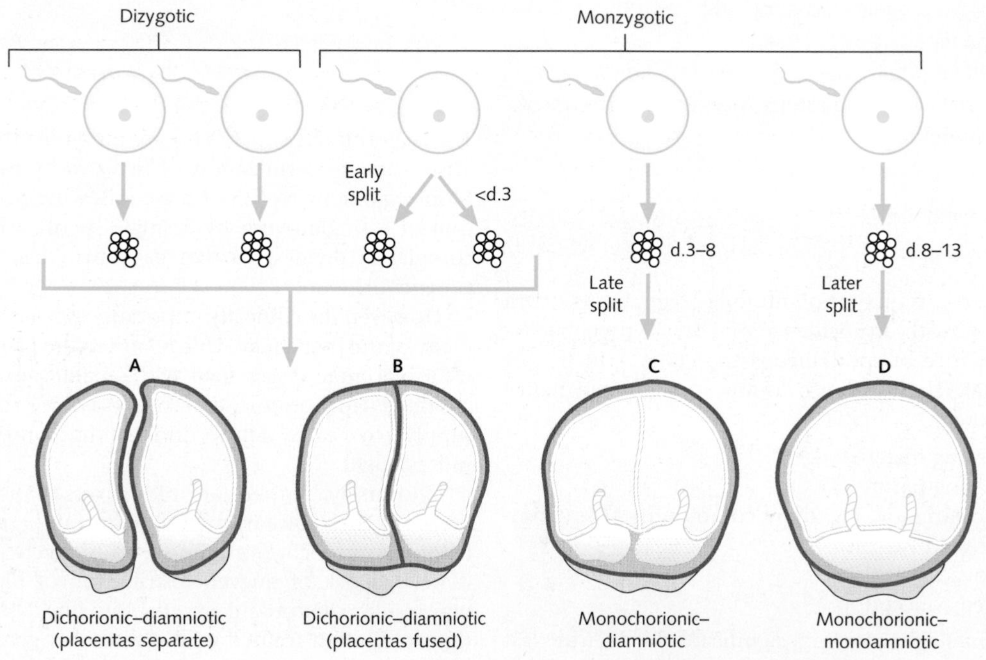

Fig. 24.1 Dizygotic and monozygotic twinning.

Diagnosis of chorionicity

Antenatally

Ultrasound assessment of the membrane dividing the amniotic sacs diagnoses the chorionicity; this must be done before 16 weeks' gestation. Figure 24.2 shows the thicker insertion of the membrane, known as the lambda sign, which is found in a dichorionic pregnancy. In contrast, the thinner T sign is seen in a monochorionic pregnancy. If there is no dividing membrane between the fetuses, they are monochorionic monoamniotic twins.

Fetal sex can also be assessed by ultrasound. If they are discordant, then the pregnancy must be dichorionic. Localization of the placental sites may also be helpful. If the placentae can be seen as being completely separate, then similarly, the pregnancy must be dichorionic.

Postnatally

At this stage, chorionicity can be determined by:

- macroscopic and microscopic examination of membranes
- analysis of red-blood-cell markers
- DNA probes.

COMPLICATIONS

A multiple pregnancy must be treated as a high-risk pregnancy. The majority of pregnancy-related complications are more common in multiple pregnancies, e.g. gestational diabetes or pre-eclampsia. There are also certain problems that are specific to multiple pregnancies.

HINTS AND TIPS

The mother is at risk of any complication associated with a singleton pregnancy but the risks are increased.

Fetal malformations

The frequency of fetal malformations is thought to be almost double in a twin pregnancy compared with a singleton pregnancy; especially for monochorionic twins (4% cf. 2%). In terms of screening for chromosomal anomalies, parents must be counselled about the possibility of a screen positive result in one baby, but a negative one in the other. With an invasive procedure, there is a greater risk of pregnancy loss than in a singleton pregnancy. Separate sampling must be performed with dichorionic twins. There is also the potential dilemma of finding an abnormality in only one fetus at the anomaly ultrasound scan. Selective fetocide can result in the miscarriage of the apparently normal fetus as well as the abnormal one.

Antenatal assessment of fetal well-being and growth

In a multiple pregnancy, antenatal care should be more frequent, managed by a hospital consultant in a unit with facilities for regular ultrasound scans to check fetal growth and neonatal care facilities in case of preterm labour and delivery

Serial ultrasounds are usually performed every 2 to 4 weeks to exclude IUGR. This is especially important in pregnancies with monochorionic placentation, which are at greater risk of discordant growth between

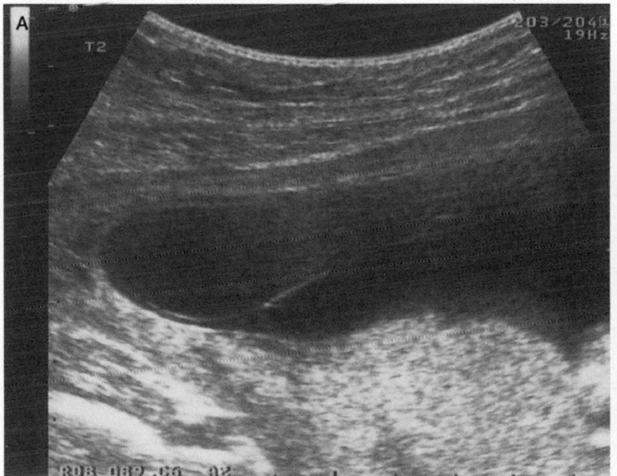

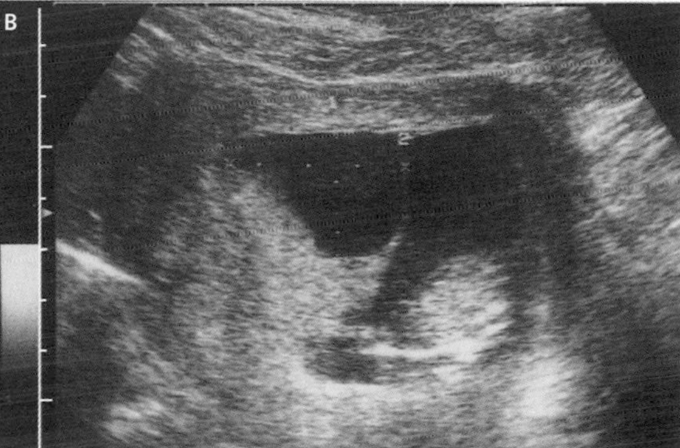

Fig. 24.2 Diagnosis of chorionicity. (A) The T sign is indicative of monochorionic diamniotic pregnancy. (B) The lambda sign is indicative of dichorionic diamniotic pregnancy.

the fetuses and the development of twin-to-twin transfusion syndrome (see below).

Preterm labour

Spontaneous preterm labour occurs in 30% of twin pregnancies. There is some evidence to suggest that cervical length screening by transvaginal ultrasound may be a useful screening tool. In higher-order multiple pregnancies, some physicians opt to put in an elective cervical suture at the start of the second trimester, to reduce the risk of preterm labour.

If pre-term labour is diagnosed, tocolytics should be considered to allow in utero transfer to a hospital with neonatal intensive care facilities and to allow time for steroids administered to the mother to improve lung maturation (see Chapter 29).

Pregnancy-induced hypertension

Hypertension is about three times more common in multiple pregnancies than in singleton pregnancies because of the larger size of the placental bed (see Chapter 22). It often develops earlier and is more severe. National guidelines recommend consideration for aspirin 75 mg daily to reduce the risk.

Antepartum haemorrhage

The incidence of placental abruption and placenta praevia is increased in multiple pregnancies.

Twin-to-twin transfusion syndrome

This occurs in 15% of monochorionic diamniotic twin pregnancies — blood is shunted across placental interfetal vascular anastomoses, such that the donor becomes anaemic and growth restricted, with oligohydramnios, and the recipient becomes fluid overloaded with polyhydramnios. This syndrome usually occurs in the second trimester. It results in fetal death in up to 80% of cases if left untreated and a 10% risk of handicap in the surviving twin. Depending on the stage of the disease at diagnosis, up to 26 weeks, laser treatment to the placental anastomoses is generally the advised treatment in order to reduce discordant blood flow between the fetuses (known as FLAP fetoscopic laser ablation of the placenta). Amniodrainage may be appropriate at later gestations.

With monochorionic placentation, fetal death of a twin in utero puts the surviving twin at risk of neurological damage and the mother at risk of developing disseminated intravascular coagulation (DIC) as thromboplastins are released into the circulation. The pregnancy can be managed conservatively until the surviving twin reaches a gestation with improved likelihood of survival. Eighty per cent of surviving twins can be delivered vaginally.

HINTS AND TIPS

The psychological sequelae of a multiple pregnancy on the mother and her family, including existing children, should be remembered.

INTRAPARTUM MANAGEMENT OF A TWIN PREGNANCY

Figure 24.3 summarizes the management of a vaginal delivery in a twin pregnancy.

Delivery of twin pregnancy

Delivery of multiple pregnancies should be managed in a unit with neonatal intensive care facilities. For a twin pregnancy, the mode of delivery depends on the presentation of the first twin; twin one is cephalic in more than 80% of pregnancies. If presentation of twin one is anything other than cephalic, caesarean section is usually the mode of choice. In the case of higher-order multiple pregnancies, delivery is almost always by caesarean section.

For a vaginal delivery, the onset of labour can be spontaneous or induced; induction might be advised for similar reasons to a singleton pregnancy (e.g. post dates) or for an indication more specific to a twin pregnancy, such as IUGR. The woman needs intravenous access and a sample of serum saved in the blood transfusion laboratory because of the risk of postpartum haemorrhage (see below). An epidural block is often recommended to allow for possible manipulation of the second twin in the second stage of labour.

Fig. 24.3 The intrapartum management of twin pregnancy.

- Neonatal unit intensive care facilities
- Allow vaginal delivery if normal pregnancy and twin 1 cephalic presentation
- IV access/full blood count/group and save
- Regional anaesthesia
- Continuous CTG monitoring ± fetal scalp electrode to twin 1
- IV syntocinon infusion to start after delivery of twin 1 to maintain contractions
- IV syntocinon infusion for third stage to reduce risk of PPH

Both fetal heart rates should be monitored continuously, either per abdomen or with a fetal scalp electrode on the first twin. If there is an abnormality in the heart rate pattern of twin one, fetal blood sampling might be appropriate (see Chapter 31). Concerns with twin two should lead to immediate delivery by caesarean section. The reasons for augmentation of labour and for instrumental delivery are similar to those in a singleton pregnancy (see Chapter 32).

Once the first twin is delivered, the lie and presentation of the second twin must be determined by abdominal palpation and ultrasound. External cephalic version can be used to establish a longitudinal lie. Intravenous syntocinon may be necessary to maintain uterine contractions and the delivery of the second twin occurs either as a cephalic presentation or by internal podalic version and breech extraction. Again the reasons for instrumental delivery or caesarean section are similar to those of a singleton pregnancy.

Complications

Post-partum haemorrhage

Post-partum haemorrhage (PPH; see Chapter 33) is more likely with a multiple pregnancy than a singleton because of the larger placental site. Uterine atony due to the increased volume of the uterine contents – two fetuses, placentae, etc. – is a contributing factor. Active management of the third stage of labour is, therefore, appropriate including routine use of a post-partum syntocinon infusion.

Locked twins

This is a very rare complication of vaginal deliveries when the first twin is breech. As the delivery proceeds, the aftercoming head of the first twin is prevented from entering the pelvis by the head of the cephalic second twin. If this is diagnosed in the first stage of labour, a caesarean section should be performed; during the second stage, general anaesthesia is necessary to allow manipulation.

HIGHER-ORDER MULTIPLE PREGNANCIES

In comparison to twin pregnancies, higher-order multiples are associated with a higher perinatal mortality rate and an increased incidence of the antenatal complications mentioned above. Fertility treatments have increased the numbers of high-order pregnancies and, in the case of IVF, guidelines in the UK now advise that a maximum of two embryos should be replaced in a woman under the age of 40 (see Chapter 18).

Selective fetocide (multifetal pregnancy reduction)

Selective fetocide is a technique in which intracardiac potassium chloride is given to one or more fetuses in a high-order multiple pregnancy under ultrasound guidance. The aim is to improve the outcome of the remaining fetuses by reducing the risks of late miscarriage and preterm labour. It is usually performed at 12–14 weeks gestation, after results of screening for Downs syndrome have been obtained if the parents wish this. Despite the procedure-related risk of miscarriage of about 6%, the incidence of complications is low. However, ethical dilemmas arise with respect to abortion in general, as well as possible miscarriage of the entire pregnancy.

Further reading

Chamberlain, G., Steer, P., 2001. Turnbull's Obstetrics, third ed. Churchill Livingstone, Edinburgh.

Enkin, M.W., Keirse, M.J.N.C., Neilson, J., et al., 2000. A Guide to Effective Care in Pregnancy and Childbirth, third ed. Oxford University Press, Oxford.

Nicolaides, K.H., Sebire, N.J., Snijders, J.M., 2004. The 11–14 Week Scan Fetal Medicine Foundation. Available online at: www.fetalmedicine.com/fmf.

NICE, 2011. Guideline Multiple Pregnancy CG129. National Institute for Health and Care Excellence, London. Available online at: www.nice.org.uk.

RCOG, 2008. Monochorionic Pregnancy, Management. Green-top Guideline No. 51. Royal College of Obstetricians and Gynaecologists, London. Available online at: www.rcog.org.uk.

Abdominal pain in the second and third trimesters of pregnancy

Objectives

By the end of this chapter, you should be able to:

- Understand the important points in the history for a patient presenting with abdominal pain in the second and third trimesters of pregnancy
- Perform an examination on this patient
- Undertake appropriate investigations on this patient in order to establish a diagnosis.

DIFFERENTIAL DIAGNOSIS OF ABDOMINAL PAIN IN PREGNANCY

The important differential diagnosis when assessing abdominal pain in pregnancy is whether the cause is obstetric or non-obstetric. Figure 25.1 shows the systems that might be involved.

Don't forget to take a history, which includes the non-obstetric causes of abdominal pain. Some of them are more common than the obstetric causes, such as a urinary tract infection.

HISTORY

With diverse differential diagnoses, the history is very important to identify the cause of the pain. Figure 25.2 gives a summary of the points elicited from the history and examination that help to make the diagnosis.

Current obstetric history

This should include the current gestation and the parity. The antenatal history may be relevant. For example, if the patient has a history of pregnancy-induced hypertension (see Chapter 22) then she is at risk of pre-eclampsia and placental abruption (see Chapter 21). She may already have been admitted earlier in the pregnancy with suspected preterm labour (see Chapter 29) or with a urinary tract infection.

Presenting symptoms

As with any history of pain, its characteristics are important:

- Nature: continuous or intermittent
- Quality: stabbing or burning or tightening
- Site: generalized or specific
- Radiation: to the pelvis or to the back
- Duration
- Exacerbating factors

It is important to ask about other symptoms, particularly gastrointestinal and genitourinary, such as frequency of bowel habit, vomiting or dysuria.

Past obstetric history

A history of pre-eclampsia or preterm labour in a previous pregnancy puts the patient at increased risk in her current pregnancy.

Past gynaecological/medical/surgical history

Ultrasound scans earlier in the current pregnancy may have diagnosed an ovarian cyst or uterine fibroids. There may be a history of peptic ulcer disease or gallstones. If the patient has previously had an appendicectomy or a cholecystectomy, these differential diagnoses can be excluded.

EXAMINATION

General examination

As with any clinical examination, the general condition of the pregnant patient should be assessed, including:

- temperature
- pulse
- blood pressure
- respiratory rate
- cardiovascular system
- respiratory system.

Fig. 25.1 Differential diagnosis of abdominal pain in 2nd and 3rd trimesters.

System involved	Pathology
Obstetric	Labour Placental abruption Symphysis pubis dysfunction Ligament pain Pre-eclampsia/HELLP syndrome Acute fatty liver of pregnancy
Gynaecological	Ovarian cyst rupture/torsion/ haemorrhage Uterine fibroid degeneration
Gastrointestinal	Constipation Appendicitis Gallstones/cholecystitis Pancreatitis Peptic ulcer disease
Genitourinary	Cystitis Pyelonephritis Renal stones/renal colic

Abdominal palpation

The abdomen should be inspected for any previous operation scars. In the presence of a gravid uterus, abdominal palpation to establish the cause of the symptoms may not be straightforward. Compared with examining a non-pregnant patient, the site of the tenderness might not be typical. For example, examining a non-pregnant patient who has an ovarian cyst torsion is likely to elicit tenderness and guarding in the iliac fossa. Depending on the gestation, this might not be so specific in a pregnant patient because the gravid uterus interferes with the usual anatomical markings. Similarly, tenderness at McBurney's point, which is typical of appendicitis (see *Crash Course in Surgery*) may be difficult to elicit in a patient who is late in the second or in the third trimester of pregnancy for a similar reason.

HINTS AND TIPS

When examining an obstetric patient, remember that she might feel faint if she lies flat on her back for too long, secondary to pressure on the large vessels reducing venous return to the heart and causing supine hypotension. She should be examined with left lateral tilt.

The uterus should be palpated to determine:

- lie, presentation and engagement of the fetus (see Chapter 3)
- presence of uterine contractions
- generalized or specific areas of uterine tenderness
- presence of uterine fibroids.

Vaginal examination

A speculum examination is appropriate to exclude cervical causes of bleeding (see Chapter 21). A digital examination may be indicated if the history and abdominal palpation suggest that the patient is in labour, in order to determine if there is cervical change (see Chapter 28).

INVESTIGATION

Figure 25.3 gives a summary of the investigations that should be considered and Figure 25.4 provides an algorithm for the investigation of abdominal pain.

Blood tests

Full blood count/clotting studies

The full blood count can show a reduced haemoglobin if the patient is bleeding, for example in the case of a placental abruption. The platelet count is usually low in association with pre-eclampsia or HELLP syndrome (haemolysis, elevated liver enzymes, low platelets). This may be associated with abnormal clotting studies. A group and save sample of serum is essential if there is ongoing bleeding, in case cross-matched blood is required for transfusion. With the non-obstetric causes of pain, the white blood cell count and C-reactive protein will be raised if there is infection, for example, with pyelonephritis or cholecystitis.

Urea/electrolytes/glucose/liver function tests

In pre-eclampsia or HELLP syndrome, urea, creatinine and the liver transaminases can be raised. Serum uric acid is also high in pre-eclampsia and in acute fatty liver. The latter is associated with hypoglycaemia.

Urinalysis/midstream urine sample

In pre-eclampsia, there is proteinuria on dipstick urinalysis. A single sample protein/creatinine ratio or 24-h urine collection will quantify the amount of protein

Fig. 25.2 Making a diagnosis from the history and examination.

Differential diagnosis	Clinical features
Labour (see Chapter 28)	Intermittent pain, usually regular in frequency, associated with uterine tightenings. The presenting part of the fetus is usually engaged. Vaginal examination shows cervical change.
Placental abruption (see Chapter 21)	Mild or severe pain, more commonly associated with vaginal bleeding.The uterus is usually tender on palpation and can be irritable or tense. There might be symptoms and signs of pre-eclampsia.
Symphysis pubis dysfunction	Pain is usually low and central in the abdomen just above the symphysis pubis, which is tender on palpation. Symptoms are worse with movement.
Ligament pain	Commonly described as sharp pain, which is bilateral and often associated with movement.
Pre-eclampsia/HELLP syndrome (see Chapter 22)	Epigastric or right upper quadrant pain, associated with nausea and vomiting, headache and visual disturbances. On examination, there is hypertension and proteinuria.
Acute fatty liver of pregnancy	Epigastric or right upper quadrant pain, associated with nausea, vomiting, anorexia and malaise.
Ovarian cyst (see Chapter 9)	Unilateral pain, which is intermittent and might be associated with vomiting.
Uterine fibroid (see Chapter 7)	Pain is localized and constant. Fibroid may be noted on palpation and is tender.
Constipation	Usually suggested by the history, can cause lower abdominal discomfort and bloating.
Appendicitis	Pain associated with nausea and vomiting. Tenderness with guarding and rebound might be localized to the right iliac fossa depending on gestation.
Gallstones/cholecystitis	Right upper quadrant or epigastric pain, which might radiate to the back or to the shoulder tip. Tenderness in the right hypochondrium, pyrexia present with cholecystitis.
Pancreatitis	Epigastric pain radiating to the back, associated with nausea and vomiting. Occurs more commonly in the third trimester.
Peptic ulcer	Epigastric pain associated with food. There might be heartburn, nausea and even haematemesis.
Cystitis	Usually suggested by history of dysuria , with pain and tenderness in the low abdomen or suprapubically.
Renal stones/renal colic/ pyelonephritis	Loin pain that might radiate to the abdomen and groin, possibly associated with vomiting and rigors. Pyrexia is present with pyelonephritis.

in order to determine the severity of the disease. Proteinuria may also be present with a urinary tract infection and may be associated with microscopic haematuria, particularly in the presence of renal stones.

Cardiotocograph

Before 26 weeks gestation, the fetal heart should be auscultated with a pinard or a sonicaid. A cardiotocograph is performed after 26 weeks' gestation (see Chapter 31) and will help determine fetal well-being, particularly in the case of placental abruption. The recording will also detect uterine activity including the presence and frequency of uterine contractions.

Ultrasound scan (uterus/ovaries/kidneys/liver/gallbladder)

Although generally a clinical diagnosis, an ultrasound scan may show a retroplacental haematoma in the case of severe placental abruption. If preterm delivery is necessary, for example in acute fatty liver, fetal well-being and growth should be assessed, and the fetal weight estimated to inform the paediatricians.

For the other systems, ultrasound examination can assist diagnosis and management. An ovarian cyst might be seen if haemorrhage, rupture or torsion of the cyst is suspected. Renal stones or gallstones can be visualized.

Fig. 25.3 Summary of investigations to be considered in a patient with abdominal pain.

- Full blood count
- Clotting studies
- Group and save (G&S) sample
- Urea/electrolytes
- Liver function tests (LFTs)
- C-reactive protein
- Glucose
- Urinalysis/midstream urine (MSU)/24-h urine collection for protein or protein-creatinine ratio
- Cardiotocograph (CTG)
- Ultrasound scan of the uterus, ovaries, kidneys, liver and gall bladder

MANAGEMENT

This depends on the cause of the pain and the gestation of the pregnancy. With regard to the obstetric causes, caesarean section or induction of labour might need to be considered. For example, in severe pre-eclampsia, the benefits of delivery to the mother's health can outweigh the risks to the fetus of preterm birth. Placental abruption might be severe enough to compromise the fetus, and then delivery should be expedited.

However, most conditions can be managed conservatively. This includes analgesia in the presence of renal stones, or antibiotics for pyelonephritis. Multidisciplinary management with other specialties is important, for example with gastroenterology in a patient suspected of having gallstones or a peptic ulcer. Depending on the clinical findings, an operation is necessary for an acute appendicitis or for ovarian torsion.

HINTS AND TIPS

Multidisciplinary team management of patients with suspected medical or surgical complications in pregnancy is essential, e.g. renal stones or cholecystitis. In the case of preterm labour, management must be in conjunction with the paediatricians. Do not forget to liaise with the anaesthetists for analgesia if delivery is indicated or for assistance with fluid replacement and airway management.

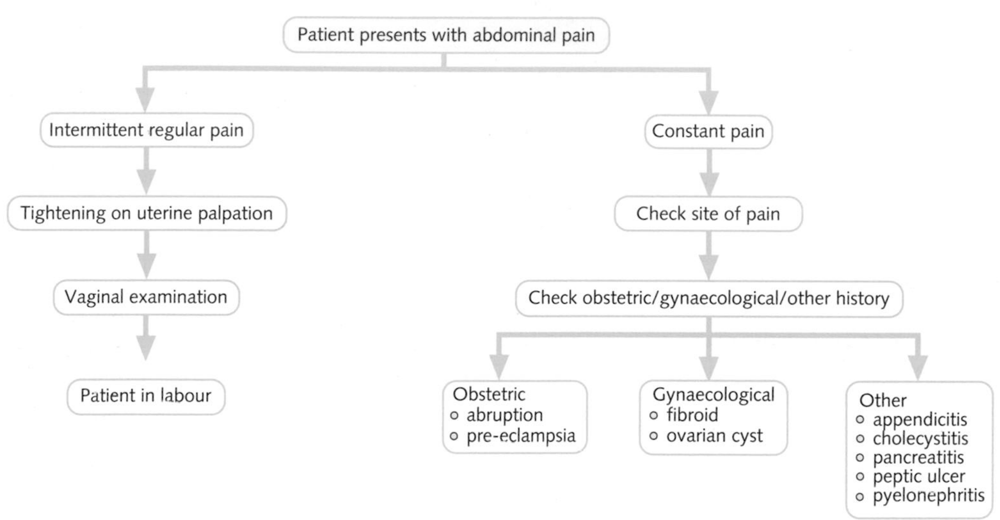

Fig. 25.4 Algorithm for abdominal pain.

Large or small for dates in pregnancy

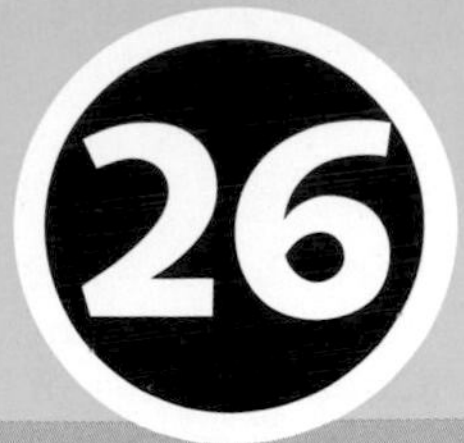

Objectives

By the end of this chapter, you should be able to:

- Understand the important points in the history for a patient presenting with a large-for-dates (LFD) or small-for-dates (SFD) uterus
- Perform an examination on this patient
- Undertake appropriate investigations on this patient in order to establish a diagnosis.

DIFFERENTIAL DIAGNOSIS

The growth of a pregnancy is estimated by measuring the symphysis–fundal height (SFH – see Chapter 3). This takes into account the size of the fetus, the liquor volume and the maternal structures, including the uterus. Ideally, every woman should have what is generally known as a dating scan between 11 and 14 weeks of pregnancy in order to establish the estimated date of delivery (EDD). Before deciding whether SFH is abnormal or not, the dates of the last menstrual period and the scan reports should be checked to confirm the gestation of the pregnancy, and also whether it is a singleton pregnancy.

The differential diagnoses of the large-for-dates (LFD) or small-for-dates (SFD) uterus can be considered in two categories:

1. Fetal/placental
2. Maternal

A fetus found to be SFD can be categorized according to its growth pattern diagnosed with serial ultrasound scans:

- Small for gestational age (SGA): the fetus is small for the expected size at a certain gestation, but continues to grow at a normal rate over time
- Intrauterine growth restriction (IUGR): the fetus is small or normal-sized for the expected size at a certain gestation, but the growth rate slows down as the pregnancy advances.

HINTS AND TIPS

The SFH measurement should be +/- 3 cm equal to the number of weeks of pregnancy after 24 weeks, i.e. at 32 weeks a normal SFH will be between 29 and 35 cm. Discrepancy of more than 3 cm is LFD, less than 3 cm is SFD.

HISTORY

Past obstetric history

With respect to the LFD uterus, a patient who had gestational diabetes in a previous pregnancy is at risk of developing the same condition again (see Chapter 23). This disorder puts the pregnancy at risk of fetal macrosomia and polyhydramnios (increased liquor volume).

A previous history of a baby that was SGA or IUGR, whether in relation to pre-eclampsia or not, increases the risk of a future pregnancy being similarly affected.

Past gynaecological history

A diagnosis of uterine fibroids or an ovarian cyst, either prior to pregnancy or in early pregnancy can cause the SFH to palpate as LFD.

Past medical history

Pre-existing diabetes increases the chance of fetal macrosomia and polyhydramnios. The abdomen will palpate LFD, as in gestational diabetes. Fetal infection with cytomegalovirus or rubella may produce polyhydramnios so the mother should be asked about recent flu-like illness or rash.

Current maternal disease increases the risk of IUGR and, therefore, a SFD uterus (see Chapter 23):

- Renal disease including renal transplantation
- Hypertension
- Congenital heart disease
- Severe anaemia
- Sickle-cell disease
- Systemic lupus erythematosus
- Cystic fibrosis
- HIV infection.

Family history

In relation to a LFD uterus, a family history of diabetes will put the patient at increased risk of developing gestational diabetes in her current pregnancy.

There is also evidence that a family history of pre-eclampsia is relevant. This disorder can be associated with IUGR (see Chapter 22).

Social history

The ethnic group of the patient can be relevant in a SFD patient. The growth charts used in most units were derived from Caucasian populations, in whom the average birthweight is greater than, for example, an Asian population. Hence some units have developed customized growth charts for each particular patient group.

Smoking in pregnancy is a major cause of a fetus being SGA, so that the abdomen palpates as SFD. It affects growth in the third trimester. Alcohol and illegal drug use are also causes of being SGA and so all these factors must be checked in the antenatal history.

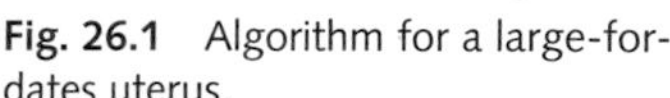

EXAMINATION

Chapter 3 discusses examination of the pregnant patient and the uterus. General examination should include checking blood pressure, and urinalysis for proteinuria or glycosuria. Body mass index should be routinely calculated at the booking visit. If it is below the normal range, the fetus is at risk of measuring SFD in the third trimester. Conversely, a raised BMI may make it difficult to assess fetal size accurately, as well as increasing the risk of gestational diabetes. In both situations, it is appropriate to arrange serial growth scans. The following should be noted on abdominal palpation in relation to LFD or SFD:

- SFH
- Number of fetuses
- Fetal lie
- Liquor volume
- Presence of uterine fibroids
- Presence of adnexal masses.

INVESTIGATION

Figures 26.1 and 26.2 provide algorithms for the investigation of the LFD and SFD uterus.

Blood tests

In the case of a LFD uterus, a glucose tolerance test should be arranged to establish whether gestational diabetes has developed (see Chapter 23). If polyhydramnios is found in the absence of diabetes, fetal infection may be the cause so maternal antibodies (IgM and IgG) to rubella and cytomegalovirus should be investigated.

Fig. 26.1 Algorithm for a large-for-dates uterus.

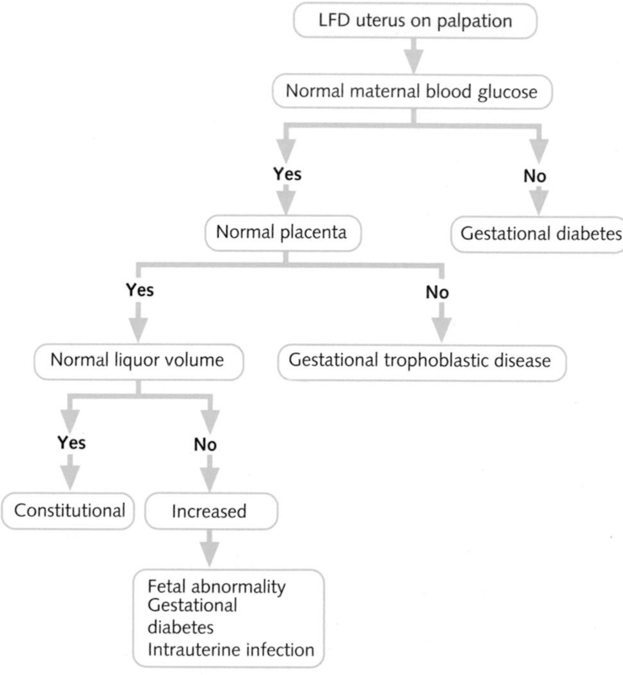

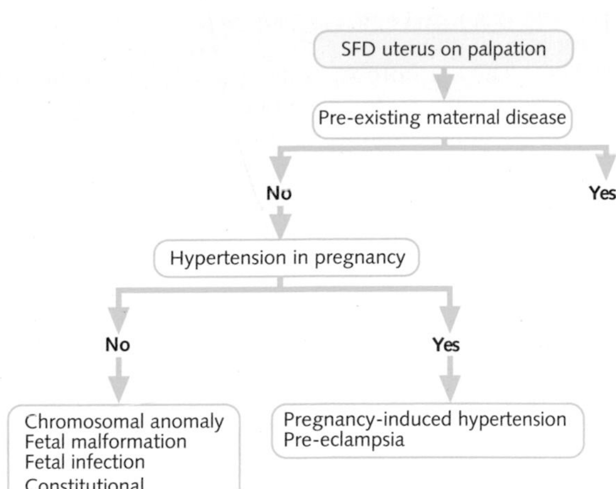

Fig. 26.2 Algorithm for a small-for-dates uterus.

A patient who is SFD and is also hypertensive should be investigated for pre-eclampsia (see Chapter 22). The blood investigations include a full blood count, liver and renal function tests, including a uric acid level.

HINTS AND TIPS

If there is no evidence of uteroplacental insufficiency, the other causes of the fetus being small-for-dates should be excluded. Ultrasound scan should examine for fetal abnormalities and check for signs of in utero infection. Prior screening for chromosomal abnormalities should be reviewed.

Ultrasound

Fetal ultrasound

Plotting ultrasound measurements of head circumference, abdominal circumference and femur length on a growth chart is the main method of monitoring fetal growth, either LFD or SFD. In the case of SFD, then serial measurements, at least 2 weeks apart, should be taken to distinguish between SGA and IUGR. The latter is often secondary to uteroplacental insufficiency.

With IUGR, the fetus preferentially diverts blood to the vital organs. There is less blood to the kidneys and, therefore, reduced production of liquor (oligohydramnios), as well as less storage of glycogen in the fetal liver. The latter results in a tailing off of the abdominal circumference measurement.

HINTS AND TIPS

The fetal causes of oligohydramnios are related to its ability to produce urine and thus liquor, e.g. renal agenesis. The fetal causes of polyhydramnios are secondary to its inability to swallow liquor, e.g. oesophageal atresia.

Placenta/liquor ultrasound

Trophoblastic disease is usually excluded at the 12-week dating scan by checking the structure of the placenta (see Chapter 20). This condition very rarely presents later in pregnancy with a uterus that palpates LFD.

A scan can also be used to measure the liquor volume objectively (Fig. 26.3). The amniotic fluid index (AFI) is the sum of the fluid pockets in the four quadrants of the abdomen. The amount varies with gestation, but the normal range is 5–25 cm.

Fig. 26.3 Causes of increased or decreased liquor volume.

Increased liquor volume	Decreased liquor volume
Diabetes	Ruptured membranes
Fetal abnormality	Fetal abnormality
Multiple pregnancy	Aneuploidy
Fetal infection	IUGR
	Fetal infection
	Maternal drugs eg atenolol

Maternal ultrasound

Ultrasound scan is useful to diagnose uterine fibroids or the presence of ovarian cysts.

Doppler studies

In conjunction with growth scans and measurement of the liquor volume, Doppler waveforms of the blood flow in the uteroplacental and fetal circulations can be used to assess the fetus. Increased placental vascular resistance, for example in pre-eclampsia, changes the pattern of the flow in the umbilical artery. There is normally flow towards the placenta during fetal diastole. However, as the placental resistance increases, diastolic flow becomes absent and then reversed. Other vessels can also be examined within the fetus, including the middle cerebral artery and the ductus venosus, to look for patterns of flow redistribution or, in severe cases, heart failure, that occur if the placental blood flow is insufficient.

Cardiotocography

The cardiotocography (CTG) can be used to assess the IUGR fetus. When not in labour, the tracing might be abnormal if the uteroplacental insufficiency is severe. The presence of the following should be excluded:

- Reduced variability
- Bradycardia
- Tachycardia
- Decelerations.

Further reading

NICE, 2008. Diabetes. Guideline CG63. National Institute for Health and Care Excellence, London. Available online at: www.nice.org.uk.

RCOG, 2013. Small for Gestational Age Fetus, Investigation and Management. Green-top Guideline No. 31. Royal College of Obstetricians and Gynaecologists, London. Available online at:www.rcog.org.uk.

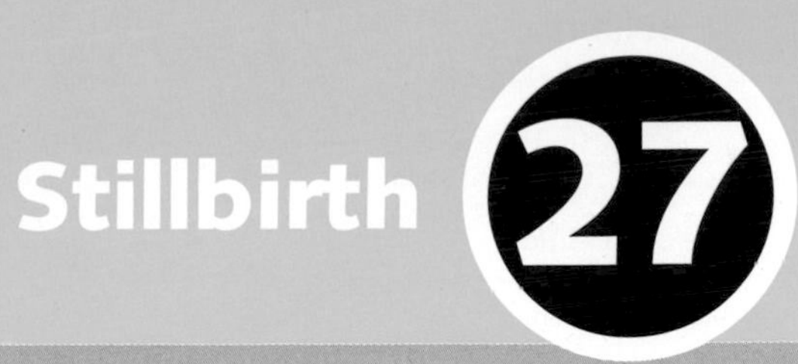

Stillbirth 27

Objectives

By the end of this chapter, you should be able to:

- Understand the definition of stillbirth and the prevalence
- Understand the diagnosis and management
- Understand the key investigations.

INTRODUCTION

Despite advances in prenatal and antenatal care, stillbirth is still a common occurrence and has a massive impact on the families affected. Investigations into the cause of stillbirth by means of maternal investigations and a post mortem are aimed at reducing the risk of this devastating situation recurring in a future pregnancy and potentially identifying causes, which may help reduce the overall incidence (Fig. 27.1).

DEFINITIONS

- Stillbirth: A baby that is born with no signs of life after 24 completed weeks of pregnancy.
- Intrauterine death: A fetus in utero **greater than 24 completed weeks** of pregnancy found to have no cardiac activity.

INCIDENCE

As mentioned above stillbirth is common, with an incidence of 1 in 200 babies. In 2007 there were 4027 stillbirths in the UK, with Scotland having the highest rate. More than 50% of stillbirths were found to be unexplained.

DIAGNOSIS

Most commonly a diagnosis of an intrauterine death is made when the patient presents with reduced fetal movements. Occasionally it will be made during a routine antenatal visit when the clinician is unable to auscultate the fetal heart. It can also present with symptoms of the event that caused the baby to die, e.g. antepartum haemorrhage and abdominal pain associated with a placental abruption.

When a patient presents with reduced fetal movements and one is unable to auscultate the fetal heart using a cardiotocography machine or handheld Doppler this should prompt rapid referral to a trained clinician to perform a real-time ultrasound. Diagnosis of an intrauterine death can only be made using ultrasound, when no fetal heart activity can be seen. Ideally, this should be verified by a second appropriately trained individual.

TELLING THE PARENTS

Conveying the diagnosis of an intrauterine death to the parents can be one of the most challenging things a clinician ever has to do. It is imperative that the parents are told straight away in a sensitive and empathetic manner using clear unambiguous terms. Occasionally, if a mother presents on her own, one should offer to call her partner or a relative to come and join her.

HISTORY

Taking a history from a patient diagnosed with an intrauterine death is aimed at:

- assessing maternal well-being
- identifying potential risk factors.

Using the handheld obstetric notes to review their past obstetric and medical history or by direct questioning of the patient, the following points should be identified:

- Maternal rhesus group – mothers that are rhesus negative should be investigated to rule out the possibility of rhesus disease as cause of the stillbirth (see Chapter 2 Antenatal Care).

Fig. 27.1 Causes of stillbirth.

Type of condition	Cause of stillbirth
Maternal condition	Diabetes (pre-existing and gestational) Pre-eclampsia Sepsis Obstetric cholestasis Acute fatty liver Thrombophilias, e.g. protein C and protein S resistance, factor V Leiden mutation, antithrombin III deficiency
Fetal condition	Infection: *Toxoplasma*, *Listeria*, *Syphilis*, parvovirus Chromosomal abnormality Structural abnormality Rhesus disease leading to severe anaemia Twin-to-twin transfusion syndrome (affects monochorionic twins only) IUGR Alloimmune thrombocytopaenia
Placental condition	Postmaturity Abruption Placenta praevia: significant bleed Cord prolapse

- Trisomy screening – trisomy screening is usually offered to patients in the first trimester, the results should be checked. In patients found to be high risk, a chromosomal abnormality may be the cause.
- Ultrasound – the anomaly ultrasound scan and any subsequent growth scans should be reviewed as any abnormality, either structural or growth related, may indicate a potential cause.
- Antepartum haemorrhage – recurrent bleeds or, indeed, a large bleed may indicate a placental abruption or vasa praevia (a situation where unprotected placental vessels course through the membranes and if ruptured can lead to rapid loss of fetal blood and fetal death.
- Ruptured membranes – any history of vaginal fluid loss may indicate a breach in the fetal membranes exposing the fetus to ascending infection (chorioamnionitis).
- Itching – itching mainly affecting the palms and soles may indicate obstetric cholestasis, which is associated with an increased risk of stillbirth.
- Signs of maternal illness – fever, rash or vomiting may indicate an intercurrent illness as the cause of the fetal demise. Listeria, toxoplasmosis and parvovirus are all possible infections with can lead to intrauterine death.

EXAMINATION

A thorough general examination is important to identify any potential signs of maternal illness. Even in the absence of a preceding maternal illness, an intrauterine death can lead to maternal sepsis and/or coagulopathy. Examination should include:

- maternal pulse
- blood pressure
- respiratory rate
- temperature
- looking for rashes (may indicate maternal infection)
- or excoriations (may indicate obstetric cholestasis)

The uterus should also be palpated to assess its size, tone and contour. A uterus which is larger than one would expect for the gestation may indicate polyhydramnios, which can be secondary to maternal diabetes. A uterus which is smaller than expected may indicate IUGR. A tender firm uterus may indicate a placental abruption whereas a tender but soft uterus may indicate chorioamnionitis.

INVESTIGATIONS

Investigations in the setting of an intrauterine death are aimed at:

1. assessing the current state of maternal well-being
2. identifying a potential cause of the stillbirth
3. possibly identifying any prognostic factors for future pregnancy.

It is important that parents are told that in around 50% of all cases, no cause will be found. However, investigation is still essential – if a cause is found, this may be vital in preventing recurrence.

Haematology and biochemistry

- Full blood count – assess maternal haemoglobin levels in the context of a haemorrhage, maternal white cells if infection is suspected and platelets if a coagulopathy is suspected
- Creatinine-reactive protein – useful in infection, although non-specific as to the site
- Urea and electrolytes – assess renal function in pre-eclampsia, haemorrhage and sepsis, also useful as a baseline
- Liver function tests – assess in pre-eclampsia, obstetric cholestasis, haemorrhage and sepsis, also useful as a baseline
- Coagulation screen – assess the possibility of coagulopathy
- Kleihauer – essential for ALL women, (not just those who are rhesus negative) in order to estimate a feto-maternal haemorrhage AND allows dose calculation of anti-D in rhesus-negative patients
- Maternal thrombophilia screen +/- antibody screen – indicated if intrauterine growth restriction or hydrops identified respectively
- Random blood sugar and HbA1c – may indicate occult gestational diabetes or indeed Type 1 or Type 2 diabetes
- Maternal thyroid function – may indicate occult thyroid disease
- Parental karyotyping – indicated if fetal karyotype indicates an unbalanced translocation or if fetal karyotyping not possible and features indicate a chromosomal cause.

Microbiology

- Urine dip plus MSU – assesses the possibility of urinary tract infection, proteinuria may indicate pre-eclampsia and ketonuria in a diabetic patient would prompt assessment to rule out ketoacidosis
- Blood cultures, vaginal swabs, cervical swabs – should be performed if sepsis is suspected as they will allow accurate identification of a pathogen and appropriate antibiotic therapy
- Maternal infection serology – parvovirus B19, toxoplasmosis, rubella, cytomegalovirus, syphilis (TORCH screen).

Pathology

A post-mortem examination should be offered to all parents where an intrauterine death has been diagnosed. It is carried out by a specialist perinatal pathologist and involves examination of the placenta and fetal karyotype, as well as the fetus. A post-mortem can also be limited to a specific organ if an abnormality was suspected antenatally. It is important to emphasize that agreeing to a post mortem will not affect any funeral arrangements.

> **COMMUNICATION**
>
> Some individuals may have religious or cultural beliefs against a post mortem and these should be respected. External examination only +/- imaging, or placental examination only may be acceptable.

MANAGEMENT

Once an intrauterine death has been confirmed and the parents have been informed, it is important to allow them the time to absorb the information, as well as starting to grieve. Subsequently, a plan of care needs to be made detailing the method of delivery.

In most cases a vaginal delivery will be the most suitable way to deliver the fetus, having less impact on mode of delivery for a subsequent pregnancy. An anti-progesterone (Mifepristone) is given orally and then after 48 hours, a course of prostaglandins (e.g. misoprostol) is administered, either orally or vaginally. For gestations nearer term, an oxytocin infusion may be used as an alternative to the prostaglandin.

Rarely, labour is contraindicated, e.g. multiple previous caesarean sections or extensive uterine surgery, and a caesarean section may be required.

AFTER DELIVERY

Most units have a specialist midwife who acts as a direct contact for the patient and ensures appropriate follow-up counselling and investigations take place. In the UK, this should include details about the Stillbirth & Neonatal Death charity (SANDS), which offers support to parents. The immediate period following a stillbirth is a very vulnerable time for the mother and she is at significant risk of postnatal depression. Mothers should be offered cabergoline to suppress lactation if they wish to do so.

> **COMMUNICATION**
>
> Following delivery the parents are encouraged to hold the baby (if they wish to do so) and mementos such as pictures and foot/hand prints are taken. Religious ceremonies can also take place if the parents wish.
>
> It is very important to arrange a follow-up appointment with the consultant in charge of their care to ensure all investigations are reviewed and a plan made for future pregnancies. As always, cases need to be handled with great sensitivity and care.

Further reading

RCOG, 2010. Late Intrauterine Fetal Death and Stillbirth. Green-top Guideline No. 55. Royal College of Obstetricians and Gynaecologists, London.

Schott, J., Henley, A., Kohner, N., 2007. Pregnancy Loss and the Death of a Baby: Guidelines for Professionals, third ed. Stillbirth and Neonatal Death Charity, London.

Labour 28

Objectives

By the end of this chapter, you should be able to:
- Define the onset of labour
- Describe the normal delivery of the fetus
- Understand that normal progress in labour is multifactorial
- Describe the benefits and side effects of pharmacological methods of analgesia in labour
- Understand the different methods used to induce labour.

Labour is divided into three stages:
- **First stage**: from the onset of established labour until the cervix is fully dilated
- **Second stage**: from full dilatation until the fetus is born
- **Third stage**: from the birth of the fetus until delivery of the placenta and membranes.

ONSET OF LABOUR

Prior to the onset of labour, painless irregular uterine tightenings, known as Braxton Hicks contractions, become increasingly frequent. As the presenting part becomes engaged, the uterine fundus descends, reducing upper abdominal discomfort, and pressure in the pelvis increases. The signs and symptoms that define the actual onset of established labour are:
- painful regular contractions
- cervical dilatation of ≥4 cm and effacement (see Fig. 3.10).

These factors diagnose labour, with or without a 'show' (passage of a mucoid plug from the cervix, often blood-stained) or ruptured membranes. Irregular contractions prior to cervical dilatation and effacement are part of the latent phase of labour, which may be very variable in duration.

The exact cause of the onset of labour is not known. To some degree it is thought to be mechanical, since preterm labour is seen more commonly in circumstances in which the uterus is overstretched, such as multiple pregnancies and polyhydramnios. Inflammatory markers such as cytokines, and prostaglandins also play a role. The latter are thought to be present in the decidua and membranes in late pregnancy and are released if the cervix is digitally stretched at term to separate the membranes (a cervical sweep).

NORMAL PROGRESS IN LABOUR

Once the diagnosis of established labour has been made, progress is assessed by monitoring:
- uterine contractions
- dilatation of the cervix
- descent of the presenting part.

The rate of cervical dilatation is expected to be approximately 0.5–1 cm/h in a nulliparous woman and 1–2 cm/h in a multiparous woman. A partogram is commonly used to chart the observations made in labour (Fig. 28.1) and to highlight slow progress, particularly a delay in cervical dilatation or failure of the presenting part to descend (see Chapter 30).

Progress is determined by three factors:
- Passages
- Passenger
- Power.

Passages

Bony pelvis

The pelvis is made up of four bones:
- Two innominate bones
- Sacrum
- Coccyx.

The passage that these bones make can be divided into inlet and outlet, with the cavity between them (Fig. 28.2). The pelvic inlet is bounded by the pubic crest, the iliopectineal line and the sacral promontory. It is oval in shape, with its wider diameter being transverse. The cavity of the pelvis is round in shape. The pelvic outlet is bounded by the lower border of the pubic symphysis, the ischial spines and the tip of the sacrum. Again the shape is oval, but the wider diameter is anteroposterior.

Fig. 28.1 A partogram showing progress and observations in labour.

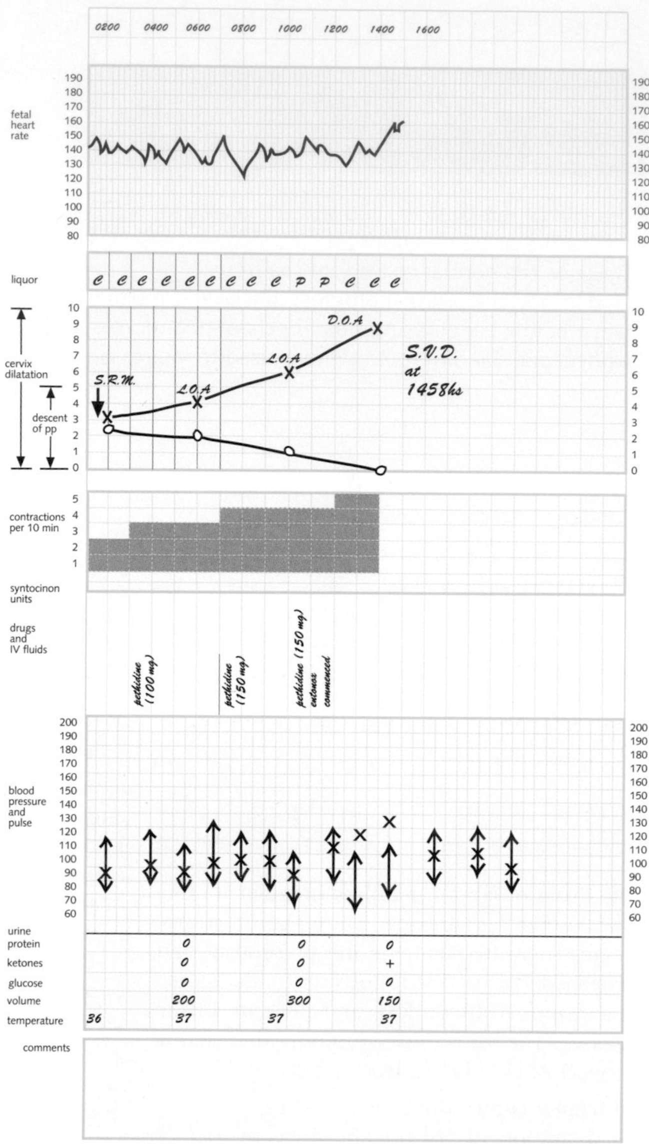

When a woman stands upright, the pelvis tilts forward. The inlet makes an angle of about 55° with the horizontal; this angle varies between individuals and different ethnic groups. The presenting part of the fetus must negotiate the axis of the birth canal with the change of direction occurring by rotation at the level of the pelvic floor muscles (see below).

Soft tissues

The soft passages consist of:

- uterus (upper and lower segments)
- cervix
- pelvic floor
- vagina
- perineum.

The upper uterine segment is responsible for the propulsive contractions that deliver the fetus. The lower segment is the part of the uterus that lies between the uterovesical fold of the peritoneum and the cervix. It develops gradually during the third trimester, and then more rapidly during labour. It incorporates the cervix as the cervix effaces, to allow the presenting part to descend.

The pelvic floor consists of the levator ani group of muscles, including pubococcygeus and iliococcygeus arising from the bony pelvis to form a muscular diaphragm along with the internal obturator muscle and piriformis muscle (see Chapter 15). As the presenting part of the

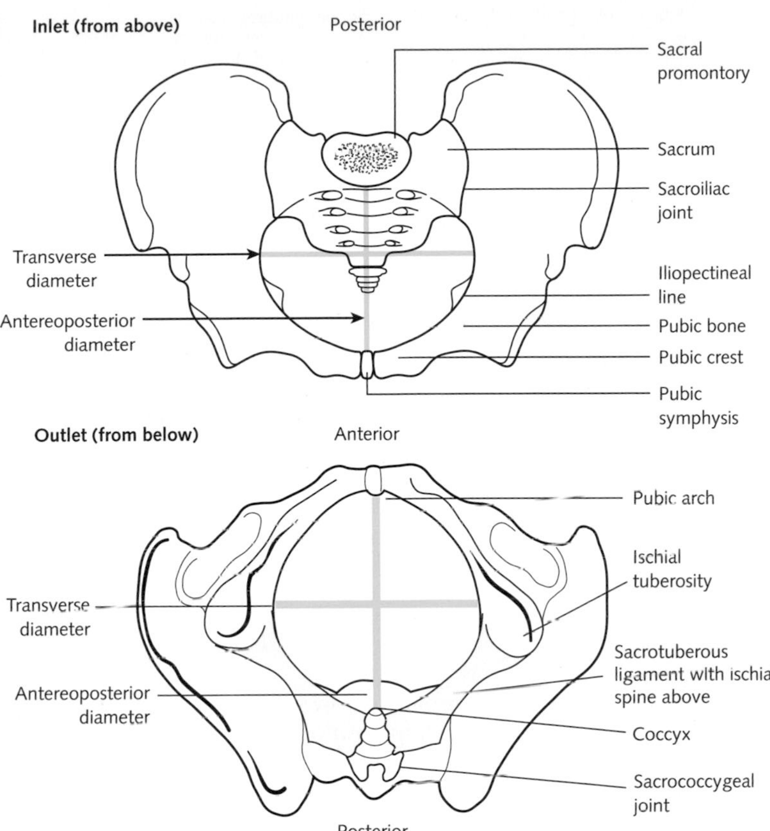

Fig. 28.2 The boundaries of the pelvic inlet and the pelvic outlet.

fetus is pushed out of the uterus it passes into the vagina, which has become hypertrophied during pregnancy. It reaches the pelvic floor, which acts like a gutter to direct it forwards and allow rotation. The perineum is distal to this and stretches as the head passes below the pubic arch and delivers.

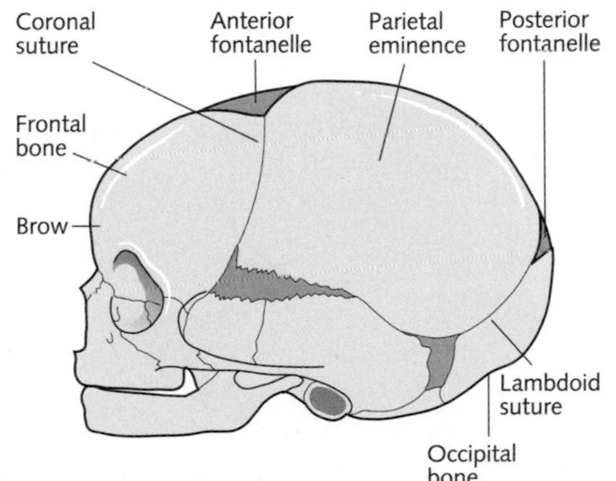

Fig. 28.3 The fetal skull showing the landmarks.

Passenger

The fetal skull consists of the face and the cranium. The cranium is made up of two parietal bones, two frontal bones and the occipital bone (see Fig. 3.13), held together by a membrane that allows movement. Up until early childhood, these bones are not fused and so can overlap to allow the head to pass through the pelvis during labour; this overlapping of the bones is known as moulding.

Figure 28.3 shows the anatomy of the fetal skull, including the sutures between the bones, and the spaces known as fontanelles. These are important landmarks that can be felt on vaginal examination in established labour and enable the position of the fetus to be assessed (see Fig. 3.14). The position is described in terms of the occiput in a cephalic presentation, and the sacrum in a breech presentation.

The degree of flexion and the position of the fetal skull determine the ease with which the fetus passes through the birth canal. Figure 28.4 shows the diameters of the fetal skull. The diameter that presents during labour depends on the degree of flexion of the head. The head usually becomes more flexed with the increasing strength of the uterine contractions. Thus the smallest diameters for

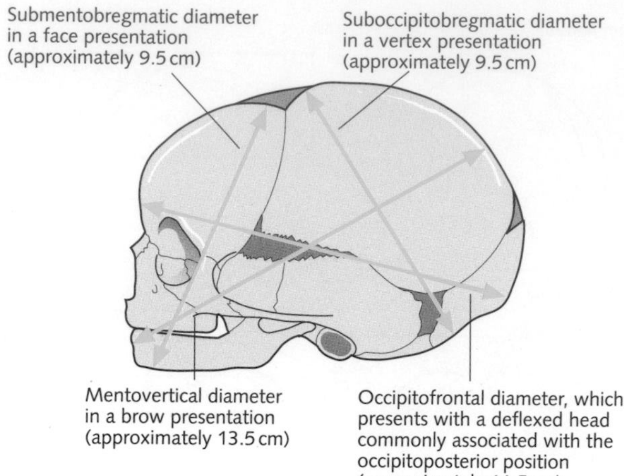

Fig. 28.4 Diameters of the fetal skull.

delivery are the suboccipitobregmatic diameter, which represents a flexed vertex presentation, and the submentobregmatic diameter, which corresponds to a face presentation. The widest diameter is mentovertical, a brow presentation, which usually precludes vaginal delivery.

Power

The myometrial component of the uterus acts as the power to deliver the fetus. It consists of three layers:

- Thin outer longitudinal layer
- Thin inner circular layer
- Thick middle spiral layer.

From early pregnancy, the uterus contracts painlessly and irregularly (Braxton Hicks contractions). These contractions increase after the 36th week until the onset of labour. In labour, a contraction starts from the junction of the fallopian tube and the uterus on each side, spreading down and across the uterus with its greatest intensity in the upper uterine segment. Like any other muscle, the myometrium contracts and relaxes, but it also has the ability to retract so that the fibres become progressively shorter. This effect is seen in the lower segment: progressive retraction causes the lower segment to stretch and thin out, resulting in effacement and dilatation of the cervix (see Fig. 3.10).

During labour, the contractions are monitored for:

- strength
- frequency
- duration.

The resting tone of the uterus is about 6–12 mmHg; to be effective in labour this increases to an intensity of 40–60 mmHg. There are usually three or four coordinated strong contractions every 10 minutes, each lasting approximately 60 s, in order to progress in labour.

In the second stage of labour, additional power comes from voluntary contraction of the diaphragm and the abdominal muscles as the mother pushes to assist delivery.

DELIVERY OF THE FETUS

Active contractions of the uterus of increasing strength, frequency and duration cause passive movement of the fetus down the birth canal. At the beginning of labour, the fetus usually engages in the occipito-transverse or occipito-anterior position, i.e. in a position appropriate to the wider transverse diameter of the pelvic inlet. As labour progresses (Fig. 28.5), the head becomes fully flexed so that the suboccipitobregmatic diameter is presenting (see above).

As descent occurs through the pelvic cavity, internal rotation brings the occiput into the anterior position as it reaches the pelvic floor. This means that the head is now in the appropriate position to negotiate the wider diameter of the pelvic outlet, which is anteroposterior. In the second stage of labour, the occiput descends below the symphysis pubis (Fig. 28.6) and delivers by

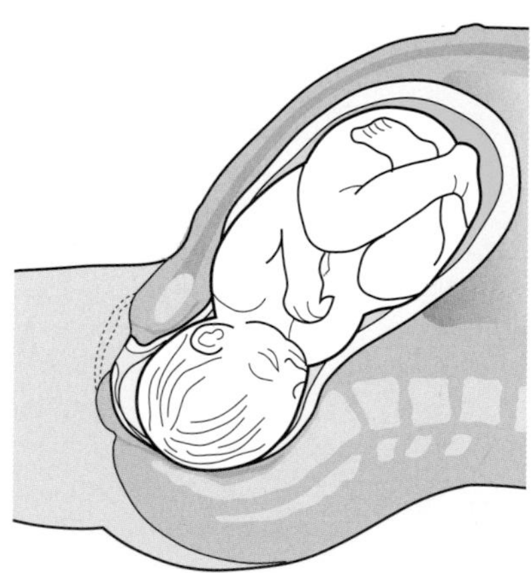

Fig. 28.5 Early labour. There has been flexion of the fetal head. The cervix is effacing and has begun to dilate.

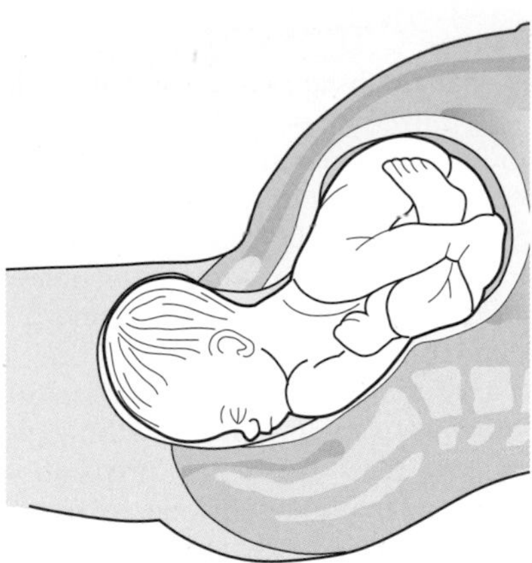

Fig. 28.6 The second stage of labour. The head has undergone internal rotation to bring the occiput into the anterior position. The cervix is fully dilated.

extension. Increasing extension round the pubic bone delivers the face (Fig. 28.7).

Delivery of the head brings the widest diameter of the shoulders (the bisacromial diameter) through the transverse diameter of the pelvic inlet into the pelvic cavity. External rotation or restitution occurs where the head rotates to a transverse position in relation to the shoulders (Fig. 28.8). This progresses with continuing descent and rotation of the shoulders to bring the bisacromial diameter into the anteroposterior diameter of the pelvic outlet. Further contractions and maternal effort enable the anterior shoulder to pass under the pubis, usually assisted by gentle downward traction on the head. Lateral flexion of the fetus delivers the posterior shoulder and the rest of the body follows (Fig. 28.9).

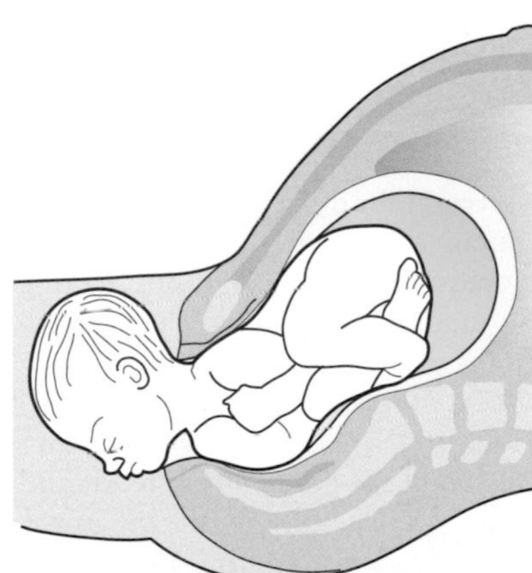

Fig. 28.7 Delivery of the head. Extension of the fetal neck occurs as the head passes under the pubic symphysis to deliver the head.

HINTS AND TIPS

The mechanism of delivery can be more easily remembered in four stages, thinking about how the head and shoulders must negotiate the different diameters of the maternal pelvis:

- Flexion of the head
- Internal rotation
- Extension
- External rotation (restitution).

A

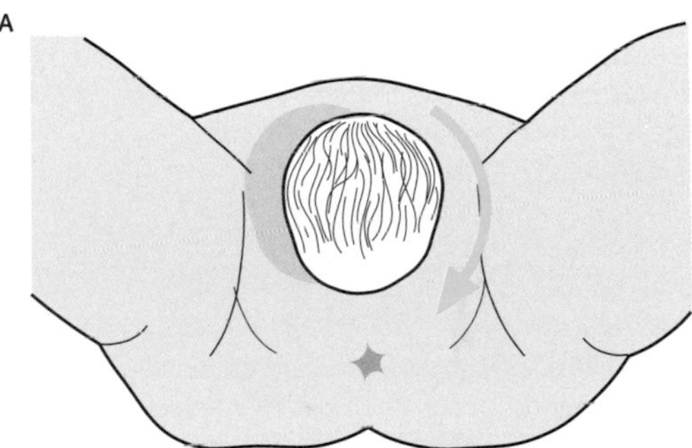

B

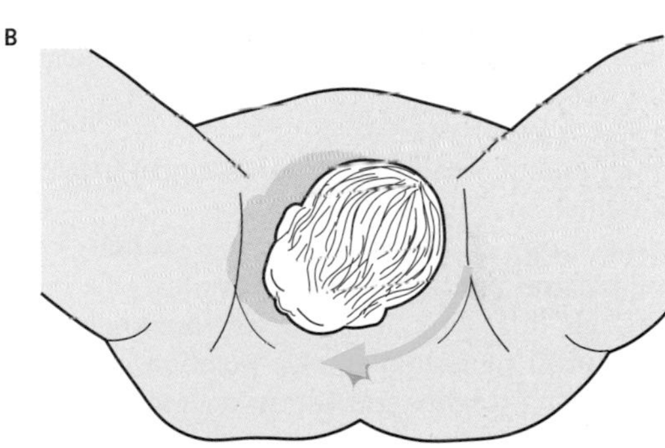

C

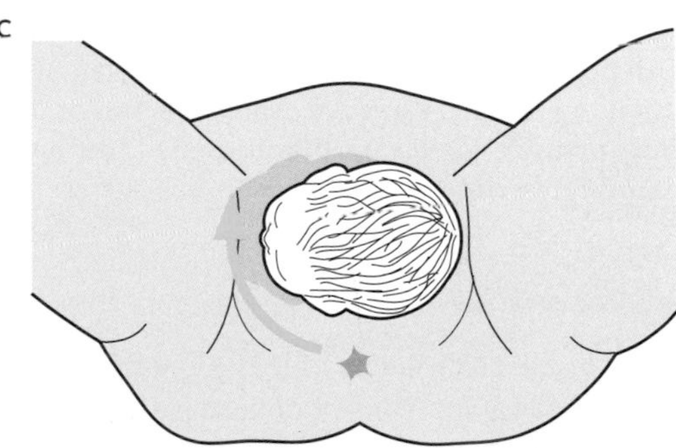

Fig. 28.8 External rotation (restitution). The head distends the perineum as it delivers in the occipitoanterior position and the external rotation occurs to allow delivery of the shoulders.

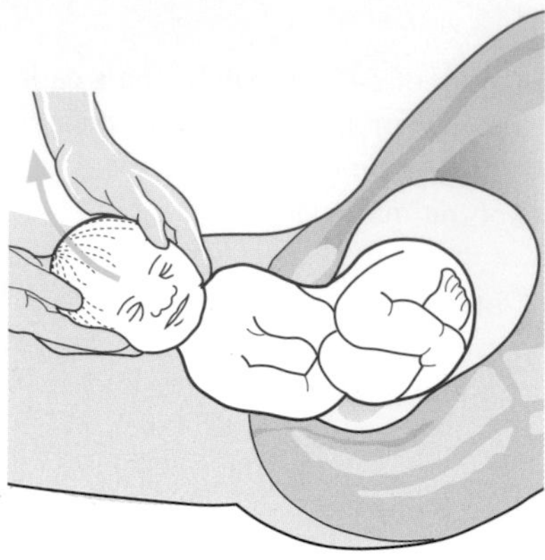

Fig. 28.9 Delivery of the shoulders. The anterior shoulder passes below the pubic symphysis, aided by downward traction of the head by the midwife or doctor. The posterior shoulder delivers as the head is gently lifted upwards.

MANAGEMENT OF THE FIRST STAGE OF LABOUR

When a patient presents in the first stage of labour, routine assessment includes the mother and fetus. Regular examination of the mother should include:

- pulse, blood pressure, respiratory rate, temperature
- urinalysis
- analgesia requirements
- abdominal palpation: symphysis-fundal height, lie, presentation, engagement
- contractions: strength, frequency, duration
- vaginal examination: degree of cervical effacement, cervical dilatation, station of presenting part in relation to ischial spines, position of presenting part, presence of caput or moulding (see Chapter 30).

The fetus must be assessed by fetal heart rate pattern, either by intermittent auscultation or electronically depending on risk factors (see Chapter 31). If the membranes are ruptured, then the liquor must be documented as clear, blood-stained or having meconium present.

HINTS AND TIPS

Descent of the presenting part is assessed by both abdominal palpation (amount of head felt above the pelvic brim expressed in fifths = **engagement**) and vaginal examination (descent in relation to level of ischial spines = **station**).

Maternal monitoring

As well as regular observations, the patient is encouraged to mobilize if possible and is allowed to eat, depending on her risk of needing an operative procedure. There is delayed gastric emptying during pregnancy and labour. Therefore, if an emergency general anaesthetic is needed, there is an increased risk of inhalation of regurgitated acidic stomach contents, causing Mendelson's syndrome.

The need for analgesia during labour varies markedly between different women, different ethnic groups and depending on their antenatal preparation. Non-pharmacological techniques include the use of psychoprophylaxis, hypnosis, massage and transcutaneous electrical nerve stimulation (TENS). The pharmacological methods are summarized in Figure 28.10.

Fetal monitoring

Intermittent or continuous fetal monitoring is appropriate, depending on the clinical picture antenatally and in labour. For example, in the presence of IUGR or if there is meconium-stained liquor, then continuous fetal monitoring is advisable (see Chapter 31). In a low-risk pregnancy, intermittent monitoring with a sonicaid or with a Pinard stethoscope is sufficient, every 15 min during and after a contraction for 60 seconds in the 1st stage of labour, and every 5 min in the 2nd stage.

In some patients, abdominal monitoring can be difficult, for example, if the patient is obese, and so a fetal scalp electrode can be applied directly to the head once the cervix dilates and the membranes are ruptured. If monitoring suggests that the fetal heart rate pattern is pathological, it may be appropriate to measure the fetal pH by taking a blood sample from the fetal scalp (see Chapter 31).

MANAGEMENT OF THE SECOND STAGE OF LABOUR

Once the cervix is fully dilated, the patient is encouraged to use voluntary effort to push with the contractions. If she has an epidural anaesthetic in situ she might be less aware of an urge to push, and so a further hour can be allowed for the presenting part to descend with the contractions alone. Without an epidural, the mother may adopt various positions for delivery of the fetus. As the head descends, the perineum distends and the anus dilates. Finally, the head crowns: the biparietal diameter has passed through the pelvis and there is no recession between contractions. The attendant can apply pressure on the perineum for support during delivery of the head. Once delivered, the neck is felt to exclude the presence of the cord.

Fig. 28.10 Pharmacological methods of analgesia in labour.

	Technique	Indication	Effectiveness	Duration of effect	Side-effects
Oxygen/ nitrous oxide	Inhalation of 50:50 mixture with onset of contraction	First stage	< 50% Takes 20–30 s for peak effect	Time of inhalation only	Does not relieve pain
Pethidine	Intramuscular injection 100–150 mg	First stage	<50% Takes 15–20 min for peak effect	Approximately 3 h	Nausea and vomiting – give with an antiemetic Respiratory depression in the neonate (this is easily reversed with intramuscular naloxone)
Pudendal block	Infiltration of right and left pudendal nerves (S2, S3 and S4) with 0.5% lidocaine	Second stage for operative delivery	Within 5 min	45–90 min	—
Perineal infiltration	Infiltration of perineum with 0.5% lidocaine at posterior fourchette	Second stage prior to episiotomy Third stage for suturing of perineal lacerations	Within 5 min	45–90 min	—
Epidural anaesthesia	Injection of 0.25% or 0.5% bupivicaine via a catheter into the epidural space (L3–4)	First or second stage Caesarean section	Complete pain relief in approximately 95% of women within 20-30 mins	Bolus injection every 3–4 h or continuous infusion	Transient hypotension – give intravenous fluid load Dural tap Risk of haemorrhage if abnormal maternal clotting Increased length of second stage because of reduced pelvic floor tone and loss of bearing-down reflex
Spinal anaesthesia	Injection of 0.5% bupivicaine into the subarachnoid space	Any operative delivery; manual removal of the placenta	Immediate effect	Single injection lasting 3–4 h	Respiratory depression

After external rotation, lateral flexion of the head towards the anus dislodges the anterior shoulder from behind the pubic symphysis with the next contraction. Lifting the head gently in the opposite direction delivers the posterior shoulder. Holding the shoulders, the rest of the body is delivered either onto the bed or the mother's abdomen. Finally, the cord is divided and cut.

MANAGEMENT OF THE THIRD STAGE OF LABOUR

Active management of the third stage has been shown to reduce the incidence of postpartum haemorrhage (PPH) (see Chapter 33). Management involves:

- using an oxytocic drug
- clamping and cutting the cord
- controlled cord traction.

In most units, syntocinon (5 units of oxytocin) or syntometrine (oxytocin with 0.5 mg ergometrine) is given intramuscularly with delivery of the anterior shoulder; it takes about 2–3 min to act. As the placenta detaches from the uterine wall, the cut cord will appear to lengthen. There is usually some bleeding and the fundus becomes hard. Brandt-Andrews' method of controlled cord traction is commonly used to deliver the placenta once it has separated to reduce the incidence of uterine inversion (Fig. 28.11). The placenta and membranes must be checked to ensure that they are complete.

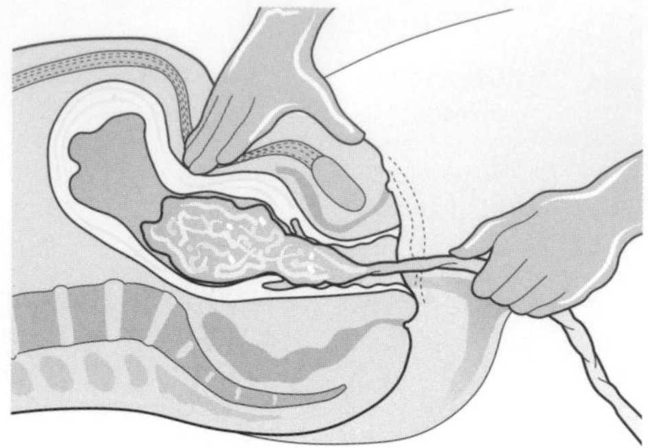

Fig. 28.11 Controlled cord traction to deliver the placenta.

Some patients choose to have a physiological 3rd stage. This means that they do not receive any routine oxytocic drugs, the attendant waits for the umbilical cord to stop pulsating before it is cut, and delivery of the placenta occurs passively. In situations where there is an increased risk of PPH or depending on parental choice, active management is advised as above.

Finally, the vagina, labia and perineum are examined for lacerations. The uterine fundus is palpated to check that it is well contracted, approximately at the level of the umbilicus. The estimated blood loss should be recorded.

INDUCTION OF LABOUR

Definition

Induction of labour is the artificial initiation of uterine contractions prior to spontaneous onset resulting in delivery of the baby.

Indications

The rate of induction varies widely between different units and even within different units. Figure 28.12 shows possible reasons for induction of labour, maternal or fetal. In the UK, the most common indication is prolonged pregnancy, more than 41 weeks' gestation.

Methods

Prior to induction of labour, the favourability of the cervix should be assessed. This is usually done by using the Bishop score (see Fig. 3.12); a higher score suggests a more favourable cervix. Complications of amniotomy and oxytocin are shown in Figure 28.13.

Fig. 28.12 Indications for the induction of labour.

Maternal	Severe pre-eclampsia Recurrent APH Pre-existing disease eg. diabetes Social
Fetal	Prolonged pregnancy Intrauterine growth restriction Rhesus disease

Fig. 28.13 Complications associated with the use of amniotomy and oxytocin.

Treatment	Complication
Amniotomy	Cord prolapse Infection Bleeding from a vasa praevia Placental separation Failure to induce efficient contractions Amniotic fluid embolism
Oxytocin	Abnormal fetal heart rate pattern Hyperstimulation of the uterus Rupture of the uterus Fluid overload

HINTS AND TIPS

With regard to the Bishop score to assess the cervix:

- Unfavourable cervix = hard, long, closed, not effaced (low Bishop score)
- Favourable cervix = soft, beginning to dilate and efface (high Bishop score).

Prostaglandins

Local application of a prostaglandin, usually prostaglandin E2, given as a vaginal gel or tablet, has been shown to ripen the cervix as part of the induction process and reduce the incidence of operative delivery when compared to use of oxytocin alone. Used locally instead of systemically, the gastrointestinal side effects are minimized. NICE guidelines have been produced to advise on the dose of prostaglandin given, in order to reduce the risk of uterine hyperstimulation.

Amniotomy

Artificial rupture of the membranes (ARM) is thought to cause local release of endogenous prostaglandins. It is done using an amnihook and may be part of the induction process or performed to accelerate slow progress in labour. It can also be done with an abnormal CTG to exclude meconium-staining of the liquor, or to allow application of a fetal scalp electrode.

Oxytocin

An intravenous infusion of synthetic oxytocin (syntocinon) is commonly used to induce labour, and to stimulate contractions after amniotomy or spontaneous rupture of membranes. The dose must be carefully titrated according to the strength and frequency of the uterine contractions, and continuous fetal monitoring is necessary.

Further reading

Enkin, M.W., Keirse, M.J.N.C., Neilson, J., et al., 2000. A Guide to Effective Care in Pregnancy and Childbirth, third ed. Oxford University Press, Oxford.

NICE, 2008. National Evidence-Based Clinical Guidelines. Induction of Labour. National Institute for Health and Care Excellence, London.

NICE, 2007. National Evidence-Based Clinical Guidelines. Intrapartum Care: Management and Delivery of Care to Women in Labour. National Institute for Health and Care Excellence, London.

RCOG, 1999. Working Party Report. Childbirth: Towards Safer Childbirth. Royal College of Obstetricians and Gynaecologists, London. Available online at: www.rcog.org.uk.

Preterm labour

Objectives

By the end of this chapter, you should be able to:

- Define preterm labour
- Discuss necessary investigations and treatments
- Be aware of the role of steroids and the importance of neonatal team involvement in counselling mothers
- Understand how preterm prelabour rupture of membranes is diagnosed and what the implications are.

PRETERM LABOUR

Preterm labour is defined as labour occurring after 24 weeks and before 37 weeks gestation, so diagnosis depends upon the accurate calculation of the estimated date of delivery at the first ultrasound scan between 11 and 14 weeks. It is important to establish whether labour is preterm for several reasons:

- Preterm labour has more risk of complications than labour at term, for example abnormal lie.
- Prematurity has potentially significant risk of morbidity to the baby – the paediatric team must be consulted.
- Up to 34 + 0 weeks' gestation, attempts should be made to stop the labour to administer corticosteroids to the mother, which will boost fetal lung surfactant production and, therefore, reduce neonatal respiratory distress.

HINTS AND TIPS

With improving standard of neonatal care it is easy to forget that prematurity is the single largest cause of neonatal mortality and long-term handicap in otherwise normal babies – preterm babies have a mortality rate of 42 per 1000 livebirths compared to 5 per 1000 livebirths overall (2005 statistics).

HINTS AND TIPS

Corticosteroids (betamethasone or dexamethasone) are given to the mother as two intramuscular injections 12–24 h apart. They have been shown to significantly reduce neonatal respiratory distress by stimulating fetal surfactant production and are recommended for any woman in threatened preterm labour between 24 + 0 and 34 + 6 weeks' gestation. Consideration should be given up to 38 + 6 weeks for women being delivered by elective caesarean section. Repeated courses of steroid administration are currently not recommended.

INCIDENCE

The incidence of preterm labour is currently around 7.6% in England and Wales, but this varies in different populations and the incidence is increasing. Risk factors for premature labour are shown in Figure 29.1, with the most significant association being a history of a previous preterm labour.

The main causes of preterm delivery are shown in Figure 29.2. Infection is thought to play a part in at least 20% of cases (Fig. 29.3 lists common pathogens implicated in preterm labour). Iatrogenic preterm delivery, accounting for one-third of preterm deliveries, occurs when obstetricians decide that delivery is necessary in the

Fig. 29.1 Risk factors for preterm labour.

- Previous preterm labour
- Smoking
- Low socio-economic group
- Body mass index <19
- Lack of social support
- Afro-Caribbean ethnicity
- Extremes of reproductive age (<20 or >35)
- Domestic violence
- Bacterial vaginosis
- Chronic medical conditions

Fig. 29.2 Causes of preterm delivery.

- Infection eg.chorioamnionitis, maternal pyelonephritis
- Uteroplacental ischaemia eg.abruption
- Uterine overdistension eg.polyhydramnios, multiple pregnancy
- Cervical incompetence
- Fetal abnormality
- Iatrogenic eg.delivery for severe IUGR caused by PET

Fig. 29.3 Pathogens implicated in preterm labour.

- Sexually transmitted: *Chlamydia, Trichomonas, Syphilis, Gonorrhoea*
- Enteric organisms: *Escherichia coli, Streptococcus faecalis*
- Bacterial vaginosis: *Gardnerella, Mycoplasma* and anaerobes
- Group B streptococcus (if a very heavy growth)

interests of fetal or maternal health, due, for example, to severe pre-eclampsia, or when scans have shown severe intrauterine growth restriction (IUGR) of the fetus.

HISTORY AND EXAMINATION

Preterm labour may be rapid in onset and progress, and is almost always unexpected. Therefore, history taking must be done as comprehensively as possible, taking into account the fact that some women will arrive in an advanced state of labour.

The history should include the timing of onset of the abdominal pain (see Chapter 25). Intermittent, but regular abdominal pain suggests uterine contractions. Frequency and intensity over time should be assessed. Preterm labour may be associated with clear watery vaginal discharge, suggesting possible rupture of the membranes, or bleeding, as with an antepartum haemorrhage (see Chapter 21). A history of normal fetal movements should be checked. With regards to possible infection, urinary and gastrointestinal symptoms should be elicited, as well as systemic symptoms such as fever. A past medical history and a social history should be taken as for the risk factors shown in Figure 29.1.

Examination must include baseline observations - pulse, blood pressure, respiratory rate and temperature - to look for possible infection. Abdominal palpation will assess:

- abdominal tenderness - site, guarding, rebound
- uterine tenderness - site
- uterine tone - soft or irritable, e.g. abruption
- uterine contractions - frequency and strength
- fetal lie, presentation and engagement.

Sterile speculum examination should be performed on a woman with abdominal pain or discharge. A vaginal swab should be taken if there is a clear watery loss suggesting ruptured membranes. Digital examination is necessary to check the dilatation of the cervix. A closed cervix in the presence of palpable uterine contractions is termed threatened preterm labour.

INVESTIGATION

As abnormal lie and presentation are far more common in preterm pregnancy, an ultrasound scan should be performed (see Chapter 30). Up to 25 + 6 weeks gestation, presence of the fetal heart beat should be confirmed with a sonicaid. After this gestation, a cardiotocograph should be performed, which will assess fetal well-being as well as indicating uterine activity.

Evidence of fetal fibronectin in the mother's cervical secretions can be checked using a specific kit; its absence suggests that delivery is less likely and this may assist with management decisions such as the need for tocolysis. Transvaginal scans may be used to examine the length of the cervix since cervical shortening is a predictor of preterm delivery (Fig. 29.4). Urinalysis must be performed to look for nitrites, which suggest a urinary tract infection.

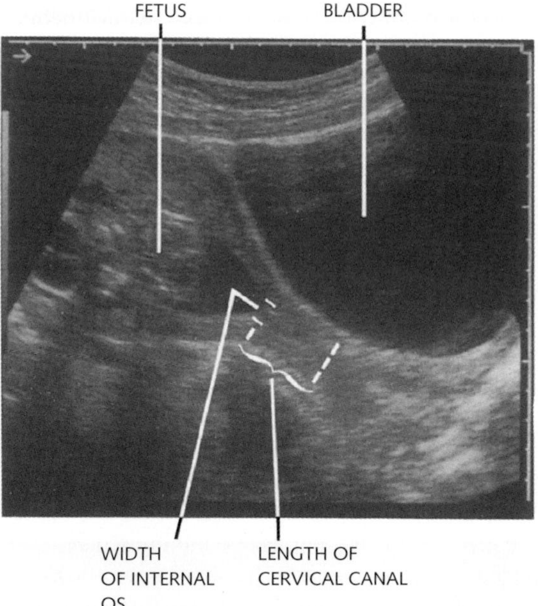

Fig. 29.4 Transvaginal scan of cervical canal. From Chudleigh 2004, with permission.

MANAGEMENT

Figure 29.5 summarizes the management plan for a woman who appears to be in preterm labour. Liaison with the neonatal team and administration of steroids are vital. Some hospitals do not have facilities for treating babies born under certain gestations and in these cases transfer to the nearest appropriate unit is made, preferably prior to delivery. If the mother is very unwell or if delivery is imminent, transfer of the baby can be arranged after delivery. Ideally, the paediatrician will have an opportunity to counsel the woman and her partner about expectations when the baby is born and some of the problems that premature babies encounter. A tour of the neonatal intensive care unit could be arranged.

HINTS AND TIPS

Parents need to be warned of problems encountered by children surviving extreme premature delivery, which may be cerebral palsy, chronic lung disease, visual and hearing deficits and learning difficulties.

Tocolysis

Administration of drugs to reduce the uterine activity should be considered depending on:

- cervical dilatation
- need to administer steroids and allow time for them to be effective
- need for in utero transfer.

Fig. 29.5 Management checklist for patient presenting in threatened preterm labour.

- Assess for signs of a precipitant of preterm labour, e.g. sepsis, polyhydramnios, abruption, severe pre-eclampsia, obstetric cholestasis. Take blood tests as appropriate. Perform urinalysis and send MSU
- Determine frequency and regularity of contractions. Monitor the fetal heart
- Perform a sterile speculum examination to examine the cervix. Take high vaginal and endocervical swabs.
- Start continuous electronic fetal monitoring (CTG) if there is cervical dilatation
- Ascertain fetal presentation (cephalic or breech)
- Give corticosteroids
- Give antibiotics if ruptured membranes or if obvious signs of sepsis
- Consider tocolysis
- Contact paediatricians and arrange transfer out if necessary and appropriate
- Discuss mode of delivery

The different drugs used to try to stop contractions are shown in Figure 29.6. They have been shown to delay the number of women who deliver within 48 hours, but there is no clear evidence that they improve perinatal morbidity and mortality overall. They allow time for corticosteroids and, if necessary, transfer to another hospital able to offer neonatal care, as above. With all drugs, the side effects on mother and fetus must be balanced against the benefit of prolonging the pregnancy. Tocolysis should not be used in the following circumstances:

- Maternal illness that would be helped by delivery, e.g. pre-eclampsia
- Evidence of fetal distress
- In the presence of chorioamnionitis
- When there has been significant vaginal bleeding, particularly if abruption is suspected
- Once the membranes have ruptured.

Antibiotic therapy

Antibiotics (erythromycin) are given prophylactically if the membranes have ruptured before term (around one-third of cases) to protect the fetus from ascending infection. If the membranes are intact the mother is screened for infection (vaginal and cervical swabs, blood cultures if pyrexial) and only given antibiotics if there are signs or confirmatory tests for sepsis.

Cervical cerclage

When there is cervical incompetence resulting in cervical dilatation but the patient is not actively labouring, a suture can be placed in the cervix to attempt to reduce the prolapse of membranes that will otherwise ensue. Once the membranes prolapse into the vagina they weaken and their rupture is likely, followed by delivery or the development of infection. The MacDonald suture, which is inserted vaginally as high in the cervix as possible, is used most commonly (Fig. 29.7). Other options are the Shirodkar suture, which is inserted vaginally, but involves the dissection of the bladder off the cervix, or a suture can be inserted into the cervix at laparotomy, which will therefore be placed higher. However, insertion of any suture can introduce infection or result in rupture of the membranes during the procedure.

Mode of delivery

In most cases of preterm labour, it is possible to plan for a normal vaginal birth. There is no firm evidence to show that caesarean section is safer for the baby than vaginal delivery, especially when the presentation is cephalic. However, the caesarean section rate is higher because of a higher incidence of low-lying placenta, fetal distress and abnormal lie in prematurity. Caesarean

Fig. 29.6 Drugs used to treat preterm labour.

Drug	Route of administration	Comments / Side effects
Oxytocin receptor antagonists eg atosiban	Intravenous	Well tolerated but expensive. 8% experience headache
Calcium-channel blockers eg. nifedipine	Oral	Block calcium channels in myometrium to reduce contractions. Not licensed in UK for this use. Side effects include headache, flushing and tremor
Beta blockers eg. ritodrine, salbutamol, terbutaline	Intravenous	Act on β receptors in myometrium to cause relaxation. Side effects are common, up to 80% of women, including tachycardia, headache, tremor, hyperglycaemia and hypokalaemia. Pulmonary oedema and myocardial ischaemia are potentially fatal. Fetal tachycardia may be seen.
Non-steroidal anti-inflammatory drugs eg. indomethacin	Oral	Act on cyclo-oxygenase enzyme that catalyses production of prostaglandin. Mild maternal side effects including heartburn and nausea. Potentially serious fetal effects including premature closure of the ductus arteriosus and reducing renal function causing oligohydramnios.
Nitric oxide donors eg. glyceryl trinitrate (GTN)	Transdermal patch	Act on myometrium in vitro to cause relaxation. Few maternal or fetal side effects.

section might have higher morbidity for the mother, particularly at very early gestations because the lower segment is less well formed increasing the necessity of having to use a classical uterine incision.

Management of future pregnancies

Any woman who has laboured prematurely is more at risk of doing so again in her next pregnancy. In many cases there will be nothing that can be done to prevent this. Exceptions are when:

- labour has been due to treatable, persistent infection, e.g. bacterial vaginosis
- there is cervical incompetence.

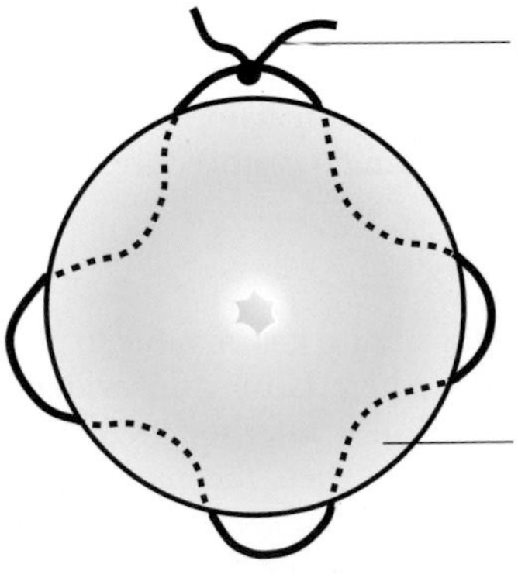

Fig. 29.7 The MacDonald suture.

Where infection has been proved it should be treated and the mother screened regularly for recurrence during subsequent pregnancies and treated as necessary.

Cervical incompetence can be treated by insertion of a cervical suture, either electively in early pregnancy (usually around 12 weeks after the high risk of early miscarriage and once results of Downs syndrome screening tests have been obtained), or, if the cervix is monitored regularly in pregnancy with transvaginal scanning, when scan shows that the cervix is shortening.

The prescription of prophylactic oral tocolytics to women at increased risk of recurrent preterm labour is not helpful, but some clinicians prescribe prophylactic corticosteroids at a point in the pregnancy before the last baby is delivered.

PRETERM PRELABOUR RUPTURE OF MEMBRANES

Preterm prelabour rupture of membranes (PPROM) occurs in only 2% of pregnancies, but is associated with 40% of preterm deliveries. The principal issue is the risk of sepsis, both maternal and fetal. Maternal sepsis with ascending uterine infection can rapidly become overwhelming if not monitored and may affect future fertility. Sepsis in the infant is one of the three leading causes of mortality in the preterm infant, along with prematurity and pulmonary hypoplasia.

Management of preterm prelabour rupture of membranes

History and examination should be performed as described above. Abdominal palpation +/- ultrasound scan should be done to check fetal lie and presentation. There is a risk of cord prolapse with an abnormal lie or with a high presenting part and ruptured membranes, particularly in a preterm infant.

Ruptured membranes are confirmed by the visualization of a pool of liquor in the posterior fornix seen on sterile speculum examination. However, a digital examination should only be performed if there are obvious signs of labour. If not, this type of examination may introduce infection higher up into the genital tract. A high vaginal swab should be taken.

Further management involves monitoring for symptoms and signs of clinical chorioamnionitis. These include:

- general feeling unwell such as fever or shivering
- abdominal pain
- change in colour of vaginal loss from clear to green or brown
- foul smelling vaginal loss
- raised maternal temperature, pulse or respiratory rate
- tender uterus on palpation.

Investigations include a cardiotocograph to exclude a fetal tachycardia. Maternal blood tests can suggest infection including a raised C-reactive protein and white blood cell count. However, chorioamnionitis should not be discounted if these tests are normal in the presence of obvious clinical signs.

Expectant management, i.e. with no symptoms or signs of infection, involves:

- administration of erythromycin to reduce chorioamnionitis
- administration of corticosteroids to improve fetal lung maturity.

Some women will start to labour within 72 hours, but for those who do not, the general principle is to aim to deliver from 34+0 weeks gestation. This will be either by induction of labour with a cephalic presentation or by caesarean section with an abnormal lie. Tocolytics are not used in PPROM.

Reference

Chudleigh, P., 2004. Obstetric Ultrasound: How, why and when. Churchill Livingstone, London.

Further reading

RCOG, 2010a. Antenatal Corticosteroids to Reduce Neonatal Morbidity. Green-top Guideline No. 7. Royal College of Obstetricians and Gynaecologists, London.

RCOG, 2010b. Preterm Prelabour Rupture of Membranes. Green-top Guideline No. 44. Royal College of Obstetricians and Gynaecologists, London.

RCOG, 2011a. Cervical Cerclage. Green-top Guideline No. 60. Royal College of Obstetricians and Gynaecologists, London.

RCOG, 2011b. Preterm Labour, Tocolytic Drugs. Green-top Guideline No. 1b. Royal College of Obstetricians and Gynaecologists, London.

Update Software Ltd. Available online at: www.update-software.com/cochrane.

Other complications of labour

Objectives

By the end of this chapter, you should be able to:

- Understand what is meant by malpresentation and how to manage different clinical situations
- Manage a breech presentation at term
- Understand the different factors that may be relevant if there is slow progress in labour
- Explain the problem with shoulder dystocia and how it is managed.

MALPRESENTATION

Any presentation other than a vertex presentation is a malpresentation. The vertex is the area between the parietal eminences and the anterior and posterior fontanelles. The most common malpresentation is the breech presentation, but others include shoulder, brow and face presentations.

Malpresentation can occur by chance, but it can also be caused by fetal or maternal conditions that prevent the vertex from presenting to the pelvis (Fig. 30.1). In all cases, management must begin by exclusion of important conditions such as fetal abnormality, pelvic masses and placenta praevia.

Breech presentation

Apart from the general causes of malpresentation, breech presentation is particularly associated with prematurity. The incidence of breech presentation increases with decreasing gestation:

- Term: 3%
- 32 weeks: 15%
- 28 weeks: 25%.

Classification of breech presentation

There are three types of breech presentation:

- Extended or frank breech approximately 50%
- Flexed or complete breech approximately 25%
- Footling breech approximately 25%.

With an extended breech, the hips are flexed and the knees extended with the feet situated adjacent to the fetal head. Flexed and footling breeches are flexed at both the hips and knees, but in the latter the feet present to the maternal pelvis not the breech (Fig. 30.2).

Diagnosis

The head can be felt as a hard lump at the uterine fundus by the examiner and the patient. Auscultation of the fetal heart at a higher level than is usual with a cephalic presentation might suggest a breech presentation, although this is not a reliable sign. Vaginal examination in labour can confirm the diagnosis, although if there is any doubt ultrasound examination is indicated, which will also determine the type of breech presentation.

Complications

There is increased perinatal mortality and morbidity associated with vaginal breech delivery when compared with cephalic presentation of comparable birthweight at term. This is usually associated with difficulty in delivering the aftercoming head. The fetal trunk is softer than the head and can pass through a borderline pelvis. Compared with a cephalic delivery, there is relatively little time for moulding to occur, which may result in entrapment of the aftercoming head. If the fetal arms become extended behind the head during delivery (known as nuchal arms) this may also reduce the available space for the head. Rapid compression and decompression of the head during delivery can produce intracranial injury. Unfortunately, no method of antenatal assessment, clinical, radiological or ultrasonic, will guarantee easy delivery of the aftercoming head.

Perinatal morbidity and mortality

Four major causes account for the increased perinatal morbidity and mortality associated with vaginal breech delivery. The relative importance of these depends on the gestational age of the fetus:

- Prematurity
- Cord prolapse
- Birth trauma
- Congenital anomaly.

Fig. 30.1 Causes of malpresentation.

Maternal	Contraction of the pelvis Pelvic tumour eg fibroid Mullerian abnormality Multiparity
Fetoplacental	Prematurity Placenta praevia Polyhydramnios Multiple pregnancy Fetal anomaly • hydrocephalus • extension of the fetal head by neck tumours • anencephaly • decreased fetal tone

HINTS AND TIPS

Those term breech presentations that are unsuccessful at external cephalic version are usually delivered by caesarean section since the perinatal morbidity and mortality following vaginal breech delivery is significantly higher. The patient must be fully counselled about the options in order for her to make an informed choice.

Cord prolapse may occur if the cervix is poorly applied to the presenting part and is most likely to occur with a footling breech and a preterm breech. Birth trauma is associated with difficulty in delivery of the aftercoming head or soft-tissue injury due to excessive traction to the fetus. The causes of morbidity and mortality associated with birth trauma following vaginal breech delivery include:

- intracranial haemorrhage/tentorial tear
- spinal cord injury
- soft tissue injury
- liver rupture
- adrenal haemorrhage
- nerve palsies, e.g. brachial plexus or facial nerve
- fractures of clavicle or humerus.

Management

There are three management options for a breech presentation:

- External cephalic version (ECV)
- Elective caesarean section
- Planned vaginal breech delivery.

All women with a term breech presentation should be offered external cephalic version, preferably at around 37 weeks gestation. If this is not successful or they decline, then the options are caesarean section or vaginal delivery. Following the publication of a large, randomized, prospective trial, the gold standard management of a breech presentation at term is delivery by caesarean section. This trial indicated a significantly lower incidence of complications in term breech babies born by caesarean section than by the vaginal route.

External cephalic version

An attempt is made to turn the fetus to a cephalic presentation by manual manipulation through the maternal anterior abdominal wall. This is usually performed at around 37 weeks gestation, in order to allow time for spontaneous version, and to minimize the number of successful versions turning back to breech. Contraindications to ECV include:

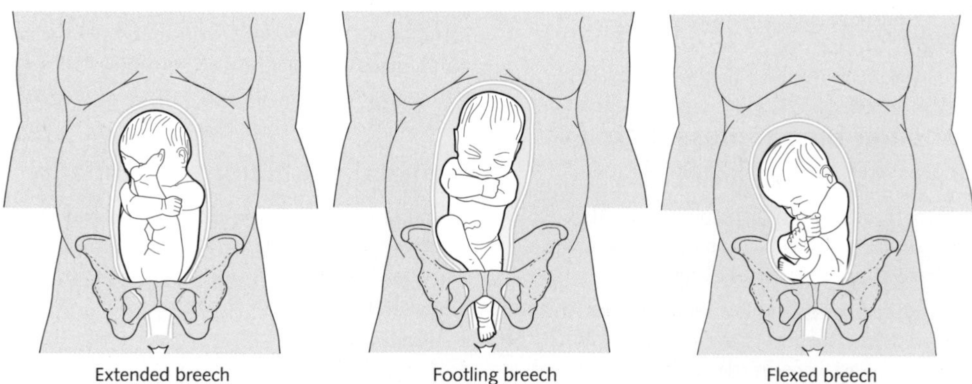

Fig. 30.2 Classification of breech presentation.

- pelvic mass
- antepartum haemorrhage
- placenta praevia
- previous caesarean section or hysterotomy
- multiple pregnancy
- ruptured membranes.

ECV can be performed with the aid of tocolytics, to reduce uterine activity, and under ultrasound control. It should be performed on the labour ward because of the small risk of fetal distress requiring immediate caesarean section (1:300). The fetus can be rolled forwards or backwards and version is successful in about half the cases. Extended breeches are more difficult to turn because the legs 'splint' the fetus. Rhesus negative women should be given anti-D immunoglobulin following attempted version because of the possibility of fetomaternal transfusion.

Antenatal assessment for vaginal breech delivery

For those women who choose to undergo a trial of vaginal breech delivery prior assessment should include fetal size. It is important to exclude a macrosomic fetus by ultrasound estimated fetal weight (EFW). A fetus with an EFW of greater than 4 kg may be best delivered by caesarean section. However, ultrasound EFW at term is associated with an error of 10–20%.

Management of labour with a breech presentation

Delivery should be in an obstetric unit with an attendant paediatrician, as vaginal breech delivery should be regarded as high risk. Management of the first stage of labour should be as for a vertex presentation, although some obstetricians do not advocate the use of syntocinon for slow progress preferring to perform a caesarean section. Continuous fetal heart rate monitoring is recommended. Exclusion of cord prolapse is mandatory when the membranes rupture or if the fetal heart rate pattern becomes abnormal. Epidural anaesthesia is recommended because of the increased level of manipulation during delivery. Approximately half of planned vaginal breech deliveries will be successful because of the lower threshold to perform caesarean section.

During the second stage, the breech should be allowed to descend onto the pelvic floor before active pushing is commenced. If descent does not occur this could indicate disproportion or an unexpectedly large fetus, and caesarean section is indicated. Delivery in the lithotomy position allows access for the attendant to perform any necessary manipulation to the fetus. Lovset's manoeuvre, as the body delivers, keeps the fetal spine anterior and aims to reduce the incidence of nuchal arms. Mauriceau-Smellie-Veit manoeuvre improves flexion of the head to allow easier delivery. Routine episiotomy is recommended to further increase access and prevent delay due to the soft tissues.

Transverse lie and unstable lie

A transverse lie occurs when the long axis of the fetus lies transverse or oblique to the long axis of the uterus, usually with the shoulder presenting (Fig. 30.3). When the fetal lie is different at each palpation, the lie is said to be unstable. The incidence of transverse lie diagnosed in labour with a single fetus is approximately 1 in 500 women but many more will have been identified and managed appropriately antenatally. On abdominal palpation, the fetal head is lateral in the maternal abdomen, and the SFH is lower than expected by gestation. Vaginal examination, which should be avoided until placenta praevia has been excluded, will reveal an empty pelvis.

The causes of transverse lie include the general causes of malpresentation shown in Figure 30.1, but there is particular association with:

- multiparity, where the tone of the uterus and anterior abdominal wall is poor
- premature labour (see Chapter 29)
- the second twin (see Chapter 24).

The most serious complication of a transverse lie is cord prolapse, and this is associated with spontaneous rupture of membranes, either antenatally or in labour.

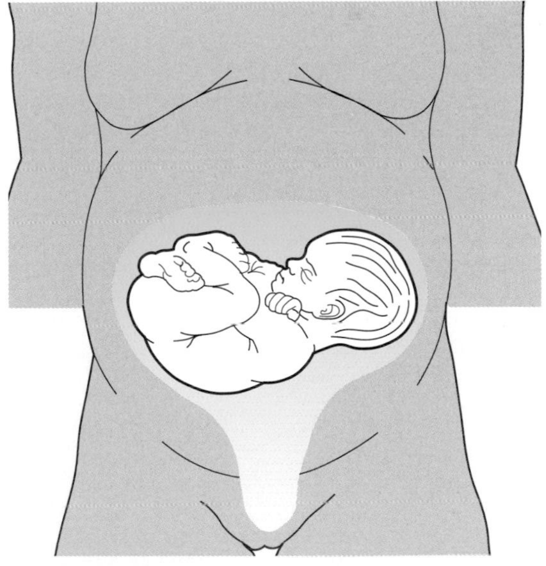

Fig. 30.3 Transverse lie.

Antenatal management

Exclusion of causes of malpresentation is important. Elective caesarean section at term is indicated in the presence of placenta praevia or a pelvic mass. In their absence, ECV can be attempted. If reversion to a malpresentation occurs, or an unstable lie is diagnosed, then admission to hospital from 37 weeks gestation is indicated when immediate delivery is possible if the membranes spontaneously rupture. At term, an unstable lie can be managed expectantly because spontaneous version to a cephalic presentation often occurs due to the increase in uterine activity. Transverse lie can be corrected by ECV followed by immediate induction of labour. If the lie remains unstable then caesarean section is indicated.

Management in labour

If a transverse lie is diagnosed in early labour, ECV may be attempted only if the membranes are intact. If successful, ARM with the head in the pelvis can stabilize the lie by inducing uterine contractions. If version is not successful or the membranes have ruptured, caesarean section is indicated. ECV of a second twin in transverse lie may be appropriate if the fetal monitoring is normal, as described in Chapter 24, with ARM once the presenting part is in the pelvis.

Face presentation

The incidence of face presentation in labour is 1 in 300 labours and occurs when the head is fully extended (Fig. 30.4). Causes include:

- normal fetus with an extended neck
- congenital tumour of neck
- anencephaly.

Diagnosis is usually made during vaginal examination in labour when the supraorbital ridges, the bridge of the nose and the alveolar margins in the mouth are palpable (Fig. 30.5). During labour, the face becomes oedematous and may be mistaken for a breech presentation.

Mechanism of labour

The chin (mentum) is the denominator and the submentobregmatic diameter is 9.5 cm (see Fig. 28.4) so vaginal delivery is possible. Flexion of the head is possible only in the mentoanterior position which occurs in 75% of cases.

HINTS AND TIPS

Face presentation will deliver vaginally if it is mentoanterior but not if it is mentoposterior.

Management of a face presentation in labour is essentially the same as for a vertex presentation. Vaginal examination should be performed when the membranes rupture to exclude a cord prolapse. Mentoposterior positions rotate spontaneously to mentoanterior in 50% of cases, usually in the second stage of labour, and in those that do not a caesarean section is indicated. Caesarean section should also be performed when the

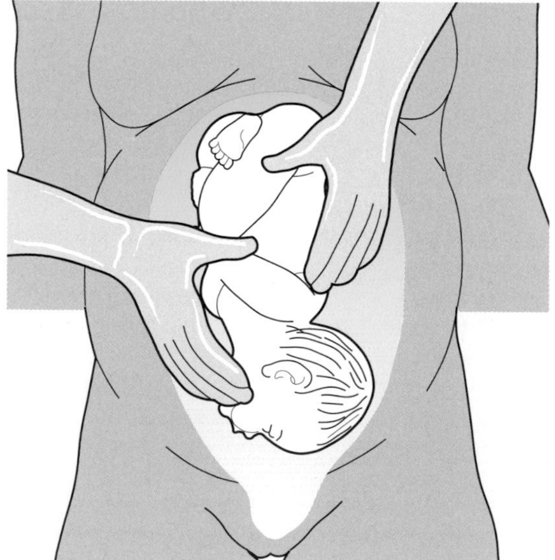

Fig. 30.4 Face presentation.

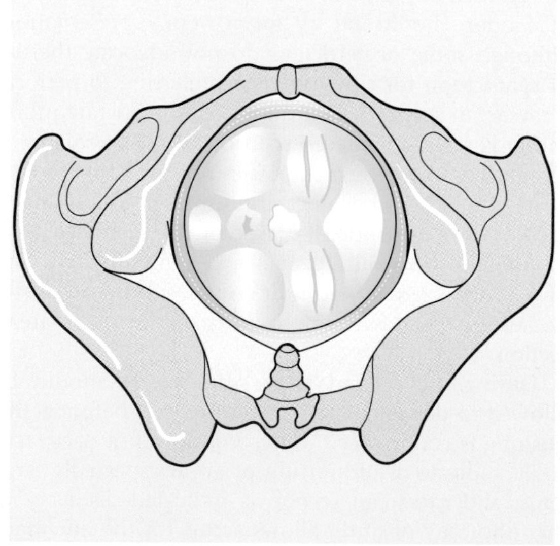

Fig. 30.5 Vaginal examination findings in face presentation.

fetal heart rate pattern is abnormal because a fetal blood sample for pH measurement should not be taken from the face. Traction forceps can be applied to a mentoanterior position to correct delay in the second stage.

The face is nearly always swollen and bruised following a face presentation and the parents should be warned about this. Care must be taken during vaginal examination because the fetal eyes can be damaged by trauma or antiseptic lotions.

Brow presentation

The incidence of brow presentation in labour is approximately 1 in 500 and the causes are the same as for a face presentation. Vaginal examination reveals a high presenting part, a palpable forehead with orbital ridges in front and the anterior fontanelle behind.

Mechanism of labour

The membranes tend to rupture early in labour and there is an increased risk of cord prolapse. With a brow presentation, the mentovertical diameter of 13.5 cm presents (Fig. 28.4). An average-sized fetus will not engage with a normal-sized pelvis and obstructed labour results. When the fetal head is small in relation to the maternal pelvis, descent might occur, allowing flexion of the head as it reaches the pelvic floor. In the absence of disproportion, labour should be allowed to continue. Further extension might occur to a face presentation or flexion to a vertex position.

FAILURE TO PROGRESS IN LABOUR

As described in Chapter 28, labour and delivery require the interaction of three components – the passages, the passenger and power – as part of a dynamic process:

- Passages: the shape and size of the hard bony pelvis and soft tissues
- Passenger: the size, presentation and position of the fetus
- Power: this is both involuntary (strength and frequency of uterine contractions) and voluntary (diaphragm and abdominal muscles).

Any of these factors can be involved in the failure of labour to progress normally, as summarized in Figure 30.6. Once the diagnosis of labour has been made, a primiparous patient is expected to progress at approximately 0.5–1 cm/h and a multiparous patient at 1–2 cm/h.

Fig. 30.6 Differential diagnoses for failure to progress in labour.

Bony passages	Abnormal shaped pelvis Cephalopelvic disproportion
Soft passages	Uterine/cervical fibroids Cervical stenosis Circumcision
Passenger	Fetal size Fetal abnormality Fetal malpresentation Fetal malposition
Power	Lack of coordinated regular strong uterine contractions

Failure to progress related to the bony pelvis

Abnormal bony shape

Antenatal X-ray pelvimetry and routine pelvic assessment by vaginal examination are no longer performed. However, certain points in a patient's history and examination can give clues to the likelihood of failure to progress in labour due to an abnormal pelvis (Fig. 30.7). Although still rare, one of the common problems is a previous pelvic fracture.

Cephalopelvic disproportion

With true cephalopelvic disproportion (CPD), the size of the pelvis is not in proportion to the fetus. It should be suspected antenatally if the head does not engage at term, particularly in a woman of short stature. Usually, a trial of labour is still appropriate, but in some cases an elective caesarean section is planned. During labour, CPD is diagnosed if the head remains unengaged on abdominal palpation. This is confirmed assessing

Fig. 30.7 Causes of abnormalities of the bony pelvis.

Congenital	Osteogenesis imperfecta Ectopia vesicae Dislocation of the hip
Acquired	Kyphosis of the thoracic or lumbar spine Scoliosis of the spine Spondylolisthesis Pelvic fractures Rickets/osteomalacia Poliomyelitis in childhood

station on vaginal examination and by the presence of caput (swelling under the fetal scalp caused by reduction in venous return) and moulding. However, these signs are more commonly found simply with malposition rather than true CPD.

Failure to progress related to the soft tissues of the pelvis

Uterus

A uterine malformation, such as the presence of a midline septum (a Mullerian or developmental abnormality), might prevent the fetus from lying longitudinally, so that a malpresentation is responsible for failure to progress. This can also be rarely caused by uterine fibroids, which may increase the SFH measurement during pregnancy and obstruct labour. The presence of a cervical fibroid might even necessitate caesarean section.

Cervix

Failure of the cervix to dilate during labour despite adequate uterine contractions is rarely secondary to cervical scarring causing stenosis. This could be the result of cervical amputation or cone biopsy.

Vagina

Congenital anomalies of the vagina rarely cause problems with respect to labour and delivery, except in patients who have had reconstructive surgery. Other types of surgery, such as a colposuspension for urinary stress incontinence or repair of a vesicovaginal fistula, generally indicates the need for an elective caesarean section at term, but more to prevent recurrent symptoms rather than because of possible slow progress in labour.

Vulva

Previous perineal tears or episiotomy should not present difficulties during delivery. More problematic is a female circumcision (FGM female genital mutilation), which may necessitate an anterior episiotomy to prevent more severe tears and the risk of fistula formation. Ideally, this patient should have been assessed antenatally in order to make the appropriate plan of care including surgery for reversal of FGM before 20 weeks gestation.

Ovary

Ovarian cysts in pregnancy are usually incidental findings at routine ultrasound. They can present with abdominal pain during pregnancy, secondary to torsion or haemorrhage (see Chapter 9). They do not cause slow progress in labour because they rise up out of the pelvis as the uterus increases in size.

Failure to progress related to the passenger

Fetal size

The possibility of a large fetus might be suggested by the patient's past medical history, for example, Type 1 diabetes or from the antenatal history, with development of gestational diabetes or hydrops fetalis, e.g. with rhesus isoimmunization or parvovirus infection (see Chapter 26). In a multiparous patient, it is useful to check the weights of previous deliveries as an assessment of ability to deliver the current infant.

Abdominal palpation is not always accurate as a method of diagnosing a large fetus, although this should be done to assess engagement of the presenting part in labour. Ultrasound is more accurate, provided that gestational age has been correctly estimated early in pregnancy.

During labour, on vaginal examination, the cervix may be felt to be increasingly oedematous. Signs of caput or moulding may be noted on the fetal head. Caput is the boggy swelling on the fetal head as subcutaneous oedema of the scalp develops. Moulding is described in Chapter 28, when the fetal skull bones overlap.

Fetal abnormality

Routine ultrasound scanning is likely to diagnose abnormalities such as a congenital goitre or a lymphangioma. These extend the neck, so that the normal process of flexion cannot take place. This may result in a face or brow presentation (see above). Abdominal enlargement caused by the presence of ascites or an umbilical hernia may make delivery difficult. Abnormalities of the fetal skull such as anencephaly should be suspected in labour if the head does not engage and the sutures feel widely spaced on vaginal examination. This condition is a type of spina bifida, again routinely diagnosed on ultrasound scan.

Fetal malposition

The fetal head normally engages with an occipitotransverse position. With descent, the head rotates to an occipitoanterior position as described in Chapter 28. Any position other than occipitoanterior can be associated with failure to progress in labour, namely:

- occipitoposterior position
- occiptiotransverse position.

Approximately 20% of vertex presentations in early labour are occipitoposterior. Diagnosis is determined by abdominal palpation:

- Maternal lower abdomen that is flattened or concave
- Fetal back cannot be palpated anteriorly
- Fetal limbs that can be palpated anteriorly.

On vaginal examination, the positions of the sutures and fontanelles are determined (see Chapter 28). If the anterior fontanelle is palpable vaginally, then the head is deflexed. If only the posterior fontanelle can be felt, then the head is flexed. This degree of flexion allows the smallest diameter of the head to present. It will, therefore, be more likely to rotate at the pelvic floor and proceed to normal vaginal delivery. The majority of OP positions will rotate during labour in the presence of adequate contractions. The minority will not rotate, but deliver vaginally in the OP position (face to pubes) if the pelvis is large enough, whilst some will need rotation either manually or with an instrument (see Chapter 32).

Fetal malpresentation

Malpresentation of the fetus is defined as a non-vertex presentation (see above). This can be:

- breech
- shoulder
- face
- brow.

Failure to progress related to the power

Uterine palpation monitors frequency, duration and strength of the contractions. The cardiotocograph checks the frequency and duration. However, the recording of the strength can be altered by position of the monitor on the abdomen and maternal obesity and so this must be assessed on palpation. In some centres, intrauterine pressure catheters are used to monitor contraction pressure. Inefficient uterine action can be diagnosed if labour is prolonged and the contractions are:

- uncoordinated
- fewer than 3–4 in 10 min
- lasting less than 60 s
- pressure less than 40 mmHg (using a pressure catheter).

After thorough abdominal and vaginal examinations, and with normal fetal monitoring, careful use of oxytocic drugs, usually intravenous syntocinon infusion, can improve the contractions. Caution must be taken to avoid too frequent contractions because this can reduce the oxygen exchange in the placental bed and lead to fetal hypoxia. Continuous electronic monitoring is advisable.

Particular care is essential in a multiparous patient because the diagnosis of inefficient uterine action is much less common than in a primiparous patient. A fetal malposition, malpresentation or increased fetal size should be considered as the cause of the slow progress; inappropriate use of oxytocic drugs is associated with uterine rupture in this group.

MANAGEMENT OF FAILURE TO PROGRESS

This depends on the cause. Contractions may be improved with:

- artificial rupture of membranes (ARM)
- use of intravenous syntocinon.

ARM is thought to release local prostaglandins and can increase the rate of labour progression. The strength and frequency of the uterine contractions can also be improved by administration of an infusion of intravenous syntocinon. However, caution must be exercised in a multiparous patient. Generally, labour proceeds more rapidly in a second pregnancy. Therefore, if progress is slow, fetal size and position must be considered so that excessive contractions do not put the patient at risk of uterine rupture with syntocinon. Regular strong contractions will help to correct a fetal malposition by rotating the head against the pelvic floor muscles, as well as improving descent. Malpresentation may be managed as described above.

The presence of good contractions over several hours but without significant progression in terms of cervical dilatation and descent of the presenting part should alert the physician to consider delivery by caesarean section.

Failure to progress in the second stage of labour should be assessed in the manner already described and instrumental delivery considered (see Chapter 32). If the head is almost crowning then an episiotomy might be all that is necessary to expedite vaginal delivery.

SHOULDER DYSTOCIA

Shoulder dystocia is a problem of the pelvic inlet preventing delivery of the shoulders once the head is out. This occurs because the shoulders fail to pass through the pelvic inlet; it is not a problem with the outlet or the perineum. The essential point is not to use excessive traction on the fetal head to facilitate delivery of the shoulders since this risks damage to the brachial plexus nerve roots in the neck. Increasing hypoxia occurs while the fetus is lodged in the vagina, with pressure on the umbilical cord. The more common injury to the fetus is Erb's palsy caused by damage to nerve roots C4, 5 and 6, which can have serious long-term neurological sequelae. Manoeuvres to aid delivery include:

- lie the patient flat
- McRoberts position — the hips are flexed in knee-chest position in order to widen the anteroposterior diameter of the pelvis
- suprapubic pressure to dislodge the anterior shoulder
- internal rotation techniques to try and rotate the anterior shoulder from under the pubic symphysis
- deliver the posterior arm.

This situation is an emergency and should therefore be practised as a regular drill by all the staff on the maternity unit. A senior paediatrician should be called to attend urgently in order to assess the baby at delivery.

Further reading

Hannah, M.E., 2000. Planned caesarean section versus planned vaginal birth for breech presentation at term: a randomized multicentre trial. Lancet. 356, 1368–1369.

NICE, 2007. Intrapartum Care. National Institute for Health and Care Excellence, London. Available online at: www.nice.org.uk.

RCOG, 2006. Breech Presentation, Management. Green-top Guidelines No. 20b. Royal College of Obstetricians and Gynaecologists, London. Available online at: www.rcog.org.uk.

RCOG, 2009. Female Genital Mutilation, Management. Green-top Guidelines No. 53. Royal College of Obstetricians and Gynaecologists, London. Available online at: www.rcog.org.uk.

RCOG, 2012. Shoulder Dystocia. Green-top Guidelines No. 42. Royal College of Obstetricians and Gynaecologists, London. Available online at: www.rcog.org.uk.

Fetal monitoring in labour

Objectives

By the end of this chapter, you should be able to:

- Understand the indications for continuous fetal monitoring in labour
- Perform an examination on a patient presenting with an abnormal cardiotocograph in labour
- Undertake appropriate investigations on a patient presenting with an abnormal cardiotocograph in labour in order to establish fetal well-being.

FETAL MONITORING IN LABOUR

The cardiotocograph (CTG) is a form of electronic fetal heart rate (FHR) monitoring used to evaluate fetal well-being antenatally and during labour. As well as the fetal heart rate, the uterine activity is recorded. It has been used increasingly in the UK since the 1970s, with the aim of detecting fetal hypoxia before it causes perinatal mortality or morbidity, in particular cerebral palsy. However, the expected reduction in hypoxia-induced intrapartum perinatal mortality has not occurred and the role of CTG monitoring has been questioned as the rate of caesarean section increases. The need to constantly educate staff about the appropriate use of the CTG and its interpretation and to audit standards in relation to patient care is essential.

Monitoring in an uncomplicated pregnancy

Intermittent auscultation of the fetal heart rate with a pinard stethoscope or a sonicaid may be appropriate for a healthy woman in labour who has had an uncomplicated pregnancy. This involves documenting the heart rate for a minimum of 60 s at least:

- every 15 min including after a contraction in the first stage of labour
- every 5 min including after a contraction in the second stage of labour.

Continuous monitoring might be recommended if intermittent auscultation is abnormal or any risk factors develop during the course of the labour, such as meconium-stained liquor.

Who should have continuous cardiotocograph monitoring?

Figure 31.1 shows the maternal and fetal indications for recommending continuous monitoring.

FEATURES OF THE CARDIOTOCOGRAPH

There are four features of the CTG, which should all be assessed individually and then taken together with the clinical picture to determine the appropriate management of the patient. For example, an antepartum haemorrhage or the presence of meconium-stained liquor should prompt more timely intervention:

HINTS AND TIPS

Use the following tool to assess the CTG:
D define
R risk
C contractions
B baseline
R rate
A accelerations
V variability
A and
D decelerations
O overall assessment

- Baseline fetal heart rate (FHR): this is the mean level of FHR over a period of 5 to 10 min. It is expressed as beats per minute (bpm) and is determined by the fetal sympathetic and parasympathetic nervous systems. The normal range is 110–160 bpm. In the preterm fetus, the baseline tends to be at the higher end of the normal range.
- Baseline variability: minor fluctuations occur in the baseline FHR at 3 to 5 cycles per minute. It is measured by estimating the difference in bpm between the highest peak and the lowest trough of change in a 1 min segment of the trace. Normal baseline variability is ≥ 5 bpm.

Fig. 31.1 Indications for recommending continuous fetal monitoring.

Maternal	Previous caesarean section Pre-eclampsia Diabetes Antepartum haemorrhage Other maternal medical disease
Fetal	Intrauterine growth restriction Prematurity Oligohydramnios Abnormal Doppler artery studies Multiple pregnancy Breech presentation
Intrapartum	Meconium-stained liquor Vaginal bleeding in labour Use of oxytocin for augmentation Epidural analgesia Maternal pyrexia Post-term pregnancy Prolonged rupture of membranes >24h Induced labour

- Accelerations: these are increases in the FHR of 15 bpm or more above the baseline rate, lasting 15 s or more. These are a feature of a normal CTG.
- Decelerations: these are falls in the FHR of more than 15 bpm below the baseline, lasting 15 s or more. Different types of decelerations can be seen, depending on their timing with the uterine contractions:
  1. Early decelerations: the FHR slows at the same time as the onset of the contraction and returns to the baseline at the end of the contraction in an identical pattern with every contraction. These are usually benign.
  2. Variable decelerations: the timing of the slowing of the FHR in relation to the uterine contraction varies within the timeframe of the contraction. A typical variable deceleration is of rapid onset and recovery, with a particular shape on the recording, known as shouldering. However, other features might make this type of deceleration more suspicious or atypical, such as loss of the normal baseline variability or loss of the shouldering.
  3. Late decelerations: the FHR begins to fall during the contraction, with its trough more than 20 s after the peak of the contraction and returning to baseline after the contraction.

The CTG can be categorized into:

- normal: all four features are reassuring
- suspicious: one feature is non-reassuring, the others are reassuring
- pathological: two or more features are non-reassuring, one is abnormal.

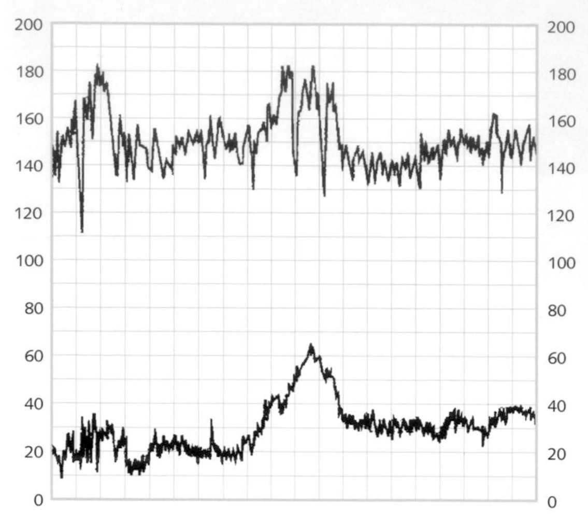

Fig. 31.2 Fetal heart acceleration during a uterine contraction with normal baseline variability.

Figure 31.2 shows a normal CTG tracing. Figure 31.3 shows how the features of the CTG are categorized. Figure 31.4 shows an abnormal CTG tracing.

HINTS AND TIPS

When presenting a CTG, note:
- patient's name
- date and time
- maternal pulse
- baseline fetal heart rate
- baseline variability
- presence or absence of accelerations
- presence or absence of decelerations.

PHYSIOLOGY

The principle of monitoring during labour is to detect fetal hypoxia and, therefore, prevent acidaemia and cell damage.

Acute fetal hypoxia

In a previously well fetus, this can occur secondary to:

- uterine hyperstimulation
- placental abruption
- umbilical cord compression
- sudden maternal hypotension, e.g. insertion of regional anaesthesia.

These conditions can result in a decrease in the fetal heart rate, with decelerations or bradycardia. This is produced by chemoreceptor-mediated vagal stimulation and then by myocardial ischaemia.

Fig. 31.3 Categorization of the features of the fetal heart rate.

Feature	Baseline (bpm)	Variability (bpm)	Decelerations	Accelerations
Reassuring	110–160	≥5	None present	Present
Non-reassuring	100–109 161–180	<5 for ≥40min	Typical variable decelerations Single deceleration 3 min	None present
Abnormal	<100 >180	<5 for ≥90min	Atypical variable decelerations Late decelerations Single deceleration >3 min	None present

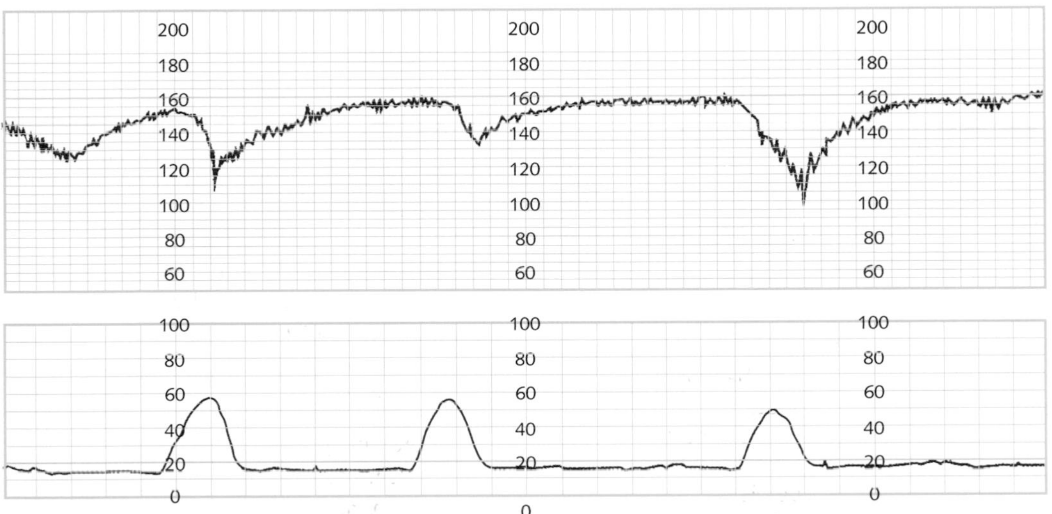

Fig. 31.4 Late decelerations occurring after uterine contractions with reduced baseline variability.

Chronic fetal hypoxia

If there has been chronic uteroplacental insufficiency during the pregnancy, for example secondary to pre-eclampsia, then the fetus is at increased risk of hypoxia during labour. Reduced intervillous perfusion during uterine contractions or maternal hypotension can exacerbate underlying reduced placental perfusion. This can result in an increase in the fetal cardiac output with an increase in the baseline heart rate, followed by reduced heart rate variability due to brainstem hypoxia. Continuing hypoxia eventually produces myocardial damage and heart rate decelerations.

MONITORING UTERINE CONTRACTIONS

As well as monitoring the FHR, the CTG also monitors the frequency of the uterine contractions. This is important, for example, if the patient is having intravenous oxytocin to stimulate the contractions. It is essential that frequency of contractions and the return to resting tone between contractions is noted.

The actual strength and the length of each contraction should be checked by palpation of the uterus, because the size of the peaks shown on the tracing may be related to positioning of the monitor on the maternal abdomen or thickness of the maternal abdominal wall.

HISTORY OF THE PATIENT WHO PRESENTS WITH AN ABNORMAL CARDIOTOCOGRAPH IN LABOUR

The need to act on an abnormal CTG in labour is influenced by maternal, fetal and intrapartum factors. Figure 31.1 gives the indications for continuous CTG monitoring as well as showing the relevant points in the patient's antenatal history that might make the staff more concerned if the CTG is suspicious. The intrapartum factors are particularly important. In the presence of meconium-stained liquor, for example, the CTG should be acted upon promptly as hypoxia may cause the fetus to gasp and inhale the meconium.

EXAMINATION OF THE PATIENT WHO PRESENTS WITH AN ABNORMAL CARDIOTOCOGRAPH IN LABOUR

Baseline maternal observations

Temperature

A raised maternal temperature might explain fetal tachycardia, for example, if there is ruptured membranes for >24 h increasing the risk of infection.

Pulse

This might be raised in conjunction with maternal pyrexia. In the presence of fetal bradycardia, maternal pulse should be checked to ensure that the monitoring is recording FHR and not the mother. This can be excluded by applying a fetal scalp electrode, provided the cervix is at least 1–2 cm dilated and the membranes are ruptured.

Blood pressure

Administering epidural anaesthesia can be associated with maternal hypotension. This results in reduced blood flow to the uterus and can cause fetal bradycardia. Therefore, intravenous fluids are administered and blood pressure regularly checked when the medication is given.

Abdominal palpation

- Uterine size
- Engagement of presenting part
- Scar tenderness in a patient with a previous caesarean section
- Uterine tone.

The size of the maternal abdomen should be assessed to check if it is large or small for dates (see Chapter 26). The engagement of the presenting part is important to assess progress in labour (see Chapter 28). In a patient who has previously had a caesarean section, the presence of scar tenderness should be elicited; scar rupture is commonly associated with an abnormal CTG and vaginal bleeding. Another cause of vaginal bleeding with an abnormal CTG is placental abruption (see Chapter 21). If this is suspected, the uterus will typically feel hard and tender.

The uterine contractions should be palpated, especially if the patient's labour is being stimulated by intravenous oxytocic agents. Hyperstimulation can cause an abnormal FHR. There should be resting tone between contractions.

Vaginal examination

As well as assessing the dilatation of the cervix to determine the progress in labour and the ability to perform a fetal blood sample, the presence of the fetal cord must be excluded. A cord prolapse, as it is known, is associated with a fetal bradycardia as the blood vessels in the cord spasm. This is an emergency situation requiring immediate delivery by caesarean section if the cervix is not fully dilated.

A vaginal examination may also be indicated to apply a fetal scalp electrode (FSE) if the CTG could be recording maternal pulse instead of fetal.

INVESTIGATING THE ABNORMAL CARDIOTOCOGRAPH

If the CTG is categorized as suspicious, the patient can be managed conservatively (Fig. 31.5), for example, by changing maternal position or reducing the dose of syntocinon.

If the CTG is pathological, fetal blood sampling (FBS) should be performed if there are the appropriate facilities. The procedure involves taking a sample of capillary blood from the fetal scalp with the mother in the left lateral position and the cervix dilated at least 2–3 cm. A sample of blood from the fetal scalp gives the fetal pH (i.e. a measure of acidosis). The result might indicate that delivery is necessary (pH ≤7.20), that the test should be repeated within 30 min (pH 7.21–7.24) or 60 min (pH ≥7.25).

If FBS is not possible, delivery should be expedited by caesarean section. Contraindications to FBS are given in Figure 31.6.

Further reading

Gibb, D., Arulkumaran, S., 2008. Fetal Monitoring in Practice, 3rd ed. Churchill Livingstone, London.

NICE, 2007. Intrapartum Care, Guideline CG55. National Institute for Health and Care Excellence, London. Available online at: www.nice.org.uk.

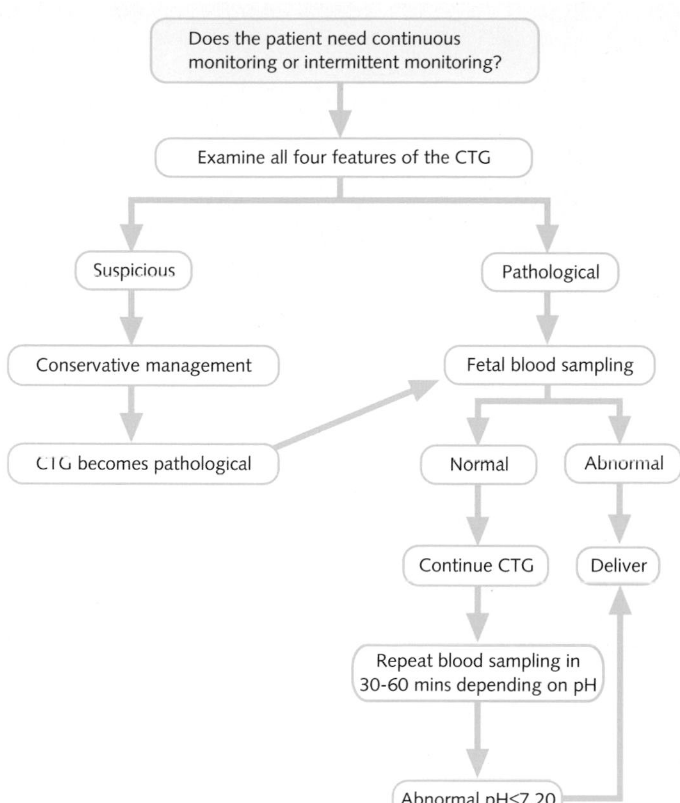

Fig. 31.5 Algorithm for cardiotocograph monitoring.

Fig. 31.6 Contraindications to fetal blood sampling.

- Maternal infection (HIV/hepatitis B/herpes simplex)
- Fetal bleeding disorder (haemophilia/thrombocytopaenia)
- Prematurity (<34 weeks)

Operative interventions in labour

Objective

By the end of this chapter, you should be able to:

- Understand the basics of repairing an episiotomy
- Describe the criteria for safe instrumental delivery
- Consider the indications for the use of forceps rather than ventouse delivery
- List the potential complications of caesarean section
- Monitor a patient undergoing vaginal birth after previous caesarean section.

HINTS AND TIPS

For all interventions in obstetrics, the following general principles apply:

- Make sure all documentation includes the time and date, a legible signature and printed name.
- Clearly record the indication for the intervention, the abdominal and vaginal examination findings as appropriate and the operative findings including any complications.
- Obtain informed consent from the patient, either verbal or written, depending on the procedure.

EPISIOTOMY

The purpose of an episiotomy is to increase the diameter of the vulval outlet by making an incision in the perineal body. Since the 1980s, the routine episiotomy rate has been reduced dramatically because studies have demonstrated its association with increased blood loss, as well as long-term morbidity such as pain and dyspareunia. However, there are still indications for its use (Fig. 32.1).

HINTS AND TIPS

To make them easier to remember, the indications for any intervention can be divided into maternal and fetal.

Two techniques are used for episiotomy (Fig. 32.2). Both should be performed with adequate analgesia, either an epidural, pudendal or perineal infiltration with local anaesthetic, and should start in the midline at the posterior fourchette:

1. Mediolateral: widely used in the UK, this type of incision is more likely to protect the anal sphincter if the incision extends during delivery.
2. Midline: this technique is widely used in the USA and, although it is easier to repair and likely to result in less postpartum pain, it is more likely to involve the anal sphincter if it extends.

Repair of an episiotomy should be performed by an experienced operator. There should be adequate light and appropriate analgesia. A three-layer technique is normally practised, with absorbable subcuticular sutures (Fig. 32.3):

- First layer – vaginal skin: identify the apex of the incision and suture in a continuous layer to the hymen to oppose the cut edges of the posterior fourchette
- Second layer – perineal body: deep sutures to realign the muscles of the perineal body
- Third layer – perineal skin: continuous subcuticular or interrupted sutures to close the skin.

At the end of the procedure, all needles and swabs should be accounted for. An examination of the vagina should be performed to ensure that the apex of the episiotomy is secure. Rectal examination should ensure that the rectal mucosa has not been broached by any deep sutures because this can result in fistula formation.

PERINEAL REPAIR

Approximately 70% of mothers who deliver vaginally will sustain some degree of perineal trauma. This can be classified as:

- 1st degree: involves skin only
- 2nd degree: involves skin and perineal muscle

Fig. 32.1 Indications for episiotomy.

Type of indication	Description
Maternal	Female circumcision Consider if previous perineal reconstructive surgery
Fetal	Instrumental delivery Breech delivery Shoulder dystocia Abnormal CTG

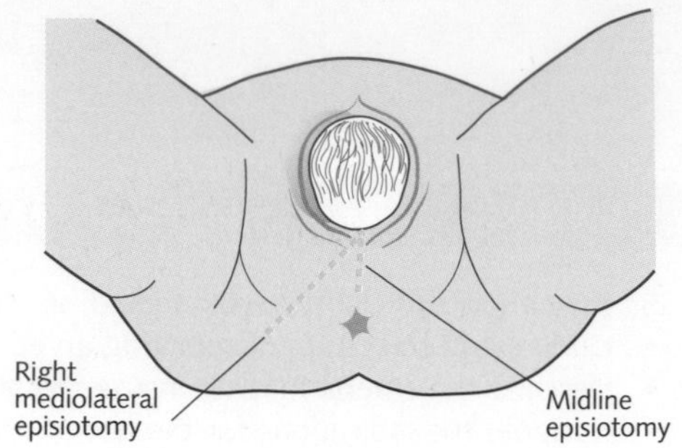

Fig. 32.2 Types of incision for episiotomy.

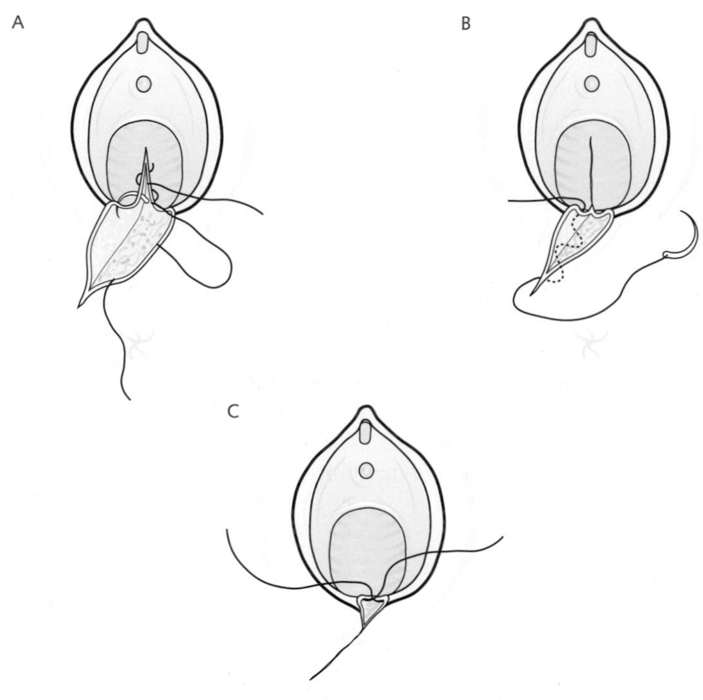

Fig. 32.3 Repair of an episiotomy. (A) Suturing the vaginal wall. (B) Suturing the perineal muscles. (C) Subcuticular sutures to the perineal skin. Tying the strands together – the knot disappears beneath the vaginal mucosa.

- 3rd degree: includes partial or complete rupture of the anal sphincter
- 4th degree: as for 3rd degree, but also involves the anal mucosa.

The principles for repair are the same as for episiotomy. Some 1st degree tears can be allowed to heal by primary or secondary intention if they are not actively bleeding. It is very important to recognize and repair appropriately any damage to the anal sphincter or mucosa; failure to do so can result in long-term morbidity, such as urgency of stool, or incontinence of flatus or faeces (this occurs in approximately 5% of women).

VENTOUSE DELIVERY

Since the 1950s, when the vacuum extractor was invented in Sweden, it has increasingly been seen as the instrument of choice for assisted vaginal delivery. Metal cups were used initially, either anterior cups or posterior cups. Subsequently silicone rubber ones were developed and more recently, the disposable hand-held KIWI cup. The metal cups are more likely to be associated with trauma to the vagina or the fetal scalp, but may be more appropriate for delivery in certain situations, such as the presence of excessive caput on the fetal head. Along with the KIWI cups, they are useful in the presence of a fetal malposition. Both the metal and silicone cups are available in different diameters depending on the gestation of the fetus. It is not an appropriate instrument at less than 34 weeks' gestation.

Indications for use of the ventouse cup are:

- maternal – delay in the 2nd stage of labour due to maternal exhaustion
- fetal – abnormal cardiotocograph (CTG) or slow progress in the 2nd stage of labour due to fetal malposition.

Technique for ventouse

The criteria shown in Figure 32.4 must be fulfilled. Instrumental delivery should not be attempted if the head is above the ischial spines because of the risks of excessive traction to the fetus – a caesarean section is indicated.

All types of cup rely on the same technique. The cup is applied in the midline over or just anterior to the occiput, avoiding the surrounding vaginal mucosa. The pressure in the connecting pump is raised to -0.8 kg/cm^2. This mechanism is 'all-in-one' with the KIWI cup.

Traction with the maternal contractions and with maternal effort should be along the pelvic curve, that is, initially in a downwards direction and then changing the angle upwards as the head crowns. This action basically mimics the passage of the fetal head during a normal delivery, but uses the vacuum pump to increase traction and flexion.

The operator should judge whether an episiotomy is needed and the procedure should be complete within approximately 15 min of cup application. The CTG should monitor the fetal heart rate throughout and, in most units, it is standard practice for a paediatrician to be present. Complications are listed in Figure 32.5.

Fig. 32.4 Criteria for instrumental vaginal delivery.

1. Adequate analgesia: perineal infiltration/pudendal block/epidural anaesthesia (see Chapter 28)
2. Abdominal examination: estimation of fetal size, head either 1/5 or 0/5 palpable
3. Vaginal examination: cervix fully dilated, head either at or below the ischial spines, known fetal position, note presence of caput or moulding
4. Adequate maternal effort and regular contractions necessary for ventouse delivery
5. Empty bladder for forceps delivery

Fig. 32.5 Complications of instrumental delivery.

Type of complication	Description
Maternal	Genital tract trauma (cervical/vaginal/vulval) with risk of haemorrhage and/or infection
Fetal	Ventouse delivery is likely to cause a chignon (scalp oedema) or, less commonly, a cephalohaematoma (subperiosteal bleed) Forceps can cause bruising if not appropriately applied, or rarely facial nerve palsy or depression skull fracture

FORCEPS DELIVERY

Over the last three to four centuries, forceps have been used for delivery. There are two main types of forceps (Fig. 32.6):

- Non-rotational or traction forceps (Simpsons, Andersons, Neville-Barnes or Wrigleys)
- Rotational forceps (Keillands).

Indications for forceps

These are shown in Figure 32.7. They differ slightly from those for the ventouse, mainly because the ventouse

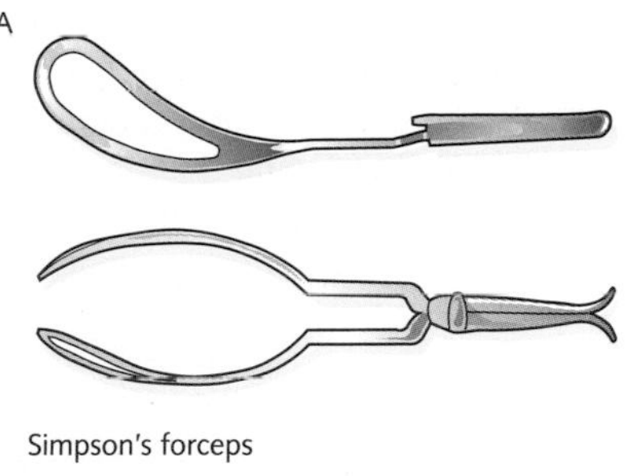

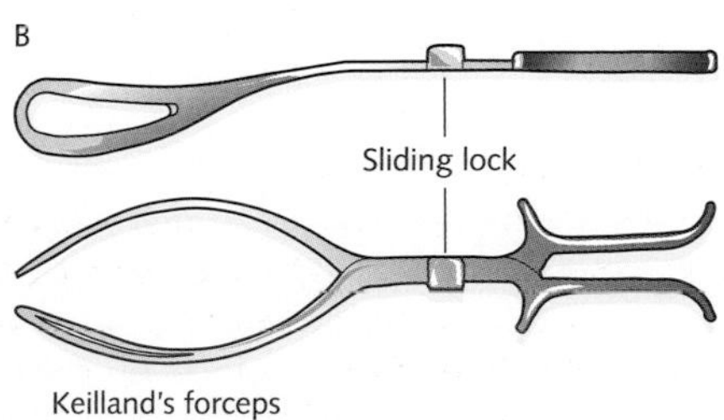

Fig. 32.6 Types of forceps.

Fig. 32.7 Indications for forceps rather than ventouse delivery.

Type of indication	Description
Maternal	Medical conditions complicating labour, e.g. cardiovascular disease Unconscious mother, i.e. conditions where the mother is unable to assist with pushing
Fetal	Gestation less than 34 weeks Face presentation Known or suspected fetal bleeding disorder After-coming head of a breech At caesarean section

requires maternal effort and adequate contractions. Non-rotational forceps are suitable only for certain positions of the fetal head – direct occipitoanterior or direct occipitoposterior. By contrast, the mode of action of the ventouse cup allows rotation to take place during traction and so it is suitable for a malposition (see Chapter 30).

With a decline in the use of rotational forceps in some units due to fetal and maternal complications such as extended vaginal wall tears, it is essential to define the fetal position before attempting delivery, so that the appropriate instrument is chosen and the correct technique used.

Technique for forceps

As for the ventouse, the necessary criteria must be fulfilled (Fig. 32.4). The blades of non-rotational forceps are applied to the head, avoiding trauma to the vaginal walls. The direction of traction is similar to that of the ventouse, with episiotomy performed when the head crowns in order to give more space (Fig. 32.8).

Use of the rotational forceps involves a slightly different technique: the knobs on the blades must always point towards the occiput; asynclitism can be corrected using the sliding mechanism of the handles and then rotation achieved prior to traction in the manner described above.

CAESAREAN SECTION

Caesarean section was first described by the ancient Egyptians. It was used increasingly throughout the twentieth century such that rates of 25% are now common in units in the UK. The lower segment procedure (lower segment caesarean section LSCS) was introduced in the 1920s and has largely replaced the 'classical' midline uterine incision. Although the latter is sometimes indicated for preterm delivery with a poorly formed lower segment or for a preterm abnormal lie, it is associated with higher rates of haemorrhage and rupture in future labours (up to 5% for midline operation, <1% for lower segment procedure).

Indications for lower segment caesarean section

These are shown in Figure 32.9.

Technique for lower segment caesarean section

An elective LSCS is usually performed at 39 or more weeks gestation. Delivery at this gestation reduces the respiratory morbidity in the infant – transient tachypnoea of the newborn (TTN). With regional analgesia more commonly than general, a low transverse skin incision is made. The rectus sheath is cut and the rectus muscles divided. The uterovesical peritoneum is incised to allow the bladder to be reflected inferiorly. The lower uterine segment is incised transversely and the fetus is delivered manually.

Intravenous oxytocin is given by the anaesthetist and the placenta and membranes are removed. The angles of the uterine incision are secured to ensure haemostasis and then the uterus is closed with an absorbable suture, usually in two layers. The rectus sheath is closed to avoid incisional hernias and, finally, the skin is closed with either an absorbable or non-absorbable suture.

HINTS AND TIPS

It is not appropriate to attempt an instrumental delivery if the fetal head is above the ischial spines. An LSCS should be performed.

Complications of lower segment caesarean section

Although LSCS has become an increasingly safe procedure, particularly with the introduction of regional anaesthesia, there is still significant morbidity associated with it:

- Haemorrhage: all patients should have a group and save sample sent; cross-match blood for certain patients, e.g. those with placenta praevia

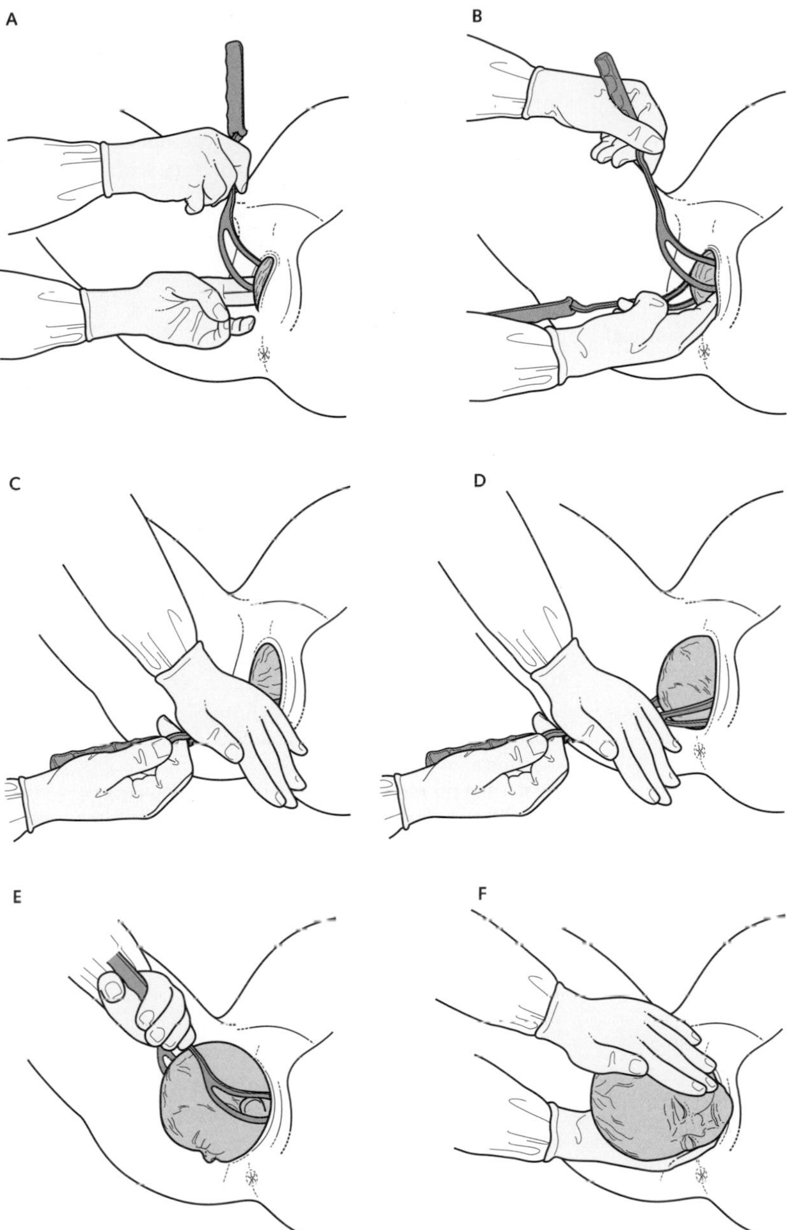

Fig. 32.8 Forceps delivery: a right medio-lateral episiotomy is cut as the head descends to the perineum (E) shown by the dashed line.

- Gastric aspiration: particularly with general anaesthetic (Mendelson's syndrome), this is reduced by routine use of antacids
- Visceral injury: damage to bladder or bowel, particularly with a history of previous abdominal surgery
- Infection: reduced by routine use of prophylactic antibiotics
- Thromboembolic disease: prophylaxis in all patients
- Future pregnancy: subject to vaginal birth after caesarean (VBAC) (see below) or repeat operation with an increasing risk of complications, e.g. placenta praevia.

Vaginal birth after caesarean

In patients who have had a pregnancy complicated by caesarean section, options for future deliveries should be discussed. In the case of a classical caesarean, the possibility of scar rupture in labour is high (up to 5%) and thus repeat LSCS would be recommended.

With LSCS for a non-repeatable cause, for example cord prolapse, then a trial of vaginal delivery is appropriate, providing the patient is fully counselled. Certain measures are advisable during labour to monitor for the

Fig. 32.9 Indications for lower segment caesarean section.

Type of indication	Description
Maternal	Two previous LSCS Placenta praevia Maternal disease, e.g. fulminating pre-eclampsia Maternal request with no obstetric indication Active primary genital herpes simplex virus HIV disease depending on viral load.
Fetal	Breech presentation Twin pregnancy if the presentation of first twin is not cephalic Abnormal CTG or abnormal fetal blood sample in 1st stage Cord prolapse Delay in first stage of labour, e.g. due to malpresentation or malposition

possibility of scar rupture, which would mean immediate recourse to caesarean section:

- Intravenous cannula
- Full blood count (FBC) and group-and-save sample available in laboratory
- Continuous CTG monitoring
- Monitor vaginal loss to exclude bleeding
- Monitor abdominal pain: scar rupture can present with continuous pain, as opposed to intermittent contractions.

With appropriate monitoring, vaginal delivery rates of approximately 70% can be expected, with a scar rupture rate of <1%.

Further reading

Enkin, M.W., Keirse, M.J.N.C., 2000. A Guide to Effective Care in Pregnancy and Childbirth, third ed. Oxford University Press, Oxford.

NICE, 2011. CG 132. Caesarean Section. National Institute for Health and Care Excellence, London.

RCOG, 2001. National Sentinel Audit Report Oct 2001. Royal College of Obstetricians and Gynaecologists, London. Available online at: www.rcog.org.uk.

RCOG, 2007. Birth after Previous Caesarean Birth. Green-top Guidelines No. 45. Royal College of Obstetricians and Gynaecologists, London. Available online at: www.rcog.org.uk.

RCOG, 2007. Third and Fourth Degree Perineal Tears: Management. Green-top Guidelines No. 29. Royal College of Obstetricians and Gynaecologists, London. Available online at: www.rcog.org.uk.

RCOG, 2011. Operative Vaginal Delivery. Green-top Guidelines No. 26. Royal College of Obstetricians and Gynaecologists, London. Available online at: www.rcog.org.uk.

Postnatal complications

Objectives

By the end of this chapter, you should be able to:

- List the more common causes of primary postpartum haemorrhage (PPH)
- Understand the important points in the history for a patient presenting with bleeding after delivery
- Perform an examination on a patient presenting with bleeding after delivery
- Undertake appropriate investigations on a patient presenting with bleeding after delivery in order to establish a diagnosis
- Discuss the initial management of a patient who presents with a primary PPH
- List the common sites for postnatal infection and how you would investigate them
- Understand the prevalence of postnatal mental health disorders and how they are managed
- Describe the diagnosis and treatment of thromboembolic disease in the puerperium.

POSTPARTUM HAEMORRHAGE

Postpartum haemorrhage (PPH) is bleeding from the genital tract of more than 500 mL after delivery of the infant. It is classified as either primary or secondary:

Primary PPH: bleeding more than 500 mL within 24 hours of delivery

Secondary PPH: bleeding more than 500 mL that starts 24 hours after delivery and occurs within 6 weeks.

In practice, blood loss of more than 1000 mL is more clinically relevant. Most units classify bleeding of more than 2000 mL as massive obstetric haemorrhage. There is usually a specific local protocol for management, in light of the *Confidential Enquiry into Maternal Deaths* (see Chapter 35).

Incidence of primary postpartum haemorrhage

The incidence of primary PPH in the developed world is about 5% of deliveries, in contrast to developing countries where it can occur in 28% of deliveries and remains the major cause of maternal mortality.

DIFFERENTIAL DIAGNOSIS

Figure 33.1 gives the differential diagnoses that should be considered. About 90% of cases of PPH are caused by uterine atony; about 7% are due to genital tract trauma.

HISTORY

Primary postpartum haemorrhage

The main causes of primary PPH are shown in Figure 33.2.

Uterine atony

Risk factors in the patient's history that suggest an increase in the risk of a primary PPH secondary to uterine atony include:

- multiple pregnancy
- grand multiparity
- fetal macrosomia
- polyhydramnios
- fibroid uterus
- prolonged labour
- previous postpartum haemorrhage
- antepartum haemorrhage.

In a multiple pregnancy, the placental site is larger than with a singleton (see Chapter 24). There is overdistension of the uterus, which is also seen in cases of macrosomia and polyhydramnios (see Chapter 26).

When the patient presents with primary PPH, always ask the midwife to check that the placenta and membranes are complete, to exclude retained products of conception.

Mode of delivery

The mode of delivery may increase risk of PPH. Genital tract trauma can occur with a normal vaginal delivery, either from an episiotomy (see Chapter 32) or from a

Fig. 33.1 Differential diagnoses of postpartum haemorrhage (see Chapter 42).

Type of PPH	Differential diagnosis
Primary	Uterine atony Genital tract trauma (cervix/vagina/perineum) Retained placenta/placenta accreta Coagulation disorders Uterine inversion Uterine rupture
Secondary	Retained products Endometritis Persistent molar pregnancy/choriocarcinoma

Fig. 33.2 Causes of postpartum haemorrhage (see Chapter 46).

Cause	Frequency (%)
Uterine atony	Approx 90%
Genital tract trauma	Approx 7%
Retained placenta/placenta accreta Coagulation disorders Uterine inversion Uterine rupture	Approx 3%

vaginal or cervical tear. Trauma is more common with an instrumental delivery especially forceps, in particular Keilland's forceps (see Chapter 31). Therefore the genital tract should always be checked for signs of trauma once the placenta has been delivered.

Average blood loss at caesarean section is 500 mL. Placenta praevia (see Chapter 21) or a prolonged labour may increase this. In the latter, the presenting part may become impacted in the pelvis, making delivery more difficult. This can cause the incision on the uterus to tear, which may increase blood loss.

Rarely, PPH is secondary to uterine inversion that occurs after delivery of the placenta (see Chapter 29). With bleeding, the patient complains of abdominal pain, which can be severe, associated with a feeling of prolapse. Rupture of the uterus is also an uncommon cause of PPH except in association with labour in a patient who has previously had a caesarean section.

Other causes

Coagulation disorders can be acute or chronic. The chronic conditions such as inherited vascular disorders are usually known about antenatally. DIC can present acutely, secondary to placental abruption or severe pre-eclampsia.

Complications of primary postpartum haemorrhage

Sheehan's syndrome

Severe PPH can lead to avascular necrosis of the pituitary gland, resulting in hypopituitarism. This can present as secondary amenorrhoea or failure of lactation.

Prevention

In the first instance, prevention of primary PPH involves treatment of anaemia during pregnancy and identifying patients who might be at risk. These women might be obvious antenatally, such as the patient with a known inherited coagulation factor deficiency or one who has had a previous PPH. Equally, PPH might be anticipated during labour, for example the patient who has a prolonged labour ending with a difficult instrumental delivery of a large baby.

Active management of the third stage of labour is routine in most obstetric units, with the patient's consent. It involves:

- use of an oxytocic drug
- controlled cord traction to deliver the placenta (Brandt-Andrews method)
- clamping and cutting the umbilical cord.

Prophylactic use of oxytocics in particular is known to reduce the incidence of PPH by 30–40%. Intramuscular syntometrine is commonly used in the UK (5 units of syntocinon and 0.5 mg ergometrine). If the patient has hypertension, syntocinon is given alone.

Secondary postpartum haemorrhage

In the presence of retained products of conception, either placenta or membranes, the common presenting complaint is prolonged heavy vaginal bleeding or persistent offensive discharge. In the presence of infection, the patient may also present with fever and lower abdominal pain.

A molar pregnancy also presents with persistent vaginal bleeding (see Chapter 20). Choriocarcinoma, though rare, may metastasize to the lungs, liver or brain. Presenting symptoms include haemoptysis and dyspnoea or neurological symptoms.

EXAMINATION

Primary postpartum haemorrhage

The blood loss must be estimated as accurately as possible to manage the patient appropriately. Examination must include the ABC (airways, breathing, circulation)

Fig. 33.3 Examination of the patient who presents with primary postpartum haemorrhage.

- ABC
- Amount of blood loss
- Pulse
- Blood pressure
- Urine output
- Uterine contraction
- Fundal height
- Placenta and membranes complete
- Genital tract trauma

of basic resuscitation (see Chapter 34), as well as pallor, pulse and blood pressure. Abdominal palpation should assess whether the uterus is contracted or not. The fundal height should be at or below the umbilicus. If it is above, there might be retained products of conception or the uterus could be filling with clots.

HINTS AND TIPS

Always remember ABC and basic examination when the patient presents with PPH.

Uterine inversion should be considered if the fundus is indented or cannot be palpated. Vaginal examination will assess the degree of inversion, either up to the cervical os or complete inversion of the uterus and vagina.

If the uterus is well contracted and the placenta is out, then the bleeding might be from trauma to the genital tract. The patient should be examined in sufficient light and with adequate analgesia (either regional or general) to exclude lacerations to the cervix, vagina and perineum.

If the placenta and membranes have been delivered, they must be carefully examined to see that the cotyledons appear complete and that there is no suggestion of a succenturiate lobe. The examination is summarized in Figure 33.3.

Secondary postpartum haemorrhage

Basic observations should include pulse, blood pressure, respiratory rate and temperature. Tachycardia and pyrexia may be present with endometritis. The height of the uterine fundus should be checked because the uterus will usually remain poorly contracted if there are retained products of conception. Tenderness should be excluded to rule out endometritis.

Speculum examination excludes vaginal discharge if there is suspicion of infection. Bimanual palpation examines the size of the uterus, because it might be bulky with retained products or with a molar pregnancy. Tenderness is present with endometritis. If the cervical os is open there might be retained products of conception.

INVESTIGATIONS

Primary postpartum haemorrhage

Having established intravenous access, blood should be sent for haemoglobin, platelets, clotting screen including fibrin degradation products and serum save. Depending on the estimated blood loss, cross-matching blood might be necessary. Urea and electrolytes should be tested if the urine output is poor.

Figure 33.4 provides an algorithm for the management of primary PPH.

Secondary postpartum haemorrhage

A full blood count should be taken to estimate haemoglobin. A raised white blood cell count is an indication of infection. Again, cross-matching blood for transfusion might be necessary, depending on the clinical situation and the haemoglobin result. A high vaginal swab should be taken to exclude endometritis.

An ultrasound scan should be arranged to check that the uterus is empty and exclude retained products, including molar tissue. Care should be taken to interpret the findings in conjunction with the clinical picture because blood clot might have a similar scan appearance.

The diagnosis of a molar pregnancy is confirmed with a persistently raised serum β-hCG level. Evacuation of the uterus will yield tissue for histological analysis to confirm the diagnosis and exclude choriocarcinoma. However, if the latter is diagnosed, liver function tests and a chest X-ray should be performed to check for metastases.

Figure 33.5 provides an algorithm for the management of secondary PPH.

Management

Treatment must start with basic resuscitation (ABC) depending on the patient's condition and the extent of the bleeding. It is important to make an accurate estimation of the blood loss; it is frequently underestimated. Intravenous access must be established. Blood is sent for haemoglobin, platelets, clotting and cross-matching. In cases of massive obstetric haemorrhage, generally classified as $>/=$ 2000 mL, a multidisciplinary approach to management is very important, involving liaison between the obstetrician, the anaesthetist and the haematologist. The cause of the bleeding must be identified so that appropriate management can be instigated.

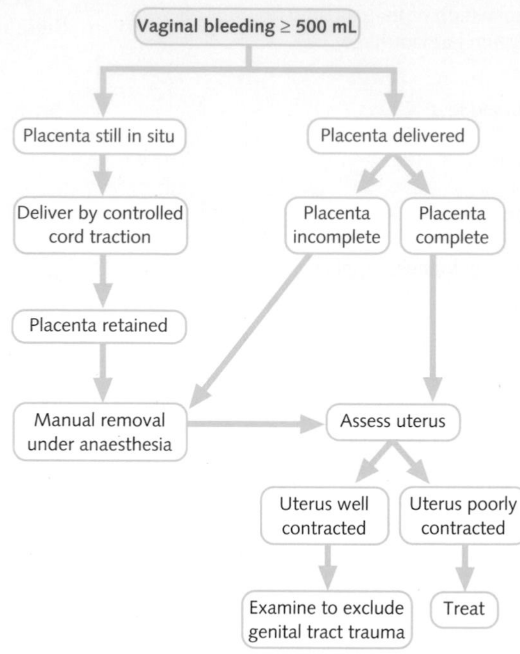

Fig. 33.4 Algorithm for the management of primary postpartum haemorrhage.

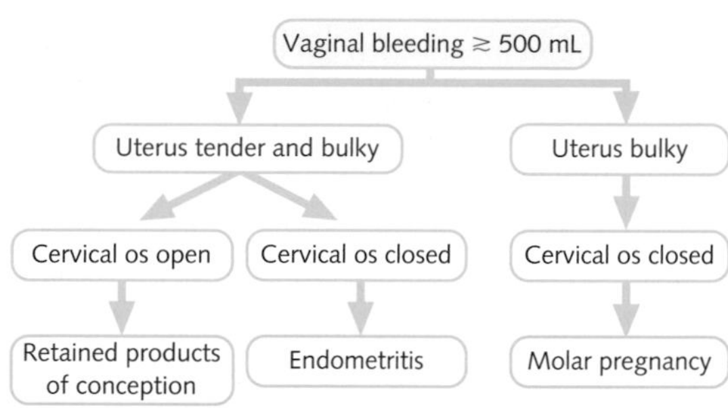

Fig. 33.5 Algorithm for the management of secondary postpartum haemorrhage.

HINTS AND TIPS

Good interdisciplinary communication is essential in obstetrics:

- haematologists in cases of massive PPH
- microbiologists in cases of sepsis of uncertain origin that does not respond to regular treatment
- psychiatrists in cases of postnatal mental illness.

All these disorders are associated with significant maternal morbidity and mortality.

Uterine atony

With uterine atony, the uterus is palpated and a contraction rubbed up by massaging the uterus abdominally. Bimanual compression may also be tried. Further oxytocic drugs are given, commonly intravenous syntocinon, initially as a single dose, then proceeding to an intravenous infusion. Prostaglandins may be beneficial, either carboprost can be injected intramuscularly or intramyometrially (also known as Hemabate®) or misoprostol can be given rectally. Use of the latter drug for this purpose is unlicensed.

In severe cases, surgery is necessary and even life-saving. This includes bilateral uterine artery ligation or bilateral internal iliac artery ligation. A B-Lynch compression suture can be performed to avoid hysterectomy and this preserves future fertility. However, prompt recourse to hysterectomy is essential to reduce maternal morbidity and mortality. This management is summarized in Figure 33.6.

Genital tract trauma

Bleeding while the uterus is firmly contracted is strong evidence of genital tract trauma or retained placenta. In the case of trauma, this should be repaired as soon

Fig. 33.6 Treatment of primary postpartum haemorrhage secondary to uterine atony.

- ABC
- Large bore IV access x 2
- Send FBC/XM/clotting/U&E
- Rub up uterine contractions by massaging the uterine fundus
- Give IV oxytocin
- Start oxytocin infusion
- Give PR/IM/intramyometrial prostaglandin
- Consider surgical options or uterine artery embolisation

as possible with appropriate analgesia (see Chapter 32 for perineal repair). There should be good light and care should be taken to minimize infection. Suturing may be necessary in theatre, for example, cervical lacerations bleed profusely and may need to be repaired under general anaesthesia.

Retained or incomplete placenta

If the placenta is still in situ, delivery should be attempted by controlled cord traction. Once delivered, the placenta must be examined to ensure that the cotyledons and the membranes are complete. If the placenta is still retained, manual removal is necessary under regional analgesia in the situation of a PPH. This is usually performed with antibiotic cover and with further doses of oxytocics.

Examination of the patient under anaesthetic allows exploration of the uterus if the placenta is thought to be incomplete. It also enables suturing of genital tract trauma such as cervical or vaginal lacerations once uterine atony is excluded as the cause of the PPH.

Placenta accreta

With routine active management of the third stage of labour, the placenta is usually delivered within minutes of the infant. If the patient is not bleeding, up to an hour can be left before undertaking manual removal under anaesthesia. Rarely, the placenta is found to be morbidly adherent to the uterine wall, known as a placenta accreta. Invasion of the myometrium by the placenta is known as placenta increta and if it is through the myometrium, it is known as placenta percreta. These conditions are associated with paucity of underlying decidua:

- Previous placenta praevia
- Uterine scar such as previous caesarean section
- Multiparity.

If the patient is not bleeding, it may be appropriate to leave the placenta in situ. Conservative management includes observation and antibiotics, as well as considering the use of the folate antagonist, methotrexate. However, more commonly, the patient has significant bleeding and surgery is necessary, including hysterectomy.

HINTS AND TIPS

The potential morbidity and mortality associated with PPH are so significant that earlier rather than delayed recourse to hysterectomy is essential.

Uterine inversion

The placenta and membranes should be delivered by controlled cord traction to prevent this rare complication of labour. It can be either complete, when the uterine fundus passes through the cervix, or incomplete, when the fundus is still above the cervix. It can occur spontaneously, for example in association with a fundal placental site or a unicornuate uterus, or it may be the result of mismanagement of the third stage.

The more serious presentation is of severe lower abdominal pain followed by collapse (due to neurogenic shock) and haemorrhage. The pain is secondary to tension on the infundibulopelvic ligaments. Treatment involves resuscitation of the patient, replacement of the uterus, either manually or hydrostatically, and oxytocin infusion.

Uterine rupture

This is seen very rarely in the UK, except in association with a previous caesarean section. It is associated with high rates of maternal and fetal morbidity and mortality. The incidence has fallen dramatically with the introduction of the lower segment procedure (<1%), as opposed to the classical vertical incision of the uterus (up to 5%). Spontaneous rupture is much less common. It is seen in a patient of high parity, associated with the use of syntocinon to augment labour.

Uterine rupture can present with an abnormal cardiotocograph (CTG) in labour (see Chapter 31), or with continuous abdominal pain and vaginal bleeding. Diagnosis is made at laparotomy and the treatment is surgical; either repair of the rupture or hysterectomy.

LACTATION

There are two main hormonal influences on breast tissue during pregnancy:

- Oestrogen increases the number and the size of the ducts
- Progesterone increases the number of alveoli.

Colostrum, which is rich in antibodies, is secreted in late pregnancy and production increases after delivery. The level of oestrogen falls in the first 48 hours after delivery so that prolactin can act on the alveoli and initiate lactation.

Suckling stimulates two reflexes:

1. The anterior part of the pituitary gland releases prolactin into the bloodstream, which induces the alveoli to secrete milk.
2. The posterior part of the pituitary gland releases oxytocin into the bloodstream, which causes contraction of the myoepithelial cells surrounding the alveoli so that the milk is ejected.

POSTNATAL INFECTION

Definition

Also known as puerperal infection, this is defined as a maternal temperature of 38 °C maintained for 4–6 hours in the first 14 days after delivery. The causative agent is commonly Group A Streptococcus.

Incidence

Infection remains a major cause of maternal mortality (see Chapter 35). However, with improved hygiene and the use of antibiotics, the incidence has fallen to 1–3%.

HINTS AND TIPS

Maternal sepsis is currently the major cause of maternal mortality and so must be investigated thoroughly and treated promptly.

Sites of infection

- Uterus
- Abdominal incision
- Perineum
- Chest
- Urinary tract
- Breast.

History

The site of infection is usually obvious from the patient's history. Dysuria and urine frequency would suggest a urinary tract infection. If there is also loin pain then there might be an ascending infection to the kidneys causing pyelonephritis. If the patient has a productive cough and complains of feeling breathless, then she may have a chest infection. This is typically a postoperative complication, seen after caesarean section.

A uterine infection is also more common after an operative intervention, such as a caesarean section or a manual removal of placenta. It typically presents with lower abdominal pain, sometimes with unpleasant-smelling vaginal discharge. Retained products of conception must be excluded. It is now routine practice to give prophylactic antibiotics at the time of a caesarean section to decrease the incidence of wound and uterine infection.

Infection in the perineum can also present with vaginal discharge, as well as localized discomfort. There is usually a history of a vaginal tear or an episiotomy. Acute mastitis, or infection of the breast, typically presents at the end of the first week after birth, as organisms that colonize the baby affect the breast. Infection presents with pain in one or both breasts associated with fever.

Examination

Examine the patient from head-to-toe, as suggested in Figure 33.7. Pyrexia, tachypnoea, hypotension and tachycardia will be present with infection.

Investigations

White blood cell count and C-reactive protein level may be high. Blood cultures are indicated if the patient's temperature is ≥38 °C.

Other investigations depend on the system that is involved:

- High vaginal swab for uterine infection
- Perineal swab
- Wound swab for caesarean section patient
- Mid-stream urine sample
- Sputum sample.

Management

The antibiotic of choice will depend on local protocol, but usually involves a broad-spectrum antibiotic and anaerobic cover with metronidazole for 5–7 days. Flucloxacillin is more appropriate for mastitis or wound infection because the usual pathogen is *Staphylococcus*.

POSTNATAL MENTAL ILLNESS

Incidence

Postnatal depression is one of the most common medical diseases of pregnancy, with 10% of women fulfilling the criteria for a depressive disorder. Psychosis is much rarer, affecting 0.2% of births. These disorders should be distinguished from the 'baby blues', which affects up to 70% of women, with a peak incidence on day 4 to 5. Tearfulness, anxiety and irritability normally settle with reassurance and support from family and friends.

History

Chapter 23 lists the risk factors for postnatal depression and some of these should be sought at the time of the antenatal booking, as recommended in the triennial report into maternal death (see Chapter 35). Puerperal psychosis in particular has associated risks: previous

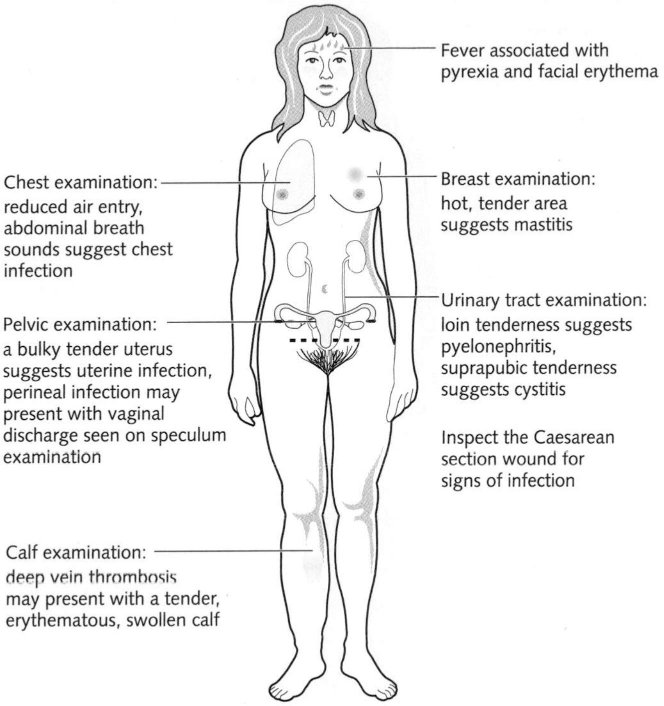

Fever associated with pyrexia and facial erythema

Chest examination: reduced air entry, abdominal breath sounds suggest chest infection

Breast examination: hot, tender area suggests mastitis

Pelvic examination: a bulky tender uterus suggests uterine infection, perineal infection may present with vaginal discharge seen on speculum examination

Urinary tract examination: loin tenderness suggests pyelonephritis, suprapubic tenderness suggests cystitis

Inspect the Caesarean section wound for signs of infection

Calf examination: deep vein thrombosis may present with a tender, erythematous, swollen calf

Fig. 33.7 Examination of the patient with postnatal pyrexia (see Chapter 35).

psychotic illness gives the woman a 1:2 chance of postnatal disease and a family history a 1:4 chance.

The common symptoms of postnatal depression and puerperal psychosis are shown in Figs 33.8 and 33.9, respectively. The peak time of onset for postnatal depression is a gradual onset 4 to 6 weeks postpartum, whereas the onset of psychosis is usually very sudden.

COMMUNICATION

Risk factors for postnatal mental illness include a previous history of mental health disorder either in or outside of pregnancy, as well as a family history of perinatal mental illness. Therefore it is essential to enquire sensitively in the antenatal period in order to aid prediction and allow early detection and management of postnatal mental illness.

Fig. 33.8 Symptoms of postnatal depression.

- Anxiety
- Low mood
- Fatigue
- Irritability
- Feelings of inadequacy
- Ambivalence towards the baby
- Reduced or absent libido

Fig. 33.9 Symptoms of puerperal psychosis.

- Insomnia or early morning wakening
- Lability of mood
- Overactivity
- Disorientation
- Lack of insight
- Hallucinations
- Persecutory beliefs, recurrent thoughts of death

Management

- Prevention
- Pharmocological
- Psychological/social.

The mainstay of management is prevention, which has improved recently as media interest increases public awareness. Early diagnosis and training of professionals to recognize the problems are also vital and has resulted in the development of the Edinburgh Postnatal Depression Scale, which is used successfully by health visitors across the UK.

Psychotherapy may be the first-line treatment for postnatal depression. Drug treatment is described in Chapter 23. As with any drug in pregnancy, use should be considered if the benefits outweigh the risks. The tricyclic antidepressants (TCAs) can be given safely both antenatally and postnatally. The newer selective serotonin reuptake inhibitors (SSRI) are probably safe, but there is less evidence to support this. Lithium is associated with cardiac anomalies, particularly Ebstein's anomaly, when used antenatally. It may be toxic to the baby and is therefore not recommended with breastfeeding. Electro-convulsive therapy is safe.

Health visitors and support groups all have an important role in helping the mother with postnatal illness.

THROMBOEMBOLIC DISEASE

Thromboembolic disease is the most common cause of pregnancy-related maternal mortality in the UK (see Chapter 34). Chapter 23 describes the risk factors, diagnosis and management in detail. Of particular importance are those women who undergo caesarean section. However, it is vital not to forget that a woman who has had a normal delivery might still have significant risk factors, such as obesity or hypertension, which necessitate thromboprophylaxis in the postpartum period of up to 6 weeks.

Further reading

Chamberlain, G., Steer, P., 2001. Turnbull's Obstetrics, third ed. Churchill Livingstone, London.

Enkin, M.W., Keirse, M.J.N.C., 2000. A Guide to Effective Care in Pregnancy and Childbirth, 3rd ed. Oxford University Press, Oxford.

Cantwell, R., Clutton-Brock, T., Cooper, G., et al., 2011. Saving Mothers' lives: reviewing maternal deaths to make motherhood safer: 2006-2008. The eighth report of the confidential enquiries into maternal deaths in the United Kingdom. BJOG. 118 (Suppl. 1), 1–203. http://dx.doi.org/10.1111/j.1471-0528.2010.02847.x.

RCOG, 2009. Reducing the Risk of Thrombosis and Embolism During Pregnancy and the Puerperium. Green-top Guideline No. 37. Royal College of Obstetricians and Gynaecologists, London.

NICE, 2007. National Evidence-Based Clinical Guideline 37. Postpartum Care. National Institute for Health and Care Excellence, London.

NICE, 2007. National Evidence-Based Clinical Guideline 45. Antenatal and Postnatal Mental Health. National Institute for Health and Care Excellence, London.

Maternal collapse

Objectives

By the end of this chapter, you should be able to:

- Understand how to assess a maternal collapse
- Understand the potential causes of maternal collapse
- Understand the initial management.

INTRODUCTION

Maternal collapse is a rare but serious event that requires prompt effective management. The Royal College of Obstetricians and Gynaecologists (RCOG) defines maternal collapse as 'an acute event involving the cardiorespiratory systems and/or brain, resulting in a reduced or absent conscious level (and potentially death), at any stage in pregnancy and up to six weeks after delivery'. In view of the serious nature of a maternal collapse and the importance of prompt management, most units in the UK run training sessions to educate clinicians on how this should be managed. The aim of this chapter is to give an overview of the main causes and initial management.

THE COLLAPSED PATIENT

The prospect of facing a collapsed patient can be very daunting for any clinician. As with any patient, the importance of summoning help and following the ABC guide of management is paramount. There are however important differences in management of the obstetric patient:

- Maintenance of a left lateral tilt during resuscitation to prevent aorto-caval compression and increase venous return (Fig. 34.1)
- The mother takes priority over the fetus and unless needed to aid maternal resuscitation, delivery of the fetus should be delayed until the mother is stable.

Figure 34.2 shows an algorithm for the initial management of the collapse patient.

CAUSES OF MATERNAL COLLAPSE

Haemorrhage

Haemorrhage has been identified as the most common cause of collapse in obstetric patients. In many cases, the bleeding will be obvious or revealed. However, in cases such as concealed placental abruption, after a caesarean or ruptured ectopic pregnancy, it may be concealed and a high index of clinical suspicion is required. In the last Centre for Maternal and Child Enquiries (CMACE) report nine women died from haemorrhage (see Chapter 35).

Major haemorrhage can be due to:

- postpartum bleeding (secondary to uterine atony or trauma)
- placenta praevia/accrete
- placental abruption
- uterine rupture or a non-obstetric intra-abdominal bleed (splenic rupture etc.).

More information on individual causes can be found in Chapter 21 (Antepartum haemorrhage).

Accurate diagnosis and resuscitation with fluids +/− blood products is imperative as these patients can rapidly deteriorate. Early involvement of senior multidisciplinary clinicians including the anaesthetic team will allow optimal management such as insertion of central intravenous access. In situations where blood is needed rapidly the use of group O negative blood may be required.

In cases of massive antepartum haemorrhage prompt delivery of the fetus and placenta should be considered to allow control of bleeding.

Thromboembolism

Although no longer the leading cause of direct maternal death according to the last confidential enquiry (2005–2008) thromboembolism remains a leading cause of maternal collapse. The use of prophylactic measures such as compression stockings, low molecular weight heparin (LMWH) and maintaining a high index of suspicion is thought to have contributed to the decline in deaths.

Pulmonary emboli (PE) can present with chest pain, tachycardia, tachypnoea and shortness of breath. Large PEs can, however, cause maternal collapse.

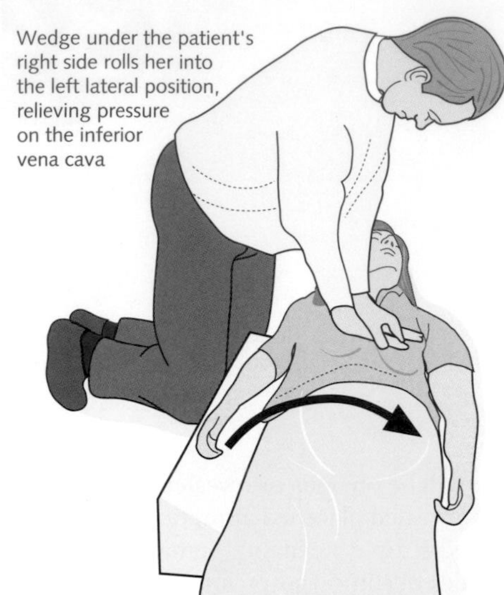

Fig. 34.1 Left tilt in the collapsed patient.

Initial management with cardiopulmonary resuscitation, oxygen and anticoagulation should be commenced until the diagnosis can be ruled out. In certain cases thrombolysis may be necessary. Chapter 23 – Medical disorders in pregnancy – deals with the topic in greater detail.

Amniotic fluid embolism

An amniotic fluid embolism (AFE) is a rare but very serious cause of maternal collapse which carries a high rate of mortality. Sadly the diagnosis is often made retrospectively at post-mortem and in patients who do survive there can be significant morbidity. Patients may present with:

- acute hypotension
- hypoxia
- respiratory distress
- seizures
- cardiac arrest.

It should be considered as a diagnosis when patients collapse during labour, caesarean section, manual removal of placenta or within 30 minutes of these.

An AFE is thought to occur when amniotic fluid enters maternal circulation and travels to distant sites such as the lungs and occludes pulmonary vessels. In addition an anaphylactic-like reaction is thought to occur. These patients then rapidly develop a coagulopathy and haemorrhage can ensue.

Management of these patients is largely supportive with maintenance of their airway, breathing and circulation. CPR may be necessary and regular blood test including clotting studies to identify any possible coagulopathy. Close liaison with the anaesthetic team and haematologists is vital and prompt correction of any coagulopathy.

Acute myocardial infarction

The last CMACE report highlighted that cardiac disease was the most common indirect cause of maternal death and, therefore, should be taken very seriously. MI must be considered in patients:

- with a history of congenital heart defects
- with a history of previous cardiac surgery
- with a history of rheumatic fever or infective endocarditis
- who smoke
- who have hypertension
- who have a high body mass index (BMI).

Patients may present collapsed or give a history of chest pain (central crushing) which radiates to the jaw +/− left arm. An electrocardiogram (ECG) should be performed in addition to other standard measures and medical advice sought as soon as possible. In obstetric patients who present collapsed, the resuscitation algorithm is identical to non-pregnant patients with the addition of conducting CPR with a left lateral tilt.

Eclampsia

Pre-eclampsia and eclampsia are both discussed in detail in Chapter 22 – Hypertension in pregnancy. In regard to the collapsed patient, eclampsia should always be considered a cause of maternal collapse. By definition, eclampsia is seizure-like activity associated with hypertension. Patients who are found collapsed may have had an eclamptic fit which may or may not have been witnessed. There may be preceding history of hypertension in association with proteinuria and if an eclamptic fit is suspected, prompt management with magnesium sulphate and antihypertensives should be started. Again it should be emphasized that stabilization of the mother in these cases takes precedence over that of the fetus.

Sepsis

Sepsis has now become the leading direct cause of maternal death (see Chapter 35) and again prompt management is essential when faced with a collapsed patient in whom sepsis is suspected. Septic patients may present with:

- pyrexia
- tachycardia
- hypotension
- rigors
- confusion
- collapse.

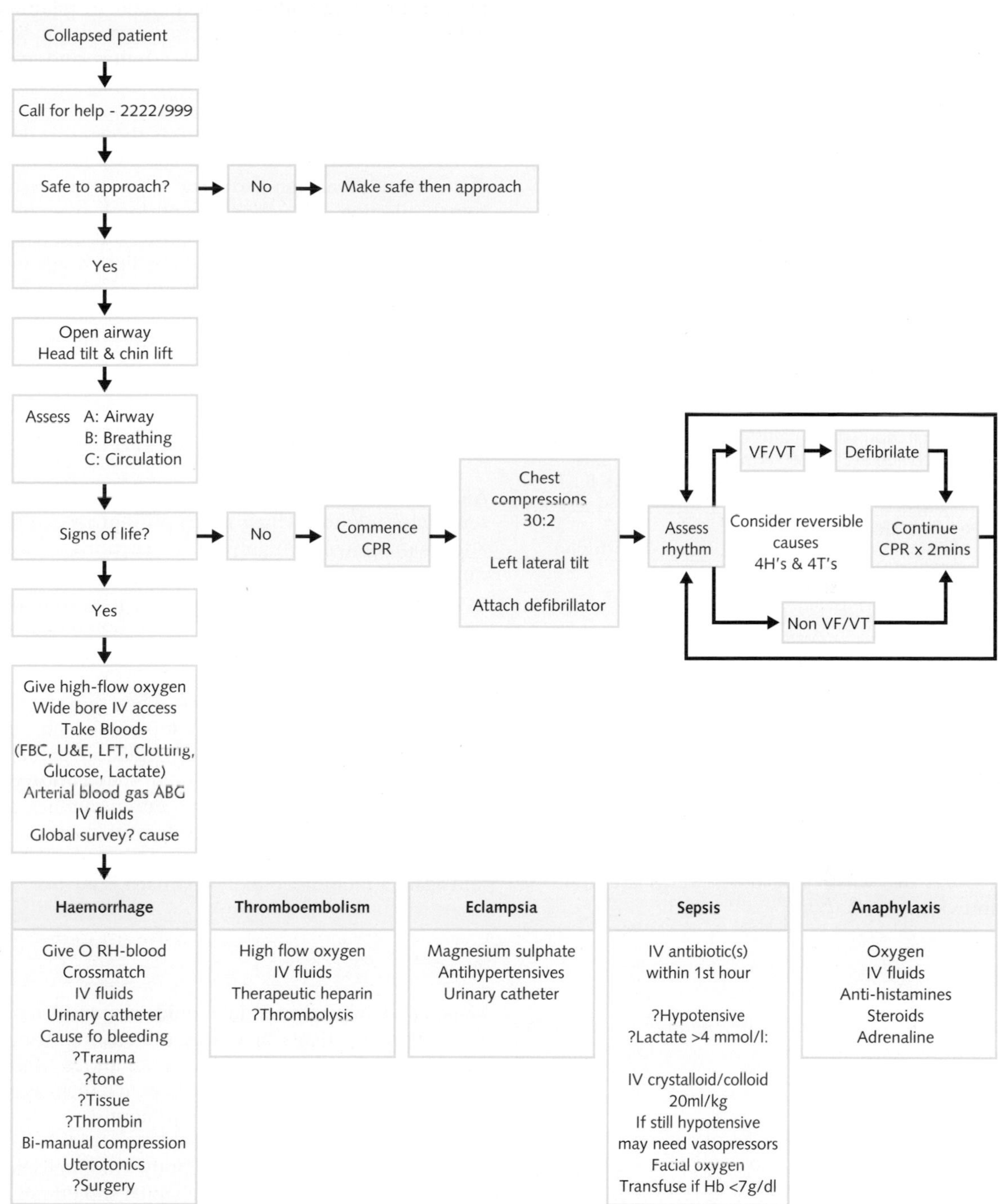

Fig. 34.2 Algorithm for the initial management of the collapsed obstetric patient.

Fig. 34.3 Sepsis care bundle.

Apply immediately or within 6 hours
1. Measure serum lactate.
2. Obtain blood cultures/culture swabs prior to antibiotics.
3. Administer antibiotic(s) within 1st hour of recognition of severe sepsis/septic shock according to local protocol
4. In the event of hypotension and/or lactate >4 mmol/l:
   a. Give an initial (min) volume of 20 ml/kg of crystalloid/ colloid
   b. Once adequate volume replacement, a vasopressor (noradrenaline, adrenaline) and/or an inotrope (e.g. dobutamine) may be used to maintain MAP > 65 mmHg.

Further management consists of:

5. In the event of hypotension despite fluid resuscitation (shock) and/or lactate over 4 mmol/l:
   a. Achieve a CVP of ≥ 8 mmHg (or ≥ 12 mmHg if mechanically ventilated) with aggressive fluid replacement
   b. Consider steroids.
6. Maintain O_2 sats with facial oxygen. Transfusion if Hb <7 g/dl.

In order to maximize the patient's chances of survival prompt treatment with IV antibiotics and IV fluids is paramount. Close multidisciplinary liaison with the anaesthetists and microbiologists is essential. The concept of the 'golden hour' during which all investigations, and management should be started has been recommended as a rule to remember. Figure 34.3 shows the Surviving sepsis guidelines, which are aimed at improving maternal care.

Drug toxicity

Drug toxicity can occur due to a number of causes and should be borne in mind when assessing a collapsed patient. Any history of the following should be considered:

- Illicit drug use
- Epidural can cause collapse due to a 'high spinal'
- Local anaesthetic may have had inadvertent intravenous administration
- Anaphylaxis.

Patients that are thought to have taken illicit drugs can present in a number of ways. Opiates such as heroine can present with reduced consciousness and respiratory depression. These patients can have pin-point pupils and will respond rapidly to treatment with naloxone. Ecstasy and cocaine users can present with seizures, hyperthermia, headaches and chest pain. Seizures can be treated with benzodiazepines such as diazepam.

A 'high-spinal' or 'total spinal' is thought to occur when there is excessive intrathecal spread of local anaesthetic. In addition it can also occur if there is inadvertent spinal injection of high doses of local anaesthetic. Depression of cervical nerves follows and the patient may complain of difficulty breathing, light headedness or collapse. Prompt recognition and supportive measures including IV fluids, intubation and vasopressors are essential as these patients can rapidly progress to cardiac arrest.

Anaphylaxis

Anaphylaxis is a very serious potentially fatal hypersensitivity reaction which needs prompt recognition and management. Anaphylactic reactions affect a number of systems and cardiac arrest can rapidly occur.

Any recent administration of drugs should be noted especially antibiotics and any known allergies identified, including to latex.

Anaphylaxis is said to be likely when there is rapid onset and progression of symptoms with life-threatening airway/breathing or circulation problems and skin/mucosal changes (RCOG). Rapid treatment with oxygen, IV fluids, steroids, anti-histamines and adrenaline is required along with removal of any potentially triggering factors. Intensive care maybe needed and again a multidisciplinary approach is advised.

Hypo or hyperglycaemia

Hypo- and hyperglycaemia should be considered in pregnancy as patients may have pre-existing diabetes or gestational diabetes. A finger prick blood glucose level should be taken for every collapsed patient as part of their assessment and acted on promptly.

Hypoglycaemia as a cause of collapse is likely to be severe and should be treated promptly with intravenous glucose (50 ml of 50% glucose), which should rapidly correct the situation.

Hyperglycaemia when presenting with a collapse can indicate diabetic ketoacidosis (DKA). Blood and urinary ketones should be measured. Prompt treatment with IV fluids and sliding scale insulin is important as well as monitoring of potassium levels.

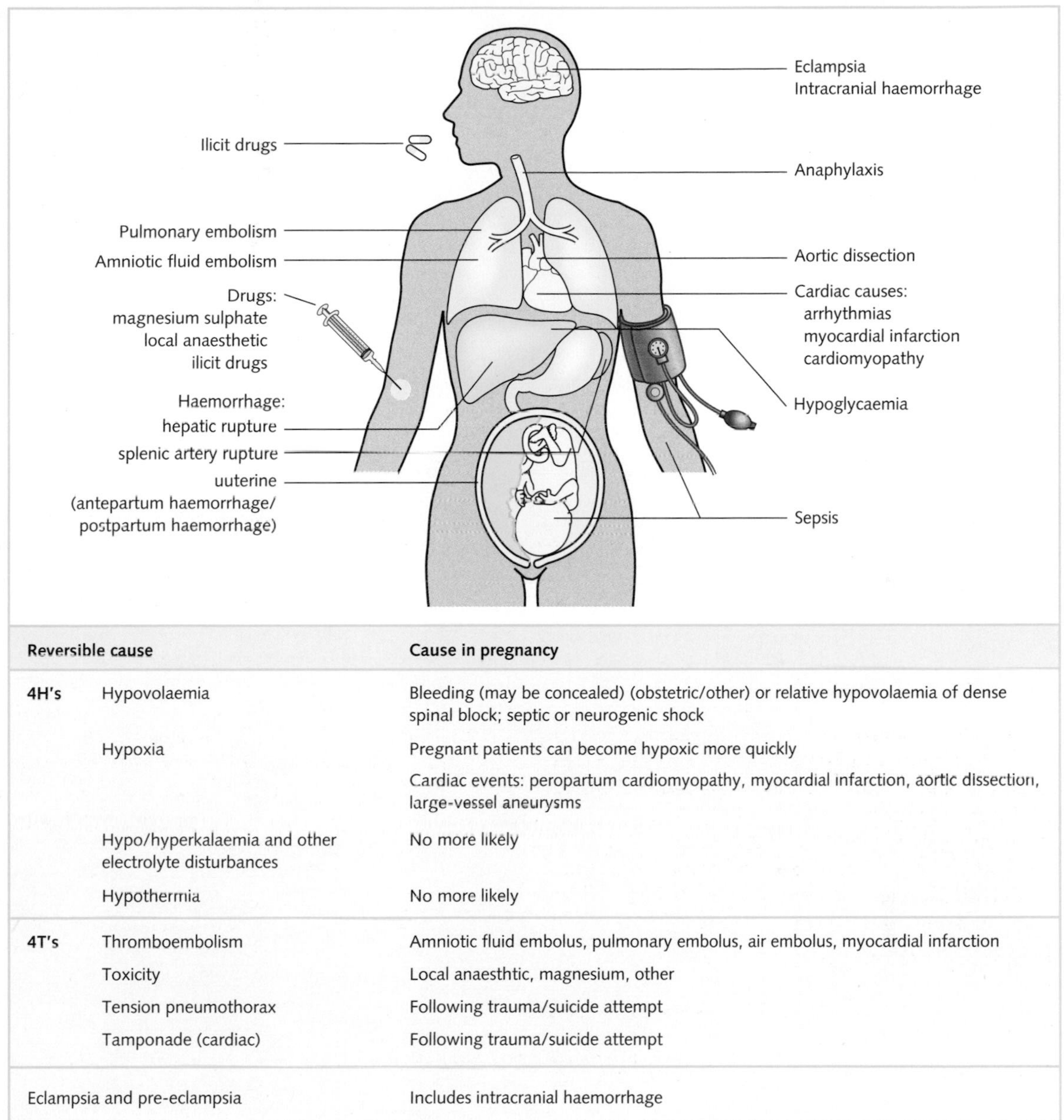

Reversible cause		Cause in pregnancy
4H's	Hypovolaemia	Bleeding (may be concealed) (obstetric/other) or relative hypovolaemia of dense spinal block; septic or neurogenic shock
	Hypoxia	Pregnant patients can become hypoxic more quickly
		Cardiac events: peropartum cardiomyopathy, myocardial infarction, aortic dissection, large-vessel aneurysms
	Hypo/hyperkalaemia and other electrolyte disturbances	No more likely
	Hypothermia	No more likely
4T's	Thromboembolism	Amniotic fluid embolus, pulmonary embolus, air embolus, myocardial infarction
	Toxicity	Local anaesthtic, magnesium, other
	Tension pneumothorax	Following trauma/suicide attempt
	Tamponade (cardiac)	Following trauma/suicide attempt
Eclampsia and pre-eclampsia		Includes intracranial haemorrhage

Fig. 34.4 Causes of maternal collapse (RCOG guideline no. 56).

Other causes

There are a huge number of other causes of maternal collapse in addition to those listed above, Figure 34.4 summarizes the main possible causes as well as the 4 H's and 4 T's which are used to remember the reversible causes of a cardiac arrest.

Further reading

RCOG, 2011. Maternal Collapse in Pregnancy and the Puerperium. Green-top Guideline No. 56. Royal College of Obstetricians and Gynaecologists, London.

Maternal death

Objectives

By the end of this chapter, you should be able to:
- Understand the prevalence of maternal death and its sub-classifications
- Understand the role of confidential enquiries into maternal deaths
- Understand the key recommendations from the reports.

INTRODUCTION

In any unit a maternal death is a traumatic and distressing experience for all involved. It has wide reaching implications not only for the family of the deceased but also the lessons that can be learned from the tragedy.

Maternal mortality rates in the UK have fallen dramatically since the early 1900s and since 1952 triennial reports have been published to report on the deaths and make recommendations about changes in practice. Maternal deaths, however, still continue to happen and the reporting and learning from these events is essential in order to further reduce the rates of maternal mortality.

Figure 35.1 shows the falling trend in maternal mortality over time.

MOTHERS AND BABIES: REDUCING RISK THROUGH AUDIT AND CONFIDENTIAL ENQUIRIES ACROSS THE UK

Mothers and Babies: Reducing Risk through Audit and Confidential Enquiries across the UK (MBRRACE), known prior to 2013 as CMACE (Centre for Maternal and Child Enquiries) and CEMACH (Confidential Enquiry into Maternal and Child Health) is an organization whose aim is to improve the care given to mothers by carrying out confidential enquiries into maternal and infant deaths.

Every 3 years, a report is published highlighting the main causes of maternal death and trends over time. Recommendations based on investigations into these deaths are also made to allow changes in local practice. Figure 35.2 shows the maternal mortality and morbidity cycle used in their work.

In the most recent report published in March 2011 the maternal mortality rate was 11.39/100 000, which was down from the previous report where the rate was 13.95/100 000. The report highlighted a welcomed fall in the maternal mortality rate in Black African women and in mothers living in the most deprived areas. Deaths from thromboembolism (previously the leading direct cause of maternal death) had also fallen, but, alarmingly, deaths from sepsis (Group A β-haemolytic Streptococcus in particular) had increased.

DEFINITIONS

When assessing maternal deaths various definitions are used to categorize them, these are listed below:

Maternal deaths: Deaths of women while pregnant or within 42 days of the end of the pregnancy from any cause related to or aggravated by the pregnancy or its management, but not from accidental or incidental causes (includes ectopic pregnancy, miscarriage and terminations of pregnancy).

Direct maternal death: Deaths resulting from obstetric complications of the pregnant state (pregnancy, labour and puerperium), from interventions, omissions, incorrect treatment or from a chain of events resulting from any of the above.

Indirect maternal death: Deaths resulting from previous existing disease, or disease that developed during pregnancy and which was not the result of direct obstetric causes, but which was aggravated by the physiological effects of pregnancy.

Late maternal death: Deaths occurring between 42 days and 1 year after abortion, miscarriage or delivery that are the result of direct or indirect maternal causes.

Coincidental: Deaths from unrelated causes, which happen to occur in pregnancy or the puerperium.

Fig. 35.1 Death rates from 1952 to the present.

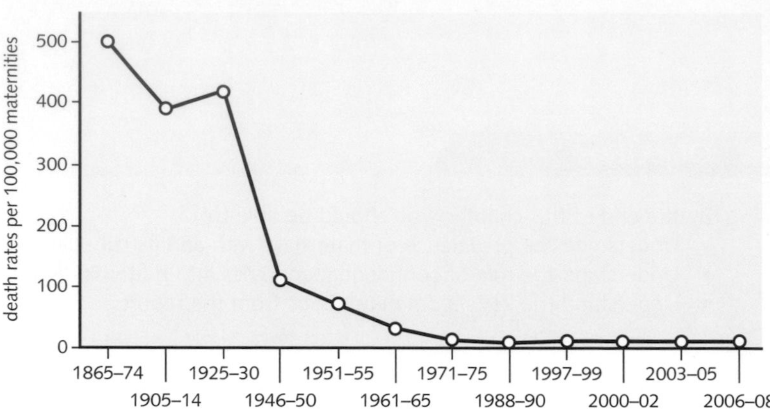

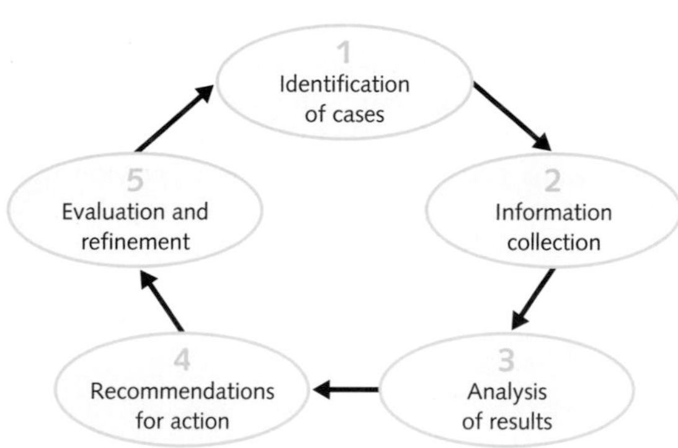

Fig. 35.2 Process cycle for the investigation of maternal deaths (CMACE Report 2008–2011)

CAUSES OF MATERNAL DEATH

Figure 35.3 displays the maternal death rates for certain direct and indirect causes from the last three confidential reports.

Direct causes

Sepsis

The last CMACE report published in March 2011 showed that sepsis, in particular secondary to Group A Streptococcus (GAS), has surpassed thromboembolism as the leading DIRECT cause of maternal death. Recommendations include:

- prompt recognition of sepsis
- treatment with broad-spectrum antibiotics
- education of patients in prevention, such as hand hygiene, perineal hygiene and seeking help if symptomatic.

These issues must be remembered in the postnatal patients as well as in antenatal patients. Chapter 34 – Maternal collapse – deals with the management of sepsis in more detail.

Young children often have sore throats which can be caused by GAS and, therefore, education of mothers in regard to hand hygiene is essential particularly if they have other children or will be in contact with them. In addition the importance of seeking medical advice early should be emphasized.

Thromboembolism

Although no longer the leading cause of direct maternal death it still remains a very important issue. Pregnancy is a prothrombotic state and, therefore, all patients should be educated about signs and symptoms as well as how to seek help. Units in the UK have robust protocols in place for the prevention of venous thromboembolism (VTE) in pregnancy and guidelines have been issued by the Royal College of Obstetricians and Gynaecologists in regard to who should receive prophylactic low molecular weight heparin (see Chapter 23).

Risk assessments should be performed:

- at booking
- on every antenatal admission
- after delivery

for all patients, but in particular those who are obese or have other risk factors such as age, family history of VTE, thrombophilia, immobility, etc.

A low threshold for investigation of symptoms of VTE is important in preventing adverse outcomes.

Pre-eclampsia and eclampsia

Pre-eclampsia and eclampsia accounted for nineteen deaths in the last CMACE report. The recognition of the importance of prompt treatment of hypertension,

	2000–2002	2003–2005	2006–2008
Direct deaths			
Sepsis	13	18	26
Pre-eclampsia and eclampsia	14	18	19
Thrombosis & thromboembolism	30	41	18
Amniotic fluid embolism	5	17	13
Ectopic	11	10	6
Haemorrhage	17	14	9
Anaesthesia	6	6	7
Other Direct	8	4	4
All Direct	106	132	107
Indirect			
Cardiac disease	44	48	53
Other Indirect causes	50	50	49
Coincidental	36	55	50

Fig. 35.3 Direct and indirect causes of maternal death from the last three confidential reports.

particularly systolic hypertension, is essential to prevent serious complications such as stroke.

Patients presenting with headaches, visual disturbances or high blood pressure should have their urine tested for the presence of protein and blood tests should be taken to exclude pre-eclampsia. Prompt identification and management will maximize the chances of a safe outcome for both mother and fetus.

Haemorrhage

Nine mothers died from haemorrhage in the last confidential report which was a decline on previous years. Management guidelines and training have helped to ensure all staff are able to deal with cases of haemorrhage including:

- use of maternity early warning charts
- prompt recognition and resuscitation
- involvement of a senior multidisciplinary team
- optimization of haemoglobin levels antenatally
- early recourse to methods such as uterine artery embolization or hysterectomy.

The latter can be life saving especially in individuals who refuse blood products.

Amniotic fluid embolism

An amniotic fluid embolism (AFE) is a rare but very serious case of maternal collapse that carries a high rate of mortality. Patients may present with acute hypotension, hypoxia, respiratory distress, seizures or, indeed, cardiac arrest. It should be considered as a diagnosis when patients collapse during labour, caesarean section, manual removal of placenta or within 30 minutes of these. In the last confidential report 13 patients died from an AFE. Chapter 34 – Maternal collapse – deals with the management of an AFE in more detail.

Ectopic pregnancy

An ectopic pregnancy can be defined as implantation of an embryo outside of the uterine cavity (see Chapter 20). However, pregnancies may implant at the site of a previous caesarean section, also referred to as scar ectopics, whilst still technically being in the uterine cavity.

Most commonly the site of implantation is the fallopian tube and if left unnoticed the pregnancy will eventually rupture. The rupture can lead to massive blood loss and, sadly, even death.

In the last confidential report six patients died from complications of an ectopic pregnancy and, therefore, the diagnosis must always be considered in women of child bearing age. In some cases, an ectopic pregnancy can present as gastro-intestinal upset and the patient may not know they are pregnant. It is for this reason that any female of reproductive age that presents with gastrointestinal symptoms should have a pregnancy test performed and if positive, an ectopic pregnancy ruled out.

A high index of suspicion is required in all patients who present with pain and bleeding in early pregnancy and education about signs and symptoms of an ectopic should be given to all patients as well as information on how to seek help. Any patient that presents with a positive pregnancy test with an intrauterine device in situ (Mirena® or copper coil) should be treated as an ectopic until proven otherwise.

Indirect causes

Cardiac disease

Cardiac disease has now become the leading cause of indirect maternal death and in the most recent report was responsible for 53 deaths. The exact causes of death included aortic dissection, myocardial infarction and cardiomyopathy.

In view of the rising trend in cardiac deaths, recommendations were made and the following highlighted:

- Those patients with a known history of cardiac disease to be referred early for consultant led care in a joint obstetric/cardiology clinic
- Low threshold for investigation of patients complaining of chest pain particularly that which radiates to the jaw, back or arm
- Be alert to those with risk factors such as obesity, smokers and those with hypertension.

Psychiatric illness

Maternal deaths from psychiatric illness accounted for 67 deaths in the latest report. This figure also includes late maternal deaths which were attributed to psychiatric illness. The majority of these deaths were due to suicide and the importance of identifying patients with a history of psychiatric illness was emphasized.

In addition it was recommended that all patients with a history of psychiatric illness should be referred to specialist services as a priority. A key finding from the report was that over half of the maternal suicides were: white, married, employed, living in comfortable circumstances and aged 30 years or older. It recommended that when assessing a patient's risk of suicide, care should be taken that this may not necessarily equate to their socio-economic status. A significant percentage of deaths from suicide were late maternal deaths indicating the importance of extended specialist postnatal follow-up in at-risk groups.

Coincidental maternal deaths

This category includes a large number of varied causes of death, with road traffic accidents and murder being the two most common. Domestic violence remains a major cause for concern to all clinicians caring for obstetric patients and should be actively screened for at each contact. Patients suffering from domestic violence are likely to be:

- late bookers
- have a poor attendance record
- have repeated admissions for seemingly trivial matters.

Partners may appear to be domineering, constantly present during all visits and those who do not let the patient answer questions should raise concerns about domestic violence. Where indicated, professional interpreters should be used rather than family members and any concerns acted upon.

Further reading

Cantwell, R., Clutton-Brock, T., Cooper, G., et al., 2011. Saving Mothers' lives: reviewing maternal deaths to make motherhood safer: 2006-2008. The eighth report of the confidential enquiries into maternal deaths in the United Kingdom. BJOG. 118 (Suppl. 1), 1–203. http://dx.doi.org/10.1111/j.1471-0528.2010.02847.x.

SELF-ASSESSMENT

Single best answer questions (SBAs)

1. Which of the following statements is incorrect?
   A. Premature menopause is defined as the last period before the age of 45 (but after 40 years) of age
   B. The average age of menopause is 51
   C. All patients should receive HRT
   D. Where there is a uterus both oestrogen and progesterone should be given as HRT
   E. Endometrial cancer is a contraindication to HRT

2. Transdermal HRT is becoming increasingly popular. Which statement regarding transdermal HRT is incorrect?
   A. Avoids first-pass metabolism
   B. Reduced risk of VTE
   C. Continuous administration
   D. Only contain oestrogen
   E. Can cause skin reactions

3. Clonidine is a centrally acting alpha-2 agonist used in the menopause, which of the following symptoms has it been shown to be useful in treating?
   A. Hair loss
   B. Loss of libido
   C. Osteoporosis
   D. Hot flushes
   E. Mood swings

4. Which of the following statistics reflects the success rate of conception for a couple trying for 1 year?
   A. 60% will conceive within 1 year with regular unprotected sexual intercourse
   B. 84% will conceive within 1 year with regular unprotected sexual intercourse
   C. 15% will conceive within 1 year with regular unprotected sexual intercourse
   D. 20% will conceive within 1 year with regular unprotected sexual intercourse
   E. 96% will conceive within 1 year with regular unprotected sexual intercourse

5. Which of the following is NOT known to cause subfertility in either the male or the female partner?
   A. Chlamydia infection
   B. Polycystic ovarian syndrome (PCOS)
   C. Epididymo-orchitis
   D. Endometriosis
   E. Varicose veins

6. Which of the following investigations should ideally be performed before a patient attends for a hysterosalpingogram?
   A. Rubella immunity
   B. Full blood count
   C. Pelvic infection screen (high vaginal and endocervical swabs)
   D. Thyroid function tests
   E. Day 21 progesterone

7. Which of the following is NOT a risk factor for cervical cancer?
   A. Human papilloma virus
   B. Smoking
   C. Multiple sexual partners
   D. Early age of first intercourse
   E. History of endometriosis

8. Mary is 55-years-old and has not had a period for 4 years. She had an ultrasound because she was feeling bloated which showed bilateral multilocular cysts and her CA125 was 80. What is her risk of malignancy index?
   A. 240
   B. 80
   C. 0
   D. 720
   E. 411

9. Agatha is 66 and underwent her last period over 15 years ago. Over the last week she has noted some blood spotting on her underwear. She has a body mass index of 34 and her GP organized an ultrasound, which showed an endometrial thickness of 12 mm. What is the most important investigation she should have next?
   A. MRI pelvis
   B. Chest X-ray
   C. Hysteroscopy and endometrial biopsy
   D. CT abdomen and pelvis
   E. Cervical smear

10. Which of the following examination findings is most suggestive of endometriosis?
    A. Cervical excitation
    B. Adnexal mass
    C. Nodules in the posterior fornix
    D. Generalized tenderness
    E. Uterine tenderness

11. Which of the following aspects of the history is most suggestive of endometriosis?
    A. Deep dyspareunia
    B. Vaginal discharge
    C. Cyclical pelvic pain
    D. Subfertility
    E. Gastrointestinal symptoms

12. A patient presents with right iliac fossa pain and cervical excitation. Her last menstrual period was 6 weeks ago. What is the most likely cause?
    A. Tubo ovarian abscess
    B. Ovarian cyst
    C. Appendicitis
    D. Fibroid
    E. Ectopic pregnancy

13. A patient gives a history of cyclical pelvic pain associated with secondary dysmenorrhoea. What is the most likely diagnosis?
    A. PID
    B. Endometriosis
    C. Fibroid
    D. Adhesions
    E. Vulval dystrophy

14. A 27-year-old woman with a known benign ovarian cyst is admitted to Accident and Emergency department with an acute abdomen. What is the most important test to do?
    A. Full blood count
    B. Group and save
    C. Mid-stream urine
    D. Pregnancy test
    E. Pelvic ultrasound scan

15. How is the RMI (risk of malignancy index) calculated?
    A. U(ultrasound score) x M (menopause score) x Ca125 level
    B. U(ultrasound score) + M (menopause score) + Ca125 level
    C. U(ultrasound score) / M (menopause score) x Ca125 level
    D. U(ultrasound score) x M (menopause score) / Ca125 level
    E. U (ultrasound score) + M (menopause score) / CA19-9 level

16. A woman diagnosed with a benign epithelial tumour presented with irregular vaginal bleeding. What is the likely diagnosis?
    A. Serous cystadenoma
    B. Mucinous cystadenoma
    C. Brenner tumours
    D. Endometrioid tumours
    E. Dermoid cyst

17. Which of the following examination findings is most suggestive of malignancy in a woman with vaginal discharge?
    A. Raised temperature
    B. Cervical excitation
    C. Tachycardia
    D. Generalized lymphadenopathy
    E. Cachexia

18. Which of the following is not a pathological cause of vaginal discharge?
    A. Cervical carcinoma
    B. Cervical ectropian
    C. Candida albicans
    D. Chlamydia trachomatis
    E. Fistula

19. A patient has been diagnosed with candida infection. Which of the following supports this diagnosis?
    A. Grey, fishy-smelling discharge
    B. Thick, itchy, white discharge
    C. Dysuria
    D. Urinary frequency
    E. Lower abdominal pain

20. A patient presents with abnormal vaginal discharge. Which aspect of her history is most helpful to rule out an infective cause?
    A. Age
    B. Weight loss
    C. Irregular vaginal bleeding
    D. Anorexia
    E. Sexual history

21. Which of the following in a patient's history is known to predispose them to Pelvic Inflammatory Disease (PID)?
    A. Monogamous relationship
    B. >25 years of age
    C. Use of Mirena IUS
    D. History of sexually transmitted infection (STI)
    E. Later onset of sexual activity

22. A patient with pelvic inflammatory disease (PID) presents with offensive, fishy smelling par vagina discharge. High vaginal swab confirms:
    A. Chlamydia
    B. Gonorrhoea
    C. Anaerobes including Gardnerella and Mycoplasma
    D. Candida
    E. Trichomonas vaginosis

23. Which of these is not an appropriate first-line investigation for pelvic inflammatory disease (PID)?
    A. White cell count (WCC)
    B. C-reactive protein (CRP)
    C. Erythrocyte sedimentation rate (ESR)
    D. Laparoscopy
    E. STD screen
    F. Pelvic ultrasound scan

24. A patient is diagnosed with acute PID. Which of the following signs does NOT support that diagnosis?
    A. Raised temperature > 37.5°C
    B. Tachycardia
    C. Vulval pruritis
    D. Abdominal tenderness
    E. Adnexal mass

25. Which of the following are not recognised risk factors for genital prolapse?
A. Connective tissue disorders
B. Prolonged labour
C. Diarrhoea
D. Increasing parity
E. Chronic cough

26. The following is an indication for the use of a vaginal pessary to manage genital prolapse:
A. The patient is post-menopausal
B. The patient prefers surgical management
C. The patient is medically fit for surgery
D. The patient is on the waiting list for surgery
E. Major degrees of prolapse with lax introitus

27. A patient has been diagnosed with genital prolapse. She has weakness in the levator ani muscles which has caused a bulge in the mid-posterior vaginal wall. This is called:
A. Cystocele
B. Procidentia
C. Vault descent
D. Uterine descent
E. Rectocele

28. A patient has prolapse of the upper anterior wall of the vagina, attached to bladder by fascia. This is called:
A. Cystocele
B. Cystourethrocoele
C. Vault descent
D. Enterocoele
E. Uterine descent

29. An 18-year-old woman seeks emergency contraception after unprotected sexual intercourse 72 hours ago. She has had two surgical terminations of pregnancy, following condom failure. Which is the most suitable method to offer?
A. Levonelle
B. Intrauterine contraceptive device (IUCD)
C. Ulipristal acetate
D. Implanon
E. Combined oral contraception

30. A 21-year-old student is requesting a reliable long-acting non-hormonal contraceptive. She has never been pregnant and is in a stable relationship. What is the most suitable option for her?
A. Condoms
B. Progesterone only pill
C. Diaphragm
D. Copper IUCD
E. Progestogen implant (Implanon)

31. A 42-year-old woman is requesting sterilization. She has completed her family, does not want to use an IUCD and her husband has refused to have a vasectomy. What is the lifetime failure rate of sterilization?
A. 1:20 000
B. 1:20
C. 1:200
D. 1: 2000
E. 1:2

32. Which of these risk factors is an absolute contraindication to combined oral contraceptive pill?
A. Family history of thrombosis
B. Hypertension
C. Migraine
D. Varicose veins
E. Pregnancy

33. Which of the following most accurately confirms molar pregnancy?
A. Ultrasound findings
B. Histology
C. Speculum findings
D. History of hyperemesis
E. Enlarged uterus, greater than gestation dates

34. Which of the following can result in an on-going, viable pregnancy?
A. Ectopic pregnancy
B. Molar pregnancy
C. Delayed miscarriage
D. Incomplete miscarriage
E. Threatened miscarriage

35. Which of the following investigations for recurrent miscarriage is best diagnosed by careful history taking?
A. Karyotyping of both partners and retained products of conception
B. Pelvic ultrasound to inspect uterine cavity and ovaries
C. High vaginal swab for bacterial vaginosis
D. Cervical weakness
E. Antiphospholipid antibodies

36. Which of the following is NOT a recognized aetiological factor of ectopic pregnancy?
A. Pelvic inflammatory disease
B. Tubal surgery
C. Combined oral contraceptive pill
D. In-vitro fertilization
E. IUCD ('coil') in situ

37. In order to perform a routine hysteroscopy the following are essential:
A. An ultrasound
B. A light source
C. Distilled water to distend the uterine cavity
D. General anaesthesia
E. A catheterized bladder

38. In order to perform a routine diagnostic laparoscopy the following are essential:
A. Normal saline to distend the peritoneal cavity
B. Indwelling catheter
C. Verress needle
D. Pregnancy test
E. Diathermy

39. In order to perform a transvaginal ultrasound scan the following are essential:
A. A full bladder
B. Bowel preparation
C. Ultrasound gel
D. A sedated patient
E. A light source

40. The following can be diagnosed during a routine hysteroscopy:
A. Endometrial polyp
B. Endometriosis
C. Polycystic ovaries
D. Meig's syndrome
E. Subserous fibroids

41. The following should be performed in the assessment of all patients with abnormal vaginal bleeding:
A. Eliciting a menstrual history
B. Coagulation studies
C. High vaginal swab
D. Thyroid function tests
E. Abdominal X-ray

42. A 55-year-old woman presents with a 3-day mild vaginal bleed. Her last menstrual period was at the age of 52 years. The following would be appropriate with regards to differential diagnosis and subsequent management:
A. The most likely cause is atrophic vaginitis so no further action is required
B. An ultrasound scan would be appropriate
C. A hysteroscopy should be performed
D. A full blood count should be taken
E. A normal pipelle excludes endometrial carcinoma

43. Which of these are the possible symptoms caused by a 3 cm submucosal fibroid:
A. Hirsutism
B. Subfertility
C. Detrusor instability
D. Deep vein thrombosis
E. Dysmenorrhoea

44. What are the commonly associated complications of fibroids in pregnancy:
A. Diabetes
B. Chorioamnionitis
C. Malpresentation
D. Intrauterine growth restriction
E. Pre-eclampsia

45. Which of these are common sites for endometriotic deposits:
A. Pouch of Douglas
B. Fallopian tube
C. Femur
D. Scars
E. Lungs

46. What are the possible medical treatments of endometriosis:
A. Ovarian drilling
B. Combined oral contraceptive pill
C. Corticosteroids
D. Tranexamic acid
E. Metronidazole

47. A 45-year-old woman presents with pruritus vulvae. The following are suggestive of an infective cause:
A. Progressively worsening symptoms over 6 months
B. Menorrhagia
C. A thick creamy white discharge
D. Red plaques in the vulval area
E. Fused labia

48. The following are important in the management of a woman with pruritus vulvae:
A. Administering antibiotics
B. A speculum examination of the cervix and smear test
C. All women should be seen in colposcopy clinic
D. Excision of the area of the discomfort
E. An abdominal X-ray

49. The following are possible methods of investigation of vulval disease:
A. CRP
B. Biopsy of vulva
C. Ultrasound scan
D. Hysteroscopy
E. Endocervical swabs

50. The following are correct about lichen sclerosis:
A. The vulval skin always appears white
B. Skin biopsy shows thinning of the epidermis
C. A biopsy is not necessary as the diagnosis is usually obvious
D. Surgical excision is first-line treatment
E. A short course of antibiotic treatment is usually required

51. A multiparous 55-year-old woman presents with a 6-month history of stress incontinence on coughing and sneezing:
A. She therefore has 'genuine stress incontinence'
B. An obstetric history is unhelpful in making the diagnosis
C. A bimanual pelvic examination is always diagnostic
D. A midstream sample of urine may help in making the diagnosis
E. Urodynamic studies are unnecessary

52. A 26-year-old woman complains of recurrent episodes of frequency, urgency and nocturia:
A. A neurological history is important
B. The likely cause is detrusor overactivity
C. A pelvic examination will usually show an abnormality

D. A high vaginal swab is mandatory to exclude infection
E. Prolapse is usually found on examination

53. Effective treatments for genuine stress incontinence in women wanting more children include:
A. Pelvic floor exercises
B. Anticholinergics
C. Behaviour therapy
D. Tension free vaginal tape
E. Antibiotics

54. Effective treatments for detrusor instability include:
A. Pelvic floor exercises
B. Antimuscarinics
C. Colposuspension
D. Treating chlamydia
E. Myomectomy

55. The following are possible causes of precocious puberty:
A. Congenital adrenal hyperplasia
B. Hyperprolactinaemia
C. Hypothyroidism
D. Turner's syndrome
E. Cystic fibrosis

56. Which of these drugs can cause hirsutism:
A. H2 antagonists, e.g. cimetidine
B. Prednisolone
C. Combined oral contraceptive pill
D. Penicillin
E. Progestogens

57. An 18-year old girl presents with a history of primary amenorrhoea. The following conditions usually present in this way:
A. Fibroids
B. Testicular feminization
C. Premature ovarian failure
D. Polycystic ovarian syndrome (PCOS)
E. Lichen sclerosis

58. A 40 year old primiparous woman attends antenatal clinic at 12 weeks gestation. She has a history of essential hypertension, with a family history of multiple pregnancy. She is allergic to penicillin. Which factor in her history is the most important in the antenatal risk assessment?
A. Maternal age 40
B. Primiparity
C. Essential hypertension
D. Family history of multiple pregnancy
E. Allergy to penicillin

59. Which of the following is not a routine booking investigation?
A. Full Blood Count
B. Blood Group
C. Hepatitis B status
D. High Vaginal Swab
E. Urine Microscopy, Culture and Sensitivity

60. Which of the following is NOT a risk factor for gestational diabetes?
A. Body Mass Index >30 kg/m^2
B. South Asian origin
C. Family history of Type 2 diabetes in a first degree relative
D. Previous gestational diabetes
E. Husband with Type 2 diabetes

61. When should an amniocentesis be performed?
A. Before 12 weeks
B. After 15 weeks but before 19 weeks
C. After 20 weeks
D. After 12 weeks but before 13 weeks
E. After 15 weeks

62. A 22 year old woman with a history of drug misuse presents to the Labour Ward at 26 weeks gestation with a 6 hour history of constant abdominal pain and some vaginal bleeding. What is the most likely diagnosis is?
A. Symphysis pubis dysfunction
B. Preterm labour
C. Uterine fibroid degeneration
D. Placental abruption
E. Acute fatty liver of pregnancy

63. A 34 year old woman is seen in antenatal clinic complaining of 2 weeks of lower abdominal discomfort. On further questioning, she has no urinary symptoms or vaginal discharge but is passing hard stools. What is the most likely diagnosis?
A. Peptic ulcer disease
B. Ligament pain
C. Constipation
D. Ovarian cyst rupture
E. Cystitis

64. A 26 year old woman with no medical or gynaecological history of note presents with a history of fresh vaginal bleeding within the last 12 hours. On further questioning, the bleeding started after sexual intercourse. What is the most likely diagnosis?
A. Cervical polyp
B. Vulval varicosities
C. Cervical ectropion
D. Cervical carcinoma
E. Vaginitis

65. Ultrasound scan is useful in the diagnosis of which of the following causes of antepartum haemorrhage?
A. Cervical polyp
B. Vasa praevia
C. Circumvallate placenta
D. Placental abruption
E. Placenta praevia

66. In a low risk primiparous woman, which of the following indications necessitates continuous fetal monitoring in labour?
A. Irregular contractions
B. Mucoid show

C. Second stage of labour
D. Pethidine analgesia
E. Meconium-stained liquor

67. A 39 year old primiparous woman has progressed spontaneously in labour to 6 cm. She is having continuous electronic fetal monitoring because she had a small antepartum haemorrhage in the latent phase of labour. The monitoring appears to have been pathological for 50 mins. What is the most appropriate course of action?
A. Fetal blood sampling
B. Intravenous fluids
C. Epidural anaesthesia
D. Check maternal blood pressure
E. Caesarean section

68. During the course of labour, abdominal palpation is the most appropriate method of assessing which of the following parameters?
A. Position of the presenting part
B. Strength of uterine contractions
C. Station of the presenting part
D. Presence of caput
E. Baseline variability of the fetal heart rate

69. Which of the following terms does NOT describe the mechanism for delivery of the fetal head?
A. Flexion
B. External rotation
C. Extension
D. Abduction
E. Internal rotation

70. A 33 year old low risk Caucasian woman in her first pregnancy is in spontaneous labour but has not progressed from 5 cm in the last 4 hours. What is the most likely diagnosis for this failure to progress in labour?
A. Incoordinate uterine activity
B. Female circumcision
C. Left ovarian cyst
D. Fetal goitre
E. Opiate analgesia

71. A 28 year old African woman is in her third pregnancy with a diagnosis of gestational diabetes. She has an amniotomy to augment the labour but at that time, there is a prolonged fetal bradycardia which is not recovering. Which is the most likely diagnosis?
A. Fetal infection
B. Uterine rupture
C. Amniotic fluid embolism
D. Umbilical cord prolapse
E. Hyperstimulation of the uterus

72. Which of the following is NOT a contraindication to external cephalic version?
A. Ruptured membranes
B. Multiparity
C. Placenta praevia
D. Previous caesarean section
E. Multiple pregnancy

73. A 25 year old Asian woman measures small for dates at 32 weeks gestation which is confirmed on ultrasound scan. Her BMI at booking was 21. She has normal blood pressure, no proteinuria and has had normal fetal anomaly ultrasound scans. Which of the following is the most likely cause for being small for dates?
A. Gestational diabetes
B. Gestational trophoblastic disease
C. Constitutional
D. Pre-eclampsia
E. Fetal chromosomal anomaly

74. A 33 year old woman has a monochorionic twin pregnancy. Ultrasound scan at 22 weeks shows discrepant growth and liquor volumes. Which is the most likely diagnosis?
A. Gestational diabetes
B. Pre-eclampsia
C. Fetal infection
D. Maternal anaemia
E. Twin-to-twin transfusion syndrome

75. A 25 year old woman in her second pregnancy is induced at 37 weeks with a twin pregnancy. The labour progresses at a normal rate and both babies are delivered normally. However, she has a heavy blood loss after delivery of approx 900 ml. Which is the most likely cause?
A. Uterine atony
B. Second degree tear
C. Placental abruption
D. Retained placenta
E. Maternal infection

76. A 31 year old primiparous woman has a forceps delivery and perineal trauma involving the perineal muscles and external anal sphincter muscle? What is the correct classification for the perineal trauma described?
A. Midline episiotomy
B. 1st degree perineal tear
C. 4th degree perineal tear
D. 3rd degree perineal tear
E. 2nd degree perineal tear

77. Which of the following is NOT indicated in the care of a woman having a vaginal delivery after caesarean section (VBAC)?
A. Continuous fetal monitoring
B. Intravenous cannula
C. Blood sent for group and save
D. Epidural anaesthesia
E. Amniotomy

78. A 19 year old woman attends the Labour Ward at 28 weeks gestation with increasingly regular tightenings every 10 mins. On cervical assessment, there is cervical effacement and dilatation of 1 cm. Which is your 1st line of management?
A. Urinalysis
B. Administration of steroids
C. Liaising with the paediatric team
D. Tocolysis
E. Caesarean section

79. In obstetric palpation, which factor is the most important for assessing progress in labour?
A. Symphysis-fundal height
B. Fetal presentation
C. Engagement
D. Fetal position
E. Liquor volume

80. In vaginal examination, which factor is the most important for assessing progress in labour?
A. Presence of caput
B. Presence of moulding
C. Fetal position
D. Cervical dilatation
E. Station

81. A 20 year old patient who is 36 weeks pregnant attends clinic with a blood pressure of 156/102. She has 2+ of protein in her urine. What investigations are required?
A. ECG, Chest X-ray and V/Q scan
B. Liver function tests, full blood count, urea & electrolytes, urine protein:creatine ratio and clotting
C. Thyroid functions tests
D. Serum cortisol
E. Renal ultrasound

82. Which of the following medications is considered as 1st line for treatment of hypertension in pregnancy in non-asthmatic patients?
A. Enalapril
B. Nifedipine
C. Methyldopa
D. Labetalol
E. Hydralazine

83. Which medication should be administered as soon as possible in a patient thought to be having an eclamptic seizure?
A. Diazepam
B. Methyldopa
C. Labetalol
D. Hydralazine
E. Magnesium Sulphate

84. Which of the following is not a known risk factor for venous thromboembolism in pregnancy?
A. Thrombophilia (Factor V Leiden, Protein C deficiency, antiphospholipid syndrome)
B. Age >35
C. BMI >30
D. Parity >3
E. Age <20

85. Anaemia in pregnancy should be identified and treated where necessary. What levels of haemoglobin are acceptable at booking and at 28 weeks?
A. >11.0 g/dl at booking and >10.5 g/dl at 28 weeks
B. >11.0 g/dl at booking and >9.5 g/dl at 28 weeks
C. >10.0 g/dl at booking and >10.5 g/dl at 28 weeks
D. >9.0 g/dl at booking and >11.g/dl at 28 weeks
E. >7.0 g/dl at booking and >10.5 g/dl at 28 weeks

86. What three steps have been shown to reduce the vertical transmission of HIV from mother to fetus?
A. Antibiotics, elective caesarean section and breastfeeding
B. Hand washing, vaginal delivery and steroids
C. Avoidance of breastfeeding, anti-retroviral medication (HAART), elective caesarean section
D. Avoidance of intercourse, avoidance of breastfeeding and antibiotics
E. Steroids, elective caesarean section and antibiotics

87. A 32 year old patient who has had type 1 diabetes since her teens comes to see you because she plans to stop the oral contraceptive pill. What advice is the most important?
A. Start taking folic acid 0.4 mg daily
B. Start aspirin 75 mg daily
C. Book an oral glucose tolerance test
D. Start taking folic acid 5 mg daily
E. Plan for midwifery-led care

88. Which of the following is NOT part of the antenatal care of patients with epilepsy?
A. Aim to control seizures with monotherapy
B. Take folic acid 5 mg daily from preconception until 12 weeks gestation
C. Prescribe vitamin K 10 mg daily from preconception until 12 weeks gestation
D. Encourage breastfeeding
E. Arrange a detailed fetal ultrasound scan to exclude cardiac defects

89. A 26 year old primiparous woman presents to the Labour Ward at 33 weeks gestation with a 2 day history of feeling increasingly unwell with nausea and vomiting. On admission, she has mildly raised blood pressure. She has blood investigations which show a raised ALT, a very high uric acid level and low blood glucose. What is the most likely diagnosis?
A. Fulminating pre-eclampsia
B. Acute fatty liver of pregnancy
C. Obstetric cholestasis
D. Pregnancy-induced hypertension
E. Cholelithiasis

90. About 2 weeks postnatally, a 36 year old multiparous woman starts to worry that her partner is spying on her as she cares for her baby. She begins to think she can hear someone telling she is doing tasks incorrectly. Her partner calls the health visitor who suspects that the most likely diagnosis is:
A. Baby blues
B. Bipolar disorder
C. Schizophrenia
D. Postnatal depression
E. Puerperal psychosis

91. Treatment of PPH must start with:
A. Identifying the cause of bleeding
B. Multidisciplinary team approach
C. Basic resuscitation ABC
D. Contacting haematology and anaesthetic specialists
E. Making an accurate estimation of the blood loss

92. The definition of secondary post partum haemorrhage (PPH) is as follows
A. > 500mls PV bleeding 24 hours after delivery, within 6 weeks
B. > 1000 mls PV bleeding post delivery
C. > 2000 mls PV bleeding post delivery
D. > 500 mls PV bleeding within 24 hours of delivery
E. < 2000 mls PV bleeding within 24 hours of delivery

93. A 29 year old primiparous, known to have fibroids, has just delivered a baby weighing 4.1 kg, after being induced and having a long 1st stage of labour. As the placenta delivers, she suddenly feels faint and passes 700 ml of blood and clot vaginally. What is the most likely cause of the postpartum haemorrhage?
A. Genital tract trauma
B. Retained placental cotyledon
C. Cervical ectropion
D. Placenta accreta
E. Uterine atony

94. A 33 year old who delivered 3 days previously by normal vaginal delivery has called her community midwife as she feels increasingly unwell with lower abdominal pain and a fever. Her 7 year old son is off school with a sore throat. The most likely possible cause of sepsis in this patient is:
A. Urinary tract infection
B. Mastitis
C. Pneumonia
D. Endometritis
E. Group A streptococcus

95. A 19 year old girl attends A&E with abdominal pain and vaginal spotting. She gives a urine sample which reveals she is pregnant. Her last period was around 7 weeks ago. She is surprised by the news and then collapses. What is the most likely cause of her collapse?
A. Appendicitis
B. Urinary Tract infection
C. Ectopic pregnancy
D. Vasovagal Syncope
E. Gastroenteritis

96. A 34 year old solicitor who is 35 weeks pregnant in her first pregnancy is at her office when she begins to feel unwell, she complains of abdominal pain and then collapses. On arrival at the hospital her BP in 76/44 and her pulse is 132. Her uterus is 'woody hard'. What is the most likely cause of collapse?
A. Sepsis
B. Placental Abruption
C. Uterine Rupture
D. Vasovagal Syncope
E. Acute myocardial Infarction

97. You are alone assessing a 40 year old lady who has just arrived from Uganda at 36 weeks and is feeling unwell. You palpate her abdomen and find she measures small for dates and she has a blood pressure of 182/122. She then appears to have a seizure and is unconscious. What is the most appropriate next line of action?
A. Start CPR
B. Put patient in recovery position and wait till she wakes up
C. Call for help, position patient with a left lateral tilt and protect airway until help arrives
D. Organise an ECG once she wakes up
E. Take an arterial blood gas

98. In the last CMACE report 2006-2008, what was found to be the leading cause of direct maternal death?
A. Pre-eclampsia and eclampsia
B. Thrombosis & thromboembolism
C. Sepsis
D. Amniotic fluid embolism
E. Ectopic

99. In the last CMACE report 2006-2008, what was found to be the leading cause of indirect maternal death?
A. Ectopic
B. Haemorrhage
C. Anaesthesia
D. Cardiac Disease
E. Murder

100. Which of the following has been highlighted as a serious, rapidly fatal infection in pregnancy which all clinicians should be aware of?
A. Toxoplasmosis
B. Group A β-haemolytic Streptococcus
C. Proteus Mirabilis
D. Escherichia Coli
E. Varicella Zoster

Extended-matching questions (EMQs)

1. Bleeding in the second and third trimesters of pregnancy:

A. Molar pregnancy
B. Vasa praevia
C. Ectopic pregnancy
D. Placenta praevia
E. Placental abruption
F. Cervical ectropion
G. Retained placenta
H. Vaginal tear
I. Uterine atony
J. Cervical tear

For each scenario described below, choose the single most likely diagnosis from the list of options given above. Each option may be used once, more than once, or not at all.

1. A 35-year-old woman, who has had two previous caesarean sections, presents with vaginal spotting and a transverse lie at 35 weeks.
2. A 22-year-old woman has artificial rupture of membranes during labour and there is heavy vaginal bleeding in association with an abnormal CTG. The uterus is soft and non-tender.
3. A 28-year-old woman has a history of 16 weeks amenorrhoea. She has severe nausea and vomiting. On abdominal palpation the uterus is 24 weeks in size. No intrauterine sac can be seen on ultrasound scan.
4. A 32-year-old woman is 28 weeks pregnant. She has a 2-hour history of vaginal bleeding. She also complains of a headache and constant abdominal pain. On examination, the uterus is firm and tender.
5. A 30-year-old woman presents with a post-coital bleed at 22 weeks' gestation.

2. Abdominal pain in the second and third trimesters of pregnancy:

A. Fibroid degeneration
B. Gastroenteritis
C. Symphysis pubis dysfunction
D. Placental abruption
E. Acute appendicitis
F. Ovarian torsion
G. Pre-eclampsia
H. Urinary tract infection
I. Gallstones
J. Labour

For each of the clinical findings below, select the pathological process most likely to account for them from the list of options given above. Each option may be used once, more than once, or not at all.

1. On abdominal palpation, hard tender uterus, difficulty defining the fetal parts.
2. Nitrites on urinalysis.
3. Regular contractions palpated on abdominal examination, cervical change on vaginal examination.
4. The uterus palpates large-for-dates, with tenderness elicited over a specific site.
5. The patient is hypertensive and hyperreflexic, with tenderness over the right hypochondrium.

3. Stillbirth:

A. Maternal ALT = 60 iu/L
B. Maternal HbA1c = 15%
C. Fetal Hb = 3 g/dL, positive Coombs test
D. Parvovirus IgM positive, IgG negative
E. Maternal rubella IgG positive
F. 24-hour urinary protein 2.1 g/L
G. Fetal karyotype 47XY
H. Fetal karyotype 45XO
I. 24-hour urinary protein 0.2 g/L

The conditions below are the underlying diagnoses of causes of stillbirth, made on the basis of investigations performed soon after delivery

For each of the diagnoses below, match the test result from the list of options given above. Each option may be used once, more than once, or not at all.

1. Fetus with Down's syndrome
2. Pre-eclampsia
3. Intrauterine fetal infection
4. Obstetric cholestasis
5. Rhesus isoimmunization
6. Maternal diabetes

4. Failure to progress in labour:

A. Cervical fibroid
B. Persistent OP position
C. Previous pelvic fracture
D. Fetal macrosomia
E. Irregular contractions
F. Breech presentation
G. OT position
H. Rickets
I. Transverse lie
J. Brow presentation

For each scenario described below, choose the single most likely diagnosis from the list of options given above. Each option may be used once, more than once, or not at all.

1. A 26-year-old woman who has been an insulin-dependent diabetic since the age of 10.
2. A primiparous patient with a term pregnancy and a cephalic presentation. Over the past 4 hours, she has remained at 4 cm dilatation on vaginal examination. She is not yet requiring analgesia.
3. A 35-year-old Nigerian woman who is in spontaneous labour. She has a history of having had a previous myomectomy for menorrhagia.
4. A 40-year-old grand multiparous woman who has attended labour ward at term with a 3 hour history of regular contractions and no PV loss. On abdominal palpation, there is nothing in the maternal pelvis.
5. On examination of a multiparous patient, the midwife is able to palpate the fetal orbital ridges and the anterior fontanelle.

5. Maternal collapse:

A. Uterine atony
B. Amniotic fluid embolism
C. Postural hypotension
D. Opiate use
E. Pulmonary embolism
F. Epileptic seizure
G. Eclampsia
H. Sepsis
I. Myocardial infarction
J. Uterine rupture

For each scenario described below, choose the single most likely diagnosis from the list of options given above. Each option may be used once, more than once, or not at all.

1. This 18-year-old had a forceps delivery of a 4.3 kg baby about 1 hour ago after a long labour that was augmented with syntocinon. She had syntometrine for the third stage. Her pulse is 100 bpm, her blood pressure is 90/45 mmHg. Her uterus is palpable above the umbilicus and feels 'boggy'. She is lying in a pool of blood.
2. This woman had her fourth caesarean section yesterday. She was kept on the labour ward overnight as the estimated blood loss at delivery was 800 mL. Her husband helped her get up to go to the shower, but then she collapsed by the side of her bed. Her pulse is 94 bpm, her blood pressure is 110/55 and her lochia is normal. There is no respiratory distress.
3. This 35-year-old, whose BMI is 38, has had frequent admissions in her pregnancy, early on with hyperemesis, now, in the third trimester, with symphysis pubis pain. When found she is tachycardic but normotensive, with cyanosis and dyspnoea.
4. This primigravid woman was aiming for home delivery, and wanted to avoid contact with the hospital if at all possible. Her membranes ruptured 3 days ago, at term, and she has had irregular contractions ever since but labour has not established. She came in because she started to feel unwell, and because fetal movements had reduced over the previous 12 hours. On examination she is tachycardic and pyrexial, and the liquor is yellowish in colour.
5. At 32 weeks, this woman had been referred in by her community midwife who found her blood pressure to be elevated and some proteinuria at a routine antenatal check. She is generally fit and well with no medical history. On arrival she is asked to provide another urine specimen. When she fails to emerge from the toilet the midwife goes in and finds her having a generalized tonic-clonic seizure.

6. Obstetric definitions:

A. Fetal presentation
B. Fetal lie
C. Position of the presenting part of the fetus
D. Station of the presenting part of the fetus
E. Perinatal mortality rate
F. Neonatal mortality rate

G. Maternal mortality rate
H. Antepartum haemorrhage
I. Labour
J. Primary postpartum haemorrhage

For each description below, choose the single most likely definition from the list of options given above. Each option may be used once, more than once, or not at all.

1. The relationship between the denominator of the presenting part and the maternal pelvis
2. Any amount of vaginal bleeding after 24 weeks gestation until delivery of the fetus
3. The number of maternal deaths per 100 000 live births
4. Regular, painful uterine contractions in the presence of cervical dilatation and effacement
5. The relationship between the presenting part of the fetus and the maternal ischial spines

7. Hypertension in pregnancy:

A. Pregnancy induced hypertension (PIH)
B. Pre-eclampsia
C. Hypertension secondary to renal disease
D. Essential hypertension
E. Essential hypertension with superimposed pre-eclampsia
F. Malignant hypertension
G. Phaeochromocytoma
H. Postural supine hypotensive syndrome
I. Severe fulminating pre-eclampsia
J. HELPP syndrome

For each scenario described below, choose the single most likely diagnosis from the list of options given above. Each option may be used once, more than once, or not at all.

1. A 19-year-old primigravida booked with a blood pressure of 90/60 mmHg at 12 weeks. She had an uneventful pregnancy until 38 weeks' gestation, when she presented with swelling of the lower legs. Her BP was noted to be 160/95 mmHg and urinalysis revealed ++ proteinuria.
2. A 39-year-old primigravida books at 13 weeks' gestation. Her blood pressure was 150/90 mmHg at booking and there was no proteinuria. She was started on methyldopa 500 mg t.d.s which maintained her BP within the normal range for the rest of the pregnancy.
3. A 25-year-old primigravida books at 16 weeks' gestation with a BP of 155/95 mmHg. She has a history or ureteric reflux and recurrent UTIs as a child requiring ureteric re-implantation surgery. Her creatinine was slightly raised.
4. A 41-year-old primigravida booked with a BP of 140/95 mmHg at 10 weeks' gestation. She was commenced on methyldopa and had a normal pregnancy until 34 weeks when she was noted to have developed proteinuria, oedema and a raised serum urate concentration.
5. A 37-year-old woman booked at 12 weeks' gestation with a BP of 95/60 mmHg. She had an uneventful pregnancy until 24 weeks' gestation when she was found to be hypertensive with oedema but normal biochemistry. She was managed conservatively with methyldopa. At 29 weeks she felt unwell and blood tests revealed a haemoglobin concentration of 8.5 g/dL with evidence of haemolysis on blood film. Her platelet concentration was 85 × 109 and her ALT concentration was raised.

8. Maternal collapse:

A. Placental abruption
B. Post-partum haemorrhage
C. Uterine rupture
D. Amniotic fluid embolism
E. Eclampsia
F. Epileptiform seizure
G. Diabetic ketoacidosis
H. Puerperal septic shock
I. Pulmonary embolism
J. Myocardial infarction

For each scenario described below, choose the single most likely diagnosis from the list of options given above. Each option may be used once, more than once, or not at all.

1. A 25-year-old woman was found collapsed at home at 8 weeks gestation. Her past history includes a deep vein thrombosis at the age of 18 years following which she was found to carry the Factor V Leiden mutation.
2. A 26-year-old woman underwent a caesarean section in her first pregnancy for fetal distress. This current pregnancy was uneventful and she went into spontaneous labour. She requested an epidural for analgesia. At 7 cm dilatation she felt unwell and collapsed at the same time that the fetal heart rate pattern became bradycardic.
3. A 34-year-old grand multiparous woman presented to the labour ward at 34 weeks gestation having experienced a small APH at home. By the time she

arrived she was experiencing severe abdominal pain. Abdominal examination revealed a tender, hard uterus and the fetal heart could not be heard with the sonicaid. During the examination she collapsed and was unresponsive.

4. An unbooked woman was admitted via ambulance unconscious. The only history available is that she was feeling unwell for the previous few days with headaches and had collapsed at home 'shaking'. On examination, she was unconscious, her BP was 180/110 mmHg and urinalysis revealed proteinuria.
5. A 35-year-old multiparous woman spontaneously ruptured her membranes at term in her third pregnancy. 48 hours later she went into labour and had a normal delivery. She went home after 6 hours. 72 hours later she started feeling unwell and feverish. She collapsed at home and was brought into hospital by ambulance. On examination she was unconscious with central cyanosis. Her temperature was 39 °C, pulse 120 beats per minute and she was profoundly hypotensive.

9. Interventions in labour:

A. Ventouse delivery
B. Lower segment caesarean section
C. External cephalic version
D. Fetal scalp electrode
E. Fetal blood sample
F. Epidural anaesthesia
G. Artificial rupture of membranes
H. Episiotomy
I. Simpsons forceps delivery
J. Intravenous syntocinon

For each scenario described below, choose the single most appropriate intervention from the list of options given above. Each option may be used once, more than once, or not at all.

1. During labour, there is difficulty monitoring the fetal heart rate in a woman with a BMI of 40.
2. In a patient with suspected intrauterine growth restriction, there is a pathological CTG in labour. Vaginal examination shows that the cervix is 7 cm dilated.
3. A primiparous patient is contracting irregularly with intact membranes. The CTG is normal and the cervix has been 4 cm dilated for the last 4 hours.
4. There is a prolonged fetal bradycardia lasting 8 minutes. The cervix is 6 cm dilated.
5. A primiparous patient has been actively pushing in the 2nd stage of labour for more than 1 hour. On examination, the fetal head is not palpable abdominally, the vertex is at +1 below the ischial spines in the right occipito-transverse position with no caput or moulding. The CTG is normal.

10. Complications of labour:

A. Failure to progress
B. Meconium-stained liquor
C. Placental abruption
D. Post-partum haemorrhage
E. Cord prolapse
F. Ruptured uterus
G. Uterine hyperstimulation
H. Shoulder dystocia
I. Face presentation
J. Fetal bradycardia

For each scenario described below, choose the single most likely diagnosis from the list of options given above. Each option may be used once, more than once, or not at all.

1. A patient who has previously had a caesarean section is having a vaginal delivery in this pregnancy. At 8 cm dilatation, the CTG suddenly shows a prolonged fetal bradycardia.
2. After a long labour, a primiparous patient with a BMI of 35 has a ventouse delivery for a prolonged second stage. The fetal head shows the turtle-neck sign as it delivers and there is difficulty delivering the baby.
3. In established labour with a breech presentation, the CTG suddenly shows a prolonged fetal bradycardia.
4. A patient who has been diagnosed with severe pre-eclampsia is having labour induced at 37 weeks. She starts to complain of constant sharp abdominal pain. The uterus is tender and hard on palpation. The CTG has become suspicious.
5. A patient on intravenous syntocinon is contracting 6 in 10. The CTG shows variable decelerations with a rise in the baseline heart rate.

11. Interventions in the antenatal period:

A. Umbilical artery Dopplers
B. Cardiotocograph
C. Membrane sweep
D. Speculum examination
E. Cervical cerclage
F. Amniocentesis
G. Chorionic villus sampling
H. Amniodrainage

I. External cephalic version
J. Fetocide

For each scenario described below, choose the single most appropriate intervention from the list of options given above. Each option may be used once, more than once, or not at all.

1. At 40 weeks' gestation, a multiparous woman is seen in antenatal clinic. Her pregnancy has been straightforward and she is keen to avoid induction of labour.
2. At 30 weeks' gestation, a primiparous woman complains of a 4-hour history of a clear watery vaginal loss. She has no abdominal pain.
3. A multiparous woman is diagnosed with a breech presentation at 37 weeks. Her pregnancy is uncomplicated.
4. A 38-year-old woman has an increased risk of trisomy 21 on serum screening testing at 16 weeks.
5. At 34 weeks' gestation, ultrasound scan shows a slowing of the fetal growth rate with a reduction in the liquor volume.

12. Complications of the antenatal period:

A. Obstetric cholestasis
B. Gestational diabetes
C. Recurrent antepartum haemorrhage
D. Symphysis pubis dysfunction
E. Iron deficiency anaemia
F. Intrauterine growth restriction
G. Pyelonephritis
H. Preterm labour
I. Preterm ruptured membranes
J. Deep vein thrombosis

For each scenario described below, choose the single most likely diagnosis from the list of options given above. Each option may be used once, more than once, or not at all.

1. A 40-year-old woman with a BMI of 36 presents to A&E at 18 weeks' gestation with unilateral calf swelling.
2. Ultrasound scan shows a macrosomic fetus with polyhydramnios.
3. At 32 weeks' gestation, a primiparous patient complains of itchy palms and soles. Her liver function tests are abnormal.
4. At 28 weeks' gestation, a multiparous patient presents with severe abdominal pain. On examination, she is pyrexial with nitrites on urinalysis.
5. At 28 weeks' gestation, a multiparous patient presents with severe abdominal pain. On abdominal examination, there are palpable uterine contractions, vaginal examination shows cervical effacement.

13. Complications of the postnatal period:

A. Puerperal psychosis
B. Postnatal depression
C. Endometritis
D. Deep vein thrombosis
E. Postpartum haemorrhage
F. Mastitis
G. Urinary tract infection
H. Pulmonary embolus
I. Dural puncture headache
J. Cerebral vein thrombosis

For each scenario described below, choose the single most likely diagnosis from the list of options given above. Each option may be used once, more than once, or not at all.

1. Vaginal bleeding more than 500 ml from 24 hours post delivery up to 6 weeks.
2. 2 weeks after delivery, a primiparous patient complains of low mood and feeling unable to cope with caring for her baby.
3. 2 weeks after delivery, a primiparous patient complains that she cannot sleep because she is worried a neighbour is trying to take her baby. On further questioning with her partner, the neighbour has simply been offering to help with babysitting.
4. 6 days after emergency caesarean section, a patient complains of increasingly constant severe lower abdominal pain. The lochia are offensive-smelling. On examination, the patient is pyrexial and the uterus is tender.
5. After a prolonged labour and delivery with epidural anaesthesia, a patient complains of being unable to sit upright because of a severe headache.

14. Postpartum haemorrhage:

A. Primary PPH
B. Secondary PPH
C. Second degree tear
D. Third degree tear
E. Uterine atony
F. Uterine rupture
G. Retained products of conception
H. Endometritis

I. Placenta accreta
J. Uterine inversion

For each scenario described below, choose the single most likely diagnosis from the list of options given above. Each option may be used once, more than once, or not at all.

1. The patient has had a forceps delivery with an episiotomy after a prolonged labour. On examination, the episiotomy has extended into the external anal sphincter and the patient is bleeding heavily from the area.
2. The patient has just had a normal vaginal delivery of a twin pregnancy. She is bleeding heavily. On examination, the uterine fundus is above the umbilicus and poorly contracted.
3. A woman has previously had two caesarean sections. At the time of caesarean section in this pregnancy, the placenta was morbidly adherent to the uterine wall.
4. Bleeding more than 500 mL within the first 24 hours of delivery of the baby.
5. At the time of controlled cord traction in the 3rd stage of labour, the patient suddenly complains of severe abdominal pain and bleeding. The uterine fundus cannot be palpated on abdominal examination.

15. Large-for-dates and small-for-dates:

A. Gestational diabetes
B. Gestational trophoblastic disease
C. Placental insuffiency
D. Twin pregnancy
E. Oesophageal atresia
F. Renal agenesis
G. Uterine fibroid
H. Trisomy 18
I. Cytomegalovirus infection
J. Maternal ovarian cyst

For each scenario described below, choose the single most likely diagnosis from the list of options given above. Each option may be used once, more than once, or not at all.

1. Fetal ultrasound scan at 20 weeks shows anhydramnios.
2. Persistant glycosuria with a macrosomic fetus on ultrasound scan.
3. IVF pregnancy with a symphysio-fundal height at the umbilicus at 14 weeks' gestation.
4. Maternal history of chronic hypertension measuring small-for-dates at 30 weeks' gestation.
5. An Afro-Caribbean woman who measures large-for-dates at 20 weeks' gestation.

16. Multiple pregnancy:

A. Consultant-led hospital care
B. Chorionicity
C. Homebirth
D. Intra-uterine growth restriction
E. Postpartum haemorrhage
F. Zygosity
G. Multiple fetal pregnancy reduction
H. Primiparity
I. Maternal age >40 years
J. Twin-to-twin transfusion syndrome

For each statement below, choose the single most appropriate option from the list given above. Each option may be used once, more than once, or not at all.

1. The most important factor in defining the risks associated with different types of twin pregnancy.
2. An essential part of counseling a couple with higher order multiple pregnancies such as triplets, in order for informed decisions regarding possible birth outcomes.
3. A complication of 15% of monochorionic pregnancies.
4. The appropriate location for care of any multiple pregnancy.
5. A risk factor in any multiple pregnancy which must be monitored by regular growth scans.

17. Antenatal investigations:

A. Serum electrophoresis
B. Serum antibody screen
C. Rubella
D. Toxoplasmosis
E. Hepatitis B
F. Glycosylated haemoglobin
G. Blood glucose level
H. HIV
I. Hepatitis C
J. Urea and electrolytes

For each scenario described below, choose the single most likely test from the list of options given above. Each option may be used once, more than once, or not at all.

1. Check the result of this test if a patient appears to have a microcytic anaemia.
2. This test should be performed at booking in a patient with established diabetes since it is associated with the risk of congenital malformations.

3. A routine test on every pregnant women regardless of any history of vaccination in childhood, because of the risk of congenital infection.
4. A good example of a screening test, since intervention can reduce the risk of vertical transmission from 25% to <1%.
5. This test is not part of the routine 1st trimester screening and would only be performed in a patient with a history of drug use.

---

18. Obstetric examination:

A. Abdominal striae
B. Body mass index
C. Symphysio-fundal height
D. Fetal lie
E. Sagittal suture
F. Linea nigra
G. Bishops score
H. Anterior fontanelle
I. Posterior fontanelle
J. Cervical effacement

For each description described below, choose the single most likely anatomical feature from the list of options given above. Each option may be used once, more than once, or not at all.

1. A fetal landmark palpable with a cephalic presentation and a deflexed head.
2. Assessment of the cervix on vaginal examination prior to induction of labour.
3. A line of pigmentation commonly seen on the maternal abdomen from the umbilicus to the pubic symphysis.
4. This essential assessment must be made at the antenatal booking visit in order to plan the appropriate level of pregnancy care.
5. A fetal landmark that can be palpated between the parietal bones.

---

19. Terminology in labour:

A. Caput
B. Extended breech
C. Shoulder dystocia
D. Meconium
E. Fetal tachycardia
F. Malpresentation
G. Malposition
H. Variability
I. Fetal bradycardia
J. Moulding

For each description below, choose the single most likely term from the list of options given above. Each option may be used once, more than once, or not at all.

1. The fetal heart rate is at a baseline level of 170 beats per minute.
2. The fetal shoulder is over the pelvic inlet in the first stage of labour.
3. The fetal occiput is palpated adjacent to the maternal sacrum at full dilatation.
4. The fetal skull bones can be felt to overlap at 6 cm dilatation.
5. The fetal heart rate differs by 5–10 beats per minute.

---

20. Medical disorders in pregnancy:

A. Take folic acid 5 mg daily
B. Organize leg venous Doppler scan
C. Check serum bile acids
D. Book a glucose tolerance test
E. Organize a chest X-ray
F. Check the peak expiratory flow rate
G. Document any known drug allergies
H. Start aspirin 75 mg daily
I. Check the body mass index
J. Arrange urgent investigations including coagulation screen and glucose level

For each scenario described below, choose the single most appropriate management plan from the list of options given above. Each option may be used once, more than once, or not at all.

1. A 32-year-old patient is referred to the obstetrician at 16 weeks' gestation because of a history of previous gestational diabetes.
2. A 25-year-old woman with a 10-year history of epilepsy sees her GP because she is planning to stop the oral contraceptive pill.
3. A primiparous patient presents to the labour ward at 34 weeks' gestation with a 24-hour history of nausea, vomiting and abdominal pain.
4. A 40-year-old multiparous woman with a BMI of 38 at booking attends A&E at 18 weeks gestation with a 48-hour history of breathlessness and chest pain.
5. A 38-year-old woman with diabetes is planning her first pregnancy. Her blood sugar levels are well controlled and she has a family history of hypertension.

21. Antenatal care:

- **A.** Serum ferritin, vitamin B12 and folate
- **B.** Glucose tolerance test
- **C.** Hepatitis B, C and HIV test
- **D.** Varicella zoster IgG
- **E.** Detailed cardiac ultrasound
- **F.** Amniocentesis
- **G.** Chorionic villous sampling (CVS)
- **H.** Routine booking investigations
- **I.** Toxoplasmosis IgG
- **J.** Varicella zoster IgM

For each scenario described below, choose the single most appropriate investigations from the list of options given above. Each option may be used once, more than once, or not at all.

1. A 21-year-old who works as a nursery nurse presents for antenatal booking at 8 weeks and has never had chicken pox. She is currently clinically well.
2. A 43-year-old presents to antenatal clinic at 16 weeks to discuss her combined screening result which shows a risk of 1:90.
3. A 25-year-old with a history of intravenous drug use attends at 11 weeks for booking.
4. A 37-year-old solicitor in her first pregnancy attends for booking at 9 weeks, she has a normal body mass index and no past medical history of note.
5. A 32-year-old Indian lady with a body mass index of 36 and a strong family history of Type II diabetes.

22. Hypertension in pregnancy:

- **A.** Postural hypotension
- **B.** Epileptic seizure
- **C.** Eclampsia
- **D.** Pre-eclampsia
- **E.** Essential hypertension
- **F.** Pregnancy induced hypertension or gestational hypertension
- **G.** HELLP Syndrome (haemolysis, elevated liver enzymes and low platelets)
- **H.** Amniotic fluid embolism
- **I.** Hyperthyroidism
- **J.** Stroke

For each scenario described below, choose the single most likely diagnosis from the list of options given above. Each option may be used once, more than once, or not at all.

1. A 31-year-old patient presents at 8 weeks for a booking visit and is found to have blood pressure of 153/92.
2. A 41-year-old patient presents at 29 weeks with proteinuria and a blood pressure of 168/103.
3. A 22-year-old patient presents at 38 weeks with a blood pressure of 144/96 with no proteinuria and no symptoms.
4. A 29-year-old patient who is 35 weeks pregnant presents with ALT of 213, platelets of 76 with a blood pressure of 180/110 complaining of a headache and epigastric pain.
5. An 18-year-old patient who is 33 weeks pregnant is brought in by ambulance fitting with a blood pressure of 205/120.
6. A 23-year-old epileptic who is in labour has a blood pressure of 132/84 has a seizure whilst pushing.

23. Medical disorders in pregnancy:

- **A.** Echocardiogram
- **B.** Antenatal and postnatal low molecular weight heparin
- **C.** Liver function tests and bile acids
- **D.** Folic acid supplementation and detailed cardiac scan
- **E.** Haemoglobinopathy screen
- **F.** Glucose tolerance test
- **G.** Thyroid function tests
- **H.** Cardiotocography
- **I.** Amniocentesis
- **J.** Fetal blood sampling

For each scenario described below, choose the single most appropriate investigation from the list of options given above. Each option may be used once, more than once, or not at all.

1. A 28-year-old Bangladeshi patient presents after an ultrasound showing polyhydramnios, fetal macrosomia and has three +++ of glucose in her urine.
2. A 19-year-old epileptic patient attends at 12 weeks for a plan of care.
3. A 27-year-old attends at 12 weeks and has a family history of PE and had an unprovoked DVT 3 years ago.
4. A 39-year-old attends at 34 weeks with itchy palms and soles but no rash.
5. A 21-year-old patient from Cyprus attends after her booking visit and is found to have a haemoglobin level of 9.1 g/dl.

24. Maternal collapse:

A. Pulmonary embolism
B. Acute myocardial infarction
C. Amniotic fluid embolism
D. Anaphylactic shock
E. Postural hypotension
F. Placental abruption
G. Eclampsia
H. Hypovolaemic shock

For each scenario described below, choose the single most likely cause of collapse from the list of options given above. Each option may be used once, more than once, or not at all.

1. A 41-year-old smoker who is 34 weeks pregnant brought in by ambulance with fresh vaginal bleeding and a 'woody hard' uterus.
2. A 19 year old, who is being induced for prolonged rupture of membranes at 40 weeks, collapses 5 minutes after being given.
3. A 24-year-old who had a caesarean section 3 hours ago for failure to progress is found collapse in her bed with a large pool of blood between her legs and a boggy uterus.
4. A 26-year-old who is in labour collapses just after delivery and is noted to be hypoxic and hypotensive, she then begins to bleed heavily and is found to have a raised INR 2.5.
5. A 36-year-old Sri Lankan patient who is in labour collapses after complaining of central chest pain which radiates to her jaw. She has a BMI of 41 and has gestational diabetes.

25. Maternal death:

A. Sepsis
B. Pulmonary embolism
C. Ruptured ectopic pregnancy
D. Postpartum haemorrhage
E. Puerperal psychosis
F. Intracranial haemorrhage
G. Amniotic fluid embolism
H. Acute myocardial infarction

For each scenario described below, choose the single most likely cause of death from the list of options given above. Each option may be used once, more than once, or not at all.

1. A 17-year-old girl who is around 6 weeks pregnant is seen by her GP complaining of lower abdominal pain and diarrhoea. She is told this may be a viral illness and is sent home. Later she is brought in collapsed by ambulance with a distended abdomen and her urine sample is βHCG positive.
2. A 36-year-old patient attends A&E with a history of fevers and rigors 3 days after a normal vaginal delivery. She is tachycardic and hypotensive and despite resuscitation has a cardiac arrest.
3. A 36-year-old patient who is 34 weeks pregnant collapses in clinic and is unresponsive. Her blood pressure prior to the collapse was 192/104 and she was complaining of a headache. She is rapidly intubated and an urgent CT scan shows a large left sided intracranial bleed with midline shift.
4. A 38-year-old patient who is 37 weeks pregnant is out walking her dog and complains to her husband of severe right sided chest pain. He calls an ambulance but she rapidly declines and her lips turn blue. Despite the best attempts, the team is unable to resuscitate her.
5. A 34-year-old who delivered 12 days ago was found collapsed at home next to an empty container of paracetamol. She was noted to be acting strangely the day before by her neighbour, saying that she was a bad mother and everybody hates her.

26. Abnormal bleeding:

A. Pelvic inflammatory disease
B. Endometriosis
C. Candida
D. Cervical intraepithelial neoplasia
E. Endometrial polyp
F. Cervical carcinoma
G. Ectopic pregnancy
H. Hypothyroidism
I. Fibroids
J. Endometritis

For each scenario described below, choose the single most likely diagnosis from the list of options given above. Each option may be used once, more than once, or not at all.

1. A 32-year-old woman complains of increasingly painful and heavy periods. The onset of pain is a few days prior to the onset of the period and lasts for 1 week after the period.
2. A 55-year-old woman presents with a 6-month history of post coital bleeding. Her last smear was abnormal and colposcopy was recommended.
3. A 22-year-old woman presents with a 3-month history of pyrexia, lower abdominal pain and irregular vaginal

discharge. On examination she is found to have lower abdominal tenderness and a purulent vaginal discharge.
4. A 45-year-old woman presents with lower abdominal pain and heavy periods. On examination she is found to have a bulky uterus.
5. A 47-year-old woman gives a 6-month history of increasingly heavy periods. During this time, she has gained 10 kg and is becoming increasingly lethargic.

27. Urinary incontinence:

A. Multiple sclerosis
B. Urinary tract infection
C. Genuine stress incontinence
D. Idiopathic detrusor overactivity
E. Sensory urgency
F. Fibroids
G. Fistula
H. Bladder tumour
I. Prolapsed disc
J. Detrusor overactivity due to menopause

For each scenario described below, choose the single most likely diagnosis from the list of options given above. Each option may be used once, more than once, or not at all.

1. A 55-year-old multiparous woman presents with a 6-month history of loss of urine on coughing and bending. Urodynamic investigations show no evidence of detrusor instability.
2. A 26-year-old woman presents with a 5-day history of worsening urinary frequency, nocturia and dysuria. Urinary testing indicates the presence of leukocytes.
3. A 60-year-old woman presents with a 6-week history of urgency nocturia and urge incontinence.
4. A 30-year-old woman, 6 weeks postpartum and recently arrived from Somalia, gives a history of continually feeling damp 'down below'.
5. A 52-year-old woman presents with a 6-week history of hot flushes, sweats and vaginal dryness and urinary frequency.

28. Primary amenorrhoea:

A. Haematocolpos
B. Androgen insensitivity syndrome
C. Hypothalamic hypogonadism
D. Constitutional amenorrhoea
E. Late-onset congenital adrenal hyperplasia
F. Anorexia nervosa
G. Premature ovarian failure
H. Polycystic ovary syndrome
I. Pregnancy
J. Turner's syndrome

For each scenario described below, choose the single most likely diagnosis from the list of options given above. Each option may be used once, more than once, or not at all.

1. A 16-year-old presents with primary amenorrhoea. On examination she has hirsuitism, acne and a BMI of 36.
2. A 17-year-old presents with primary amenorrhoea. On examination she has short stature and an increased carrying angle.
3. A 16-year-old presents with primary amenorrhoea. She is training to be a ballerina and has a BMI of 16.
4. A 17-year-old presents with primary amenorrhoea. On examination she is obese, has male pattern balding and signs of virilism.
5. A 16-year-old presents with primary amenorrhoea. On examination she has normal secondary sexual characteristics, a BMI of 23 and a normal hormone profile.

29. Pruritus vulvae:

A. Candidal infection
B. Contact dermatitis
C. Lichen sclerosus
D. Carcinoma of the vulva
E. Herpetic lesion
F. Psoriasis
G. Vulval intraepithelial neoplasia
H. Enterobius
I. Trichomonas vaginalis
J. Bechets syndrome

For each scenario described below, choose the single most likely diagnosis from the list of options given above. Each option may be used once, more than once, or not at all.

1. A 65-year-old presents with pruritus vulvae. She has noticed a lump growing on the vulva for the last 6 months. Examination confirms an ulcerated, hard, raised lesion 1 cm in diameter.
2. A 16-year-old has recently become sexually active. She complains of intense pruritus vulvae associated with an offensive discharge with a fishy odour. On examination she has a marked vulvo-vaginitis and a frothy greenish vaginal discharge.
3. A 60-year-old presents with intermittent episodes of pruritus vulvae. On examination the labia have fused, the tissues are thin and leukoplakia is present.

4. A 35-year-old has developed pruritus vulvae since changing her soap and bubble bath. Examination reveals vulvitis with no discrete lesion visible.
5. A 42-year-old develops an itchy lesion of the left vulva. Examination reveals an erythematous plaque on the left labium majora and scaly plaques on her elbows.

30. Gynaecological definitions:

A. Postmenopausal bleeding
B. Menorrhagia
C. Total abdominal hysterectomy
D. Sub-total abdominal hysterectomy
E. Endometriosis
F. Threatened miscarriage
G. Inevitable miscarriage
H. Total abdominal hysterectomy and bilateral salpingo-oophorectomy
I. Intermenstrual bleeding
J. Pelvic inflammatory disease

For each scenario described below, choose the single most likely definition from the list of options given above. Each option may be used once, more than once, or not at all.

1. The loss of more than 80 mL blood per period
2. The surgical removal of the uterus and the cervix through via laparotomy
3. The presence of functioning endometrium outside the uterine cavity
4. Vaginal bleeding in pregnancy before 24 weeks' gestation
5. Vaginal bleeding occurring more than 1 year after the last period

31. Treatment of heavy periods:

A. Mefenamic acid
B. Tranexamic acid
C. Combined oral contraceptive pill
D. Mirena inter-uterine system
E. Endometrial ablation
F. Vaginal hysterectomy
G. Total abdominal hysterectomy
H. Sub-total abdominal hysterectomy
I. Total abdominal hysterectomy and bilateral salpingo-oophorectomy
J. Hysteroscopic myomectomy

For each scenario described below, choose the single most likely treatment from the list of options given above. Each option may be used once, more than once, or not at all.

1. A 49-year-old woman who is para 9 presents with heavy periods and a genital prolapse. Her GP has treated her with mefenamic acid with some improvement. The prolapse is interfering with her sex life. On examination she has a bulky uterus with desent and the cervix is protruding through the vaginal introitus.
2. A 24-year-old nulligravid woman presents with a short history of irregular heavy periods. She is otherwise fit and well with no significant family history. She has just started a new relationship and is currently using condoms as contraception. Examination is normal.
3. A 39-year-old woman has had a 6-year history of heavy periods. Tranexamic acid has not helped. She had a Mirena IUS fitted by the GP 6 months ago, but is still getting erratic and prolonged bleeding. She has a family history of thrombo-embolism and does not want any more children. Pelvic examinations normal.
4. A 41-year-old woman has a 10-month history of heavy periods associated with iron deficiency anaemia. Hysteroscopy reveals a 3 cm submucous fibroid.
5. A 48-year-old woman has had a long history of heavy periods. One year ago she underwent an endometrial ablation, which has not improved her periods significantly. She has a strong family history of ovarian cancer. Her uterus is enlarged to the equivalent of a 12 weeks' gestation.

32. Gynaecological investigations:

A. Pelvic ultrasound scan
B. Abdominal X-ray
C. Urodynamics investigation
D. Hysterosalpingogram
E. Hysteroscopy
F. Laparoscopy
G. Laparotomy
H. Hysterosonography
I. MRI scan
J. Lateral X-ray pelvimetry

For each scenario described below, choose the single most relevant investigation from the list of options given above. Each option may be used once, more than once, or not at all.

1. A woman is referred to the gynaecologist for removal of her IUCD. She reports that when it was inserted

she experienced a lot of pain. On examination the IUCD strings were not visible. An ultrasound scan of the pelvis showed no evidence of the IUCD in the uterine cavity.
2. A 63-year-old woman presents with postmenopausal bleeding. She is not taking HRT and clinical examination is normal.
3. A 23-year-old woman presents with a history of secondary dysmenorrhoea and deep dyspareunia. Clinical examination reveals pelvic tenderness and an ultrasound scan of the pelvis is normal.
4. A 55-year-old woman presents with frequency and urgency of micturition and having to get up at night many times. She also notices that she leaks urine if she coughs or sneezes or does not get to the lavatory quickly enough. A mid-stream specimen of urine is negative on culture.
5. A 35-year-old woman and her husband present with 2 years' subfertility. Semen analysis is normal and a day-21 progesterone suggests ovulation.

33. Secondary amenorrhoea:

A. Kallman's syndrome
B. Athleticism
C. Prolactinoma
D. Sheehan's syndrome
E. Polycystic ovary syndrome
F. Radiotherapy/chemotherapy
G. Ashermann's syndrome
H. Wertheim's hysterectomy
I. Diabetes mellitus
J. Turner's syndrome

For each scenario described below, choose the single most likely diagnosis from the list of options given above. Each option may be used once, more than once, or not at all.

1. A 35-year-old woman has not experienced a period since the delivery of her first child 9 months ago. During childbirth, she lost 2 L blood. She is not breastfeeding.
2. A 20-year-old gymnast has not experienced a period for 9 months, since starting to train fulltime.
3. A 38-year-old lady has not experienced a period for 1 year, following treatment for stage III ER positive breast cancer.
4. A 19-year-old student notices that her periods have become increasingly erratic following weight gained in her first year at university, and has noticed an increase in her peripheral hair distribution.
5. A 39-year-old woman notices headaches, a change in her peripheral vision when driving and milky nipple discharge. Pregnancy test is negative.

34. Treatment for gynaecological disorders:

A. Blood transfusion
B. Metronidazole
C. Corticosteroids
D. Tranexamic acid
E. Oral contraceptive pill
F. Endometrial ablation
G. Mirena coil
H. Myomectomy
I. Transcervical resection of fibroids
J. Total abdominal hysterectomy and bilateral salpingo-oophorectomy

For each scenario described below, choose the single most likely diagnosis from the list of options given above. Each option may be used once, more than once, or not at all.

1. A 40-year-old lady with known submucosal fibroids presents with a history of menorrhagia and a haemoglobin of 9.1. She is keen to get pregnant.
2. A 56-year-old lady is diagnosed to have lichen sclerosis and is requesting treatment to soothe her pruritus.
3. A 34-year-old woman complains of fishy-smelling vaginal discharge and is diagnosed to have bacterial vaginosis.
4. A 17-year-old lady with irregular heavy periods is keen to regulate her cycle.
5. A 37-year-old multiparous lady with severe endometriosis is admitted in pain. She has had multiple admissions for endometriosis-related pain and has completed her family. Hormonal treatment has previously been unsuccessful and she would like definitive treatment for her endometriosis.

35. Initial management:

A. Resuscitation
B. FBC
C. High vaginal swab
D. Pregnancy test
E. Mid-stream urine
F. LH:FSH ratio
G. Transvaginal ultrasound
H. Pipelle biopsy
I. Laparoscopy
J. Laparotomy

For each scenario described below, choose the single most relevant management plan from the list of options given above. Each option may be used once, more than once, or not at all.

1. A 24-year-old woman complains of weight gain over the last 5 months with intermittent lower abdominal pain. She cannot remember the exact date of her last period.
2. A 19-year-old woman presents with a history of irregular periods and hirsutism. Her BMI is 33.
3. A 64-year-old woman presents to Accident and Emergency with a history of a heavy menstrual bleed. She is not on hormone replacement therapy and underwent the menopause at the age of 55.
4. A 32-year-old woman presents with severe abdominal pain with some vaginal bleeding. Her heart rate is 108 bpm and blood pressure is 70/40. She is lying flat and unable to move because of the pain. Pregnancy test is positive.
5. A 37-year-old woman presents with a two year history of deep dyspareunia. She has not changed her partner and a STI screen has been reported as normal. She has previously been treated for chlamydia and has had two caesarean sections.

---

36. Early pregnancy complications:

A. Inevitable miscarriage
B. Molar pregnancy
C. Ectopic pregnancy
D. Retained products of conception
E. Recurrent miscarriage
F. Heterotopic pregnancy
G. Possible normal pregnancy
H. Septic miscarriage
I. Threatened miscarriage
J. Complete miscarriage
K. Hyperemesis gravidarum

For each scenario described below, choose the single most likely diagnosis from the list of options given above. Each option may be used once, more than once, or not at all.

1. A 40-year-old executive has conceived with IVF and is currently 10 weeks gestation. She has been referred by her GP complaining of a 2 week history of feeling unwell, lethargic and dizzy. The GP referral letter mentions significant 'ketonuria'. You see her in the Accident and Emergency and she explains that her GP had been giving her oral medication but now is unable to tolerate this. On your assessment, she is mildly tachycardic (pulse 104 beats/min), has reduced skin turgor and some epigastric tenderness. An ultrasound scan shows 2 fetal heartbeats.
2. Miss M, a mother of 2 children, is 9 weeks pregnant and complaining of a 2 day history of heavy PVB and suprapubic pain. She had a scan 1 week ago and a fetal heartbeat was seen. Her observations are stable. She is afebrile, mildly tachycardic and anxious. The bleeding has now settled and the cervical Os is closed. Urinanalysis shows haematuria and a positive pregnancy test. An ultrasound scan showed multiple 'hyperechoeic areas' within the endometrium.
3. A 37 year old woman presents with vaginal bleeding at 7 weeks, 3 days' gestation. This is her first pregnancy. She noticed bright red par vaginum (PV) spotting for the last 5 days. She has also been complaining of excessive vomiting, struggling to keep food or fluids down. On examination her abdomen is soft and non-tender. Speculum reveals a normal closed cervix with a small amount of fresh blood in the posterior fornix. Bimanually the uterus feel bulky and soft, approximately 14 weeks size. There is no cervical excitation or adenexal tenderness or masses. BP 110/70mmHg, Pulse=72/min. TV USS shows 'bunches of grapes' appearance.
4. A 21 year old woman presents to the A&E department with a 4 hour history of abdominal pain, initially in the lower abdomen but now generalized. She feels nauseous, dizzy and constipated. She has not had any vaginal bleeding or discharge. She was treated for Chlamydia 2 years ago which was diagnosed when she attended for a surgical termination of pregnancy. She cannot recall her LMP – she thinks it was 5 weeks ago. She has a positive pregnancy test today. BP 94/52mmHg, Pulse 120 b/min. On examination, her abdomen is rigid with guarding and generalized rebound tenderness. She is pale, clammy and looks unwell.
5. Miss Smith is 13 weeks gestation and has presented to the accident and emergency department with a 2 day history of lower abdominal pain, diarrhoea, vomiting and offensive, brownish PV discharge. She is a single mother with a 4 year old son who is recovering from tonsillitis. She is febrile and tachycardic. She has uterine tenderness on palpation and USS shows no FH.

---

37. Contraception, sterilization and unplanned pregnancy:

A. Combined oral contraception
B. Mirena
C. Progestogen only pill

D. Male condoms
E. Copper IUCD
F. Essure
G. Depot provera
H. Implanon
I. Laparoscopic sterilization
J. Postcoital contraception (emergency contraception)

For each scenario described below, choose the most appropriate contraception choice from the list of options given above. Each option may be used once, more than once, or not at all.

1. A 31-year-old woman had a spontaneous delivery of her sixth child 2 days ago. She is breast feeding and would like an effective form of contraception as soon as possible. Her body mass index (BMI) is 29.5 kg/m^2
2. A 19-year-old woman attends the family planning clinic for contraception. She has had three surgical terminations of unwanted pregnancies due to missing the oral contraceptive pill and was unable to tolerate the Mirena coil. She is in a steady relationship.
3. A divorced 48-year-old woman has just started a new relationship and wants to use a long-acting reversible contraception. She is needle phobic, does not like taking pills and hates the idea of 'putting hormones in her body'.
4. A 36-year-old mother of 5 children is requesting contraception. Her youngest child is 18 months. She is certain that she has completed her family and has tried various forms of long-acting contraceptives to no avail and now just 'wants this sorted out once and for all'. She has known endometriosis but is otherwise fit and well. Her partner will not consider a vasectomy. Her BMI is 32.
5. A 28-year-old, nulliparous woman who suffers migraines and has a raised BMI (44) is requesting contraception. She wants to take the combined oral contraceptive pill.

38. Urogynaecology:

A. Sacral colpopexy
B. Vaginal hysterectomy
C. Sacrospinous fixation
D. Anterior colporrhaphy
E. McCall culdoplasty
F. Anterior and posterior repair
G. Manchester repair (Fothergill procedure)
H. Posterior repair with mesh
I. Vaginal hysterectomy with posterior repair
J. Ring/shelf pessary
K. Pelvic floor exercises (physiotherapy)

For each scenario described below, choose the single most appropriate management of genital prolapse from the list of options given above. Each option may be used once, more than once, or not at all.

1. An 82-year-old woman complains of a dragging sensation in the lower abdomen and lower back when standing and walking. She has chronic constipation and can feel a lump in the vagina. She has had five vaginal deliveries and used HRT for 5 years to treat menopausal symptoms. On examination, the cervix is at the level of the introitus and there is a large rectocele and minimal anterior wall descent.
2. A 25-year-old woman is 3 months postnatal following a spontaneous vaginal delivery of her daughter who was 4.3kg. She was complaining of 'feeling a lump coming down' prior to the pregnancy and this sensation has got worse. On examination, there is evidence of a mild (grade 1) cystocele. She is planning more pregnancies in the future but is worried that the prolapse will get worse. What do you advise?
3. A 56-year-old woman attends urogynaecology clinic complaining of voiding dysfunction and prolapse symptoms. She is para 4, having had spontaneous vaginal deliveries. All her children had birthweights between 4-4.4kg. She has a BMI of 38 and is chronically constipated. She has noticed worsening symptoms of double micturition and 'dragging' sensation. Her symptoms are disrupting her quality of life and she wants definitive management, pelvic floor exercises are not effective. On examination she has a grade 3 cystocele.
4. A 76-year-old widow is complaining of a feeling of 'something coming down'. She wants to avoid surgery, as she has chronic respiratory disease, COPD. She is not sexually active.
5. A 51-year-old woman with a previous history of rectocele is complaining of a sensation of a lump in the vagina and difficulty opening her bowels. She explained that she has notice a lump in the vagina and she sometimes has to reduce this lump digitally to enable effective bowel motion. On examination, a recurrence of the rectocele that was previously treated was noted. What will you offer her?

39. Pelvic pain and dyspareunia:

A. Adenomyosis
B. Bacterial vaginosis

C. Candida infection
D. Cervical cancer
E. Endometriosis
F. Urinary tract infection
G. Chlamydia
H. Gonococcal infection
I. Cervical ectopy

For each scenario described below, choose the single most likely diagnosis from the list of options given above. Each option may be used once, more than once, or not at all.

1. A 37-year-old woman presents with deep dyspareunia, menorrhagia and dysmenorrhoea. The uterus is fixed and tender on bimanual examination. At laparoscopy, 'powder burn' areas were seen in the pouch of Douglas.
2. At laparoscopy on a 24-year-old woman with pelvic pain and dyspareunia, adhesions around the liver are seen.
3. A 38-year-old woman, para 3+1, presents with secondary dysmenorrhoea. She reports increase in pelvic pain mid-cycle with climax at the onset of menses. She also complains of lower back 'dragging' pain. On examination she has a bulky, anteverted mobile uterus with a doughy consistency. No discrete masses can be felt. Pelvic ultrasound scan confirms the diagnosis.
4. A 26-year-old diabetic woman complains of 2 week history superficial dyspareunia. She has noticed that this has been associated with increasing amounts of PV discharge and itching. She has just recovered from a chest infection for which she was on antibiotics. On speculum examination there is a copious amount of thick vaginal discharge with a 'cottage cheese' consistency.
5. A 31-year-old woman, 19 weeks pregnant, presents to her GP with a 3 day history of pelvic pain. On direct questioning she has noticed increased urinary frequency which she attributed to the pregnancy and dysuria. No PV bleeding or constitutional symptoms. Urine analysis is nitrate positive and showed some haematuria.

40. Vaginal discharge:

A. Bacterial vaginosis
B. Candida albicans
C. Trichomonas vaginalis
D. Chlamydia trachomatis
E. Neisseria gonorrhoea
F. Cervical carcinoma
G. Retained tampon

For each scenario described below, choose the single most likely diagnosis from the list of options given above. Each option may be used once, more than once, or not at all.

1. A 20-year-old woman who is 8 weeks pregnant presents with a 2 week history of fishy smelling PV discharge. It is non-itchy and creamy coloured. She has had previous episodes outside of pregnancy which resolved spontaneously. She is in a monogamous relationship with the same partner for 5 years. On speculum examination there is a small amount of smooth grey discharge seen coating the vaginal walls.
2. A 14-year-old girl presented to the accident and emergency department with her mother. She has been feeling unwell with abdominal pain, high temperature, rigors, nausea and vomiting and an offensive PV discharge. She has been busy and stressed with exams at school. Her period started 4 days ago and she has been using tampons.
3. A 35-year-old lady has been referred from her GP to colposcopy clinic. She has recently arrived in the UK from Sub-Saharan Africa and the GP is concerned that she has never had a smear and has been complaining of an offensive blood stained PV discharge. On speculum examination there is a fungating, bleeding cervical mass that was biopsied.
4. A 26-year old woman presents to Gynaecology Clinic with a history of postcoital PVB mixed with discharge. She is up to date with her cervical smears which have been normal. She is in a new relationship and is using the COCP for contraception. She recalls feeling unwell 3 days ago with right upper quadrant discomfort which has now resolved. Speculum examination showed an inflamed 'strawberry appearance' of cervix, consistent with cervicitis. An endocervical swab was taken.
5. A 6-year-old girl is seen in GOPD with her parents. She has been having persistent vaginal discharge on her underwear and the GP has not found a cause. An abdominal ultrasound scan has been unremarkable. She is an only child and has a good relationship with both her parents and is especially close to her mother who she wants to be like 'when she grows up'. There is no suspicion of abuse. The parents comment that she is usually very talkative and inquisitive and likes exploring around the house. However, she recently has not been herself and appears to be in intermittent discomfort in the suprapubic region. She has been booked on an elective list for an examination under anaesthetic.

SBA answers

1. C. Patients should only take HRT if clinically indicated.
2. D. Transdermal patches provide both oestrogen and progesterone.
3. D. Clonidine is a useful second line agent for hot flushes.
4. B. 84% of couples will conceive within one year if the woman is under 40 years old and they have regular unprotected sexual intercourse.
5. E. Varicose veins of the legs do not affect fertility.
6. C. It is important to exclude infections such as Chlamydia, which can lead to secondary infertility.
7. E. Endometriosis may increase CA125 levels, and most commonly affects the ovaries, pouch of douglas, uterosacral ligaments and ovarian fossae. However, it does not increase the risk of cervical cancer.
8. D. RMI is calculated by multiplying the CA125 level by menopausal status and ultrasound score.
9. C. Hysteroscopy and Biopsy is important to visualise the endometrial cavity and obtain a tissue sample to exclude endometrial cancer.
10. C. All the other options are not specific to endometriosis. Nodular deposits in the posterior fornix are highly suggestive of endometriosis and should be sought at speculum examination and digital vaginal examination within the context of a consistent clinical history.
11. C. All the other options are recognized features of several differential diagnoses, e.g. PCOS, PID. Cyclical pelvic pain is unique to endometriosis, reflecting the hormonal influence of the menstrual cycle on disease activity.
12. E. Although all the other options have these symptoms, an ectopic pregnancy is relatively more common and a life-threatening condition that must be ruled out first. Always work on the assumption that all women of child-bearing age with pelvic pain have an ectopic pregnancy until proven otherwise. The presence of cervical excitation suggests peritonism, which makes the diagnosis most likely.
13. B. Cyclical pelvic pain is characteristic of endometriosis.
14. D. It is essential to rule out ectopic pregnancy in the first instance in a woman of child-bearing age with an acute abdomen. Other possible gynaecological differentials include miscarriage, sepsis or cyst accident/haemorrhage.
15. A. Risk of malignancy index is an important tool used to triage women with ovarian cysts to the most appropriate place for further investigation and management.
16. C. Brenner tumours can secrete oestrogen, causing irregular vaginal bleeding.
17. E. All the other options are not specific to malignancy and may be seen in cases of sepsis. Cachexia is more specific to malignancy and other catabolic states.
18. B. An ectropian is not pathological. It is simply an extension of endocervical columnar epithelium, which bleeds easily, onto the ectocervix and is common in pregnancy due to the influence of oestrogen. No treatment is necessary unless a co-existing infection is proven.
19. B. The thick, white discharge of Candida infection has a typical appearance of 'cottage cheese' noted on speculum examination. It is treated easily with Clotrimazole pessary or cream.
20. E. A detailed sexual history is imperative to exclude sexually transmitted infections.
21. D. Most common organisms held responsible for PID are Chlamydia and Gonorrhoea neisseria, both sexually transmitted infections. Hence any history of previous STI would predispose a patient to PID.
22. C. This describes Bacterial vaginosis, which is treated with a course of antibiotics (metronidazole).
23. D. Although described as a gold standard investigation for making the diagnosis of PID – it is not the first-line investigation in view of surgical risks. There are less invasive, effective alternatives available as listed above. The aim should be to effectively diagnose and treat PID without going into the operating theatre, unless it is absolutely necessary, e.g. diagnosis not clearly defined (possibility of ectopic pregnancy/appendicitis), clinical condition deteriorating, failed initial medical management.
24. C. Vulval pruritis is not characteristically associated with PID.
25. C. Diarrhoea is not a recognized risk factor for genital prolapse. Constipation is. Options B & E cause prolonged periods of raised intra abdominal pressure hence risk of prolapse. Options A & D cause laxity in the pelvic floor supporting the pelvic organs.
26. D. Vaginal pessaries can be used as definitive management or as a temporary measure by patients on an elective waiting list for surgery. They can remain in situ for up to 6 months before they need to be changed.
27. E. None of the other options indicate deficiency in the posterior vaginal wall. Management will depend on the severity and impact on the patient's

quality of life, as well as patient's choice. Sometimes reassurance and a good explanation of this benign condition is all that is required.

28. A. Patients will often present with urinary symptoms in association with the prolapse. These can include voiding difficulty and recurrent UTIs.
29. B. The IUCD is the ideal form of emergency contraception here, as it not only prevents a third unplanned pregnancy, but also can remain in situ as an effective contraception for a further 5 years. It can be inserted upto 120 hours (5 days) after the earliest episode of unprotected sexual intercourse.
30. D. This is the best option for a woman in stable relationship who specifically wants to avoid hormonal contraception. Trained practitioners are required to insert the coil. Since she has never been pregnant, a narrow cervical canal may impede the smooth transit of the copper coil into the uterus causing some discomfort and requiring local anaesthetic.
31. C. Interestingly this is the same risk quoted when counselling women who want to use Levonorgestrel (Mirena). IUS which avoids surgery altogether and has the added advantage of being reversible and making menstrual periods lighter.
32. E. It is vitally important that a detailed history and pregnancy test is taken prior to commencing any contraception.
33. B. Molar pregnancy is a histological diagnosis.
34. E. PV bleeding in early pregnancy with a closed cervix (threatened miscarriage) is managed conservatively. Cause is not known – there is some suggestion that undiagnosed marginal placental bleeds are responsible.
35. D. History of late miscarriages, previous (repeat) cervical surgery are risk factors for cervical weakness. If there is a high clinical suspicion of cervical weakness patients can have serial cervical length measurements in pregnancy.
36. C. The progesterone-only pill is a recognized aetiological factor of ectopic pregnancy, not combined oral contraceptive pill.
37. B. A light source is essential to view the inside of the uterine cavity. Not all patients need to have an ultrasound before undergoing hysteroscopy. The media used to distend the uterine cavity include normal saline or glycine. Distilled water is not normally used. Outpatient hysteroscopy under local anaesthesia is possible. There is no need to catheterize – it does not facilitate insertion of telescope.
38. D. A pregnancy test must be performed prior to undertaking a laparoscopy or hysteroscopy. CO_2, rather than saline, is inserted into the peritoneal cavity to avoid injury to organs and facilitate view. The bladder must be emptied to avoid injury to the bladder, but an indwelling catheter is not indicated. Direct insertion of the trocar is possible by dissection under direct vision. A diathermy is not usually required for diagnostic laparoscopy.
39. C. Ultrasound gel to allow transmission of sound waves. A full bladder is only required for transabdominal ultrasound. Bowel preparation is not a usual requirement and the procedure does not usually cause discomfort. As ultrasound relies on sound waves and not light, a light source is not required.
40. A. Endometrial polyps can be diagnosed during a routine hysteroscopy. These have a typical polypoid appearance. By definition, endometriosis is aberrant uterine tissue lying outside of the uterine cavity and, therefore, will not be seen on hysteroscopy. Polycystic ovaries and the peritoneal fluid/pleural effusions and benign ovarian tumours of Meigs' syndrome cannot be seen via hysteroscopy. Submucous fibroids can be diagnosed via hysteroscopy, but subserous fibroids cannot.
41. A. A menstrual history is essential in a patient with abnormal bleeding. Coagulation studies should only be performed if a clotting disorder is suspected. Although useful in investigating intermenstrual and post-coital bleeding, a high vaginal swab is not clinically indicated in menorrhagia. Thyroid function tests are not an essential part of the routine work up for the investigation of abnormal periods unless other symptoms suggest a thyroid disorder. An abdominal X-ray is not usually required for investigation of abnormal genital tract bleeding. Caution should be exercised if one is ordered as the patient could be pregnant.
42. B. An ultrasound scan is the standard investigation for postmenopausal bleeding for endometrial thickness. Action is always required for postmenopausal bleeding. Hysteroscopy should only be performed if clinically indicated or if ultrasound reveals pathology. A full blood count is only indicated in a symptomatic patient or heavy bleeding. A pipelle sample of the endometrium is reassuring, but does not absolutely exclude malignancy.
43. B. A 3 cm submucosal fibroid may be the cause of due interference with implantation mechanism. Fibroids are not associated with hirsutism. They may press on the bladder leading to urinary frequency or stress incontinence, not detrusor instability. Subserous or large submucosal fibroids may cause deep vein thrombosis. Fibroids may cause menorrhagia, but are not associated with dysmenorrhoea.
44. C. Malpresentation can be due to obstruction by fibroid in the lower segment/cervix. There is no association between fibroids and pre-eclampsia. Both fibroids and pregnancy may cause urinary

frequency, but there is no association between fibroids and chorioamnionitis. Intrauterine growth restriction and pre-eclampsia are not recognized complications of fibroids.

45. A. The Pouch of Douglas is a common site common sites for endometriotic deposits. Fallopian tubes, femur, scars, lungs are all rare.

46. B. The combined oral contraceptive pill provides ovulation suppression plus continuous progestogenic activity. Ovarian drilling is a surgical intervention used to treat polycystic syndrome. Corticosteroids have no known benefits for endometriosis. Tranexamic acid is used to treat menorrhagia. There are no known benefits for antibiotics in treating endometriosis.

47. C. A thick creamy white discharge supports a diagnosis of infection, possibly candida. An acute onset, rather than progressively worsening symptoms over 6 months suggests infection. There is no association between menorrhagia and pruritus vulvae. Red plaques in the vulval areas suggest psoriasis or eczema. Fused labia suggest lichen sclerosis.

48. B. CIN is often associated with VIN. Antibiotics should only be prescribed where infection is found. Women should be referred to colposcopy only where clinically indicated. Surgical intervention is not common practice. Abdominal X-ray is not a usual part of the routine work-up for pruritus vulvae.

49. B. Biopsy of vulva for histological diagnosis. CRP does not identify a cause, but provides a marker for infective causes only. Ultrasound is not commonly used to investigate vulval disease; CT and MRI are more sensitive when considering vulval malignancy. Hysteroscopy alone does not identify vulval pathology, but an examination under anaesthetic may. Endocervical swabs will exclude endocervical infection only.

50. B. The epidermis is usually thin and hyalinized. Lichen sclerosis can appear as white or reddish plaques. A skin biopsy is mandatory to exclude malignant change. 50% of symptoms of pruritus vulvae can recur following surgical excision. A long course of steroids is often required.

51. D. A midstream urine sample will exclude a urinary tract infection as the cause of the urinary symptoms. The diagnosis of genuine stress incontinence can be made only in the absence of detrusor overactivity on urodynamic investigation. An obstetric history indicating traumatic deliveries of large infants would support a diagnosis of genuine stress incontinence. Occasionally, stress incontinence can be due to pressure from a large pelvic tumour, e.g. fibroid, ovarian cyst, but this may not always be the case. Urodynamic studies are essential to exclude detrusor overactivity as a cause for the symptoms.

52. A. A neurological examination is important to exclude causes such as multiple sclerosis. In this age group the likely diagnosis is sensory urgency where DO is absent. It is unlikely that a pelvic abnormality will be found. A midstream urine will exclude a urinary tract infection as the cause of the symptoms. Genital prolapse is unlikely to be found in this scenario.

53. A. Pelvic floor exercises improve the tone of pelvic floor muscles to prevent loss of urine. Anticholinergics are indicated for detrusor instability to prevent involuntary muscle contraction. Bladder drills are used to treat detrusor instability. Tension free vaginal tape may be used in women who have completed their families. Antibiotics are only helpful for detrusor instability caused by a urinary tract infection.

54. B. Antimuscarinics to relax the detrusor muscle. Pelvic floor exercises are used to treat GSI. Colposuspension is indicated for GSI. Treating urine tract infections may improve detrusor instability, but pelvic infections do not affect detrusor instability. A myomectomy is performed to remove fibroids. This may help relieve stress incontinence.

55. A. Congenital adrenal hyperplasia due to adrenal hyperandrogenism. Hyperprolactinaemia causes amenorrhoea. Hypothyroidism, Turner's syndrome and cystic fibrosis cause delayed puberty.

56. E. Most synthetic progestogens can have androgenic side effects due to stimulation of androgen receptors. H2 antagonists can cause gynaecomastia in men. Prednisolone, although a steroid, is not associated with hirsutism. The combination of oestrogen and progesterone in the combined oral contraceptive pill counteract the androgenic side effects of progesterone alone. There is no link at all with progestogens!

57. B. The genotype for testicular feminization is XY, therefore, by definition there is primary amenorrhoea. Fibroids cause menorrhagia. Premature ovarian failure can occur at this age, but it usually presents as secondary amenorrhoea. Polycystic ovary syndrome usually presents as secondary amenorrhoea. Lichen sclerosis is a vulval skin condition, which does not cause primary amenorrhoea.

58. C. A history of essential hypertension is the most important factor since this, in conjunction with a and b, increases the risk of developing pre-eclampsia.

59. D. There is currently no recommendation by the National Screening Committee to perform a high vaginal swab at booking. However, it is currently being considered, in order to diagnose Group B Streptococcus infection.

60. E. The husband's medical history is not relevant to his partner's risk of gestational diabetes.
61. E. Amniocentesis can be performed from 15 to approx 22 weeks, or possibly later in the pregnancy after 32 weeks. There is a 1% risk of miscarriage associated with the procedure.
62. D. A placental abruption classically presents with vaginal bleeding associated with abdominal pain. It can occur at any stage in pregnancy. It is associated with cigarette smoking and cocaine use.
63. C. The effect of increasing serum progesterone in pregnancy causes a slowing of gastrointestinal motility, commonly resulting in symptoms such as heartburn and constipation.
64. C. During pregnancy, the normal tube-like shape of the cervix everts to expose the columnar epithelium within the cervical canal. This type of epithelium is prone to bleeding from pressure during intercourse.
65. E. Placental abruption and vasa praevia are more commonly clinical diagnoses which necessitate urgent delivery rather than awaiting scans . A scan for placental location will diagnose placenta praevia and determine the grading, either major or minor.
66. E. Provided the course of the pregnancy antenatally and during delivery has been normal, meconium-stained liquor is the only indication given for continuous fetal monitoring. It can occur post-term or it can be associated with fetal hypoxia.
67. A. In the absence of contraindications such as maternal hepatitis or HIV infection, or prematurity, a fetal blood sample should be performed if fetal monitoring is diagnosed as pathological.
68. B. Strength of contractions is determined by palpation rather than electronic monitoring. The latter is can assess the frequency of contractions. The other answers are determined by vaginal examination.
69. D. Abduction of the mother's legs is usually necessary to allow delivery of the baby but this is not part of the mechanism that occurs with the maternal pelvis for delivery of the head.
70. A. It is not uncommon for uterine contractions to be inco-ordinate in a primiparous labour resulting in the need for augmentation with intravenous syntocinon.
71. D. With the possibility of a big baby secondary to gestational diabetes, the fetal head may not be engaged in the maternal pelvis until late in labour in this woman and therefore, there is a risk of cord prolapse at the time of amniotomy. If it occurs, it results in a fetal bradycardia.
72. B. External cephalic version is more likely to be successful in a multiparous patient since the maternal abdominal wall muscles are usually more relaxed.
73. C. Although a fetal chromosomal anomaly can be associated with low birth weight, the more common reason for being small for dates in an Asian woman is constitutional. The standard growth charts used in the UK are based on a Caucasian population.
74. E. TTTS complicates 15% of monochorionic twin pregnancies. Therefore scans should be performed every 2 weeks from 16 weeks. Stage 1 disease presents with discrepant liquor volumes.
75. A. Due to the larger placental site in a multiple pregnancy, postpartum haemorrhage is more common and therefore a prophylactic syntocinon infusion should be used for the third stage.
76. D. A 3rd degree tear involves the external anal sphincter and may also involve the internal anal sphincter. A 4th degree tear goes through to the anal mucosa.
77. E. Any intervention in labour, including amniotomy, has been shown to increase the risk of scar rupture. Answers a-c are all indicated, whilst d is optional depending on the woman's choice.
78. B. Although a-d are all part of the management plan, steroids should be given first since the woman already appears to be in labour.
79. C. Assessment of whether the widest diameter of the presenting part has entered the pelvic brim is essential in monitoring the progress of labour to vaginal delivery.
80. E. All answers a-e are important in assessing progress in labour, but station is the most important – even at full dilatation, vaginal delivery is not possible if the presenting part does not descend past the ischial spines.
81. B. The history and examination findings suggest that this patient may have pre-eclampsia. This must be urgently investigated further with liver function tests, a platelet count, clotting studies and urine protein quantification.
82. D. Labetalol is recommended by NICE guidelines as 1st line treatment for hypertension in pregnant non-asthmatic patients.
83. E. An international multicentre study (MAGPIE trial) recommended that magnesium sulphate should be used in the immediate management of an eclamptic seizure.
84. E. Older age, rather than younger age, is associated with an increased risk of venous thromboembolism in pregnancy.
85. A. These indices are generally agreed as appropriate normal values for these gestations.
86. C. These 3 factors have been proven to reduce HIV vertical transmission, although with an undetectable viral load, there is increasing evidence that vaginal delivery has a similar risk to caesarean section.

87. D. Folic acid 5 mg is recommended from pre-conception until 12 weeks gestation in order to reduce the incidence of neural tube defects. Overall, fetal anomalies are increased in patients with diabetes.
88. C. Vitamin K should be prescribed in the 3rd trimester of pregnancy, usually from 36 weeks gestation and should be advised for the neonate.
89. B. The history and the investigations, with the very high uric acid and hypoglycaemia, are in keeping with a diagnosis of acute fatty liver of pregnancy.
90. E. The history fits with a diagnosis of puerperal psychosis. Treatment should involve admission to a mother and baby unit and antipsychotic medication.
91. C. Although all the options are required to manage postpartum haemorrhage, the first, most important step is to ensure that the woman's airway (A), breathing (B) and circulation(C) are intact and maintained. Make sure you are well acquainted the ABC of basic resuscitation - the essential first response in every emergency situation.
92. A. Maintain a high index of clinical suspicion for secondary PPH if a woman presents several weeks postpartum with heavy PV bleeding. Causes include retained products of conception, endometritis and molar pregnancy or choriocarcinoma.
93. E. The history is in keeping with uterine atony with the risk factors including a fibroid uterus, prolonged labour and a large baby. This primary postpartum haemorrhage needs urgent treatment to improve the uterine contractility.
94. E. The key to diagnosis in this patient is the history of her unwell son – the patient should have a throat swab sent to exclude Group A streptococcus infection and appropriate antibiotics.
95. C. The history, in conjunction with the positive pregnancy test, are strongly suggestive of an ectopic pregnancy. The patient must be resuscitated and taken to theatre urgently as this may have ruptured requiring urgent salpingectomy.
96. B. The history and examination indicate a likely placental abruption. The examination suggest severe internal bleeding - the patient needs resuscitation and urgent transfer to theatre for caesarean section.
97. C. The patient is likely to be having an eclamptic seizure. She needs urgent stabilisation when help arrives.
98. C. The leading cause of direct maternal death in 2006-08 was sepsis, in contrast to previous reports which showed thromboembolic disease.
99. D. Cardiac disease, a combination of congenital and acquired, was the leading cause of indirect maternal death.
100. B. The CMACE report 2006-08 highlighted maternal deaths in the pueperium from Group A Streptococcus, and clinicians should be viligant especially with a history of illness such as a sore throat in the patient's other children.

EMQ answers

1.

1. D Placenta praevia.
2. B Vasa praevia.
3. A Molar pregnancy.
4. E Placental abruption.
5. F Cervical ectropion.

2.

1. D Placental abruption.
2. H Urinary tract infection.
3. J Labour.
4. A Fibroid degeneration.
5. G Pre-eclampsia.

3.

1. G A normal karyotype is 46XX or 46XY. This analysis shows 47XY, indicating that the fetus is male and has an extra chromosome – trisomy 21 is seen in Down's syndrome.
2. F Proteinuria of greater than 0.3 g/L is significant and can point to a diagnosis of pre-eclampsia.
3. D Parvovirus infection can pass across the placenta and cause fetal anaemia, leading to cardiac failure and fetal death. Positive IgM and negative IgG confirms recent infection.
4. A Transaminases are often raised in cholestasis, as are bile acids. However, the levels of liver function tests alone do not make the diagnosis, which must also be based on the clinical picture and the absence of hepatitis.
5. C Rhesus disease causes fetal haemolysis, and therefore anaemia. Coombs test proves the presence of antibodies.
6. B This level of glycosylated haemoglobin indicates poor control, which predisposes to congenital anomalies and intrauterine death.

4.

1. D Fetal macrosomia.
2. E Irregular contractions.
3. A Cervical fibroid.
4. I Transverse lie.
5. J Brow presentation.

5.

1. A A long labour, the need for syntocinon augmentation and a big baby all predispose to poor uterine contraction after delivery leading to post-partum haemorrhage.
2. C This multipara is predisposed to anaemia, which will have been exacerbated by her blood loss at caesarean section. The standing up has led to her fainting.
3. E Pregnancy, obesity and immobility are all risk factors for thromboembolic disease.
4. H This woman has developed chorioamnionitis, with infection ascending up and around the baby, producing a systemic illness. She needs antibiotic treatment and delivery.
5. G Hypertension and proteinuria raise suspicion of pre-eclampsia, which can rapidly deteriorate into an eclamptic episode. Fits in pregnancy, even in those previously labeled epileptic, should always be suspected of being related to pre-eclampsia.

6.

1. C Position of the presenting part of the fetus.
2. H Antepartum haemorrhage.
3. G Maternal mortality rate.
4. I Labour.
5. D Station of the presenting part of the fetus.

7.

1. B Pre-eclampsia.
2. D Essential hypertension.
3. C Hypertension secondary to renal disease.
4. E Essential hypertension with superimposed pre-eclampsia.
5. J HELPP syndrome.

8.

1. I Pulmonary embolism.
2. C Uterine rupture.
3. A Placental abruption.
4. E Eclampsia.
5. H Puerperal septic shock.

9.

1. D Fetal scalp electrode.
2. E Fetal blood sample.

3. G Artificial rupture of membranes.
4. B Lower segment caesarean section.
5. A Ventouse delivery.

10.

1. F Ruptured uterus.
2. H Shoulder dystocia.
3. E Cord prolapse
4. C Placental abruption
5. G Uterine hyperstimulation.

11.

1. C Membrane sweep.
2. D Speculum examination.
3. I External cephalic version.
4. F Amniocentesis.
5. A Umbilical artery Dopplers.

12.

1. J Deep vein thrombosis.
2. B Gestational diabetes.
3. A Obstetric cholestasis.
4. G Pyelonephritis.
5. H Preterm labour.

13.

1. E Postpartum haemorrhage.
2. B Postnatal depression.
3. A Puerperal psychosis.
4. C Endometritis.
5. I Dural puncture headache.

14.

1. D Third degree tear.
2. E Uterine atony.
3. I Placenta accreta.
4. A Primary PPH.
5. J Uterine inversion.

15.

1. F Renal agenesis.
2. A Gestational diabetes.
3. D Twin pregnancy.
4. C Placental insuffiency.
5. G Uterine fibroid.

16.

1. B Chorionicity.
2. G Multiple fetal pregnancy reduction.
3. J Twin-to-twin transfusion syndrome.
4. A Consultant-led hospital care.
5. D Intra-uterine growth restriction.

17.

1. A Serum electrophoresis.
2. F Glycosylated haemoglobin.
3. C Rubella.
4. H HIV.
5. I Hepatitis C.

18.

1. H Anterior fontanelle.
2. G Bishops score.
3. F Linea nigra.
4. B Body mass index.
5. E Sagittal suture.

19.

1. E Fetal tachycardia.
2. F Malpresentation.
3. G Malposition.
4. J Moulding.
5. H Variability.

20.

1. D Book a glucose tolerance test.
2. A Take folic acid 5 mg daily.
3. J Arrange urgent investigations including coagulation screen and glucose level.
4. E Organize a chest X-ray.
5. H Start aspirin 75 mg daily.

21.

1. D Varicella zoster IgG.
2. F Amniocentesis
3. C Hepatitis B, C and HIV test.
4. H Routine booking investigations.
5. B Glucose tolerance test.

22.

1. E Essential hypertension.
2. D Pre-eclampsia.
3. F Pregnancy induced hypertension or gestational hypertension.

4. G HELLP Syndrome (haemolysis, elevated liver enzymes and low platelets).
5. C Eclampsia.
6. B Epileptic seizure.

23.

1. F Glucose tolerance test.
2. D Folic acid supplementation and detailed cardiac scan.
3. B Antenatal and postnatal low molecular weight heparin.
4. C Liver function tests and bile acids.
5. E Haemoglobinopathy screen.

24.

1. F Placental abruption.
2. D Anaphylactic shock.
3. H Hypovolaemic shoc.
4. C Amniotic fluid embolism.
5. B Acute myocardial infarction

25.

1. C Ruptured ectopic pregnancy.
2. A Sepsis.
3. F Intracranial haemorrhage.
4. B Pulmonary embolism.
5. E Puerperal psychosis.

26.

1. B One of the classic ways in which endometriosis presents is with increasingly heavy and painful periods. The pain typically commences before the period and/or lasts for a few days after the period (secondary dysmenorrhoea).
2. F Cervical carcinoma typically presents with painless post-coital bleeding and is particularly likely in this age group.
3. A Lower abdominal pain and tenderness (typically bilateral) associated with a temperature and vaginal discharge are commonly due to PID.
4. I A bulky uterus in this age group associated with heavy periods is often due to uterine enlargement secondary to fibroids.
5. H This must not be forgotten as a possible medical cause of menorrhagia, particularly in the perimenopausal era. Two of the commonest symptoms are increasing tiredness and weight gain.

27.

1. C It is essential that urodynamic investigations have been performed to exclude detrusor overactivity as a cause of incontinence during laughing, sneezing, etc.
2. B Symptoms of frequency, dysuria and nocturia are often due to a urinary tract infection and this diagnosis is supported by presence of protein in the urine.
3. D Symptoms of urgency, nocturia and urge incontinence in this age group are often due to detrusor overactivity – the diagnosis should be confirmed with urodynamics.
4. G This is a recognized complication of prolonged obstructed labour and leads to continuous incontinence due to the presence of a urinary fistula, often connecting to the vagina. It is a particular problem in Somalia where women often have to walk miles to reach the nearest hospital.
5. J Detrusor overactivity (DO) symptoms are common in the menopause due to deterioration of the collagen in the urethra and bladder from oestrogen deficiency.

28.

1. H Polycystic ovary syndrome.
2. J Turner's syndrome.
3. C Hypothalamic hypogonadism.
4. E Late-onset congenital adrenal hyperplasia.
5. D Constitutional amenorrhoea.

29.

1. D Carcinoma of the vulva.
2. I Trichomonas vaginalis.
3. C Lichen sclerosus.
4. B Contact dermatitis.
5. F Psoriasis.

30.

1. B Menorrhagia.
2. C Total abdominal hysterectomy.
3. E Endometriosis.
4. F Threatened miscarriage.
5. A Postmenopausal bleeding.

31.

1. F Vaginal hysterectomy.
2. C Combined oral contraceptive pill.
3. E Endometrial ablation.
4. J Hysteroscopic myomectomy.
5. I Total abdominal hysterectomy and bilateral salpingo-oophorectomy.

32.

1. B Abdominal X-ray.
2. A Pelvic ultrasound scan.

3. F Laparoscopy.
4. C Urodynamics investigation.
5. D Hysterosalpingogram.

33.

1. D Sheehan's syndrome typically presents post-pregnancy and is associated with massive blood loss at the time of delivery.
2. B Athleticism and stress can induce amenorrhoea. This is reversible.
3. F Radiotherapy/chemotherapy can cause iatrogenic amenorrhoea. Therefore, all women of child-bearing age should be counselled on this prior to commencing treatment.
4. E Polycystic ovarian syndrome can cause irregular periods or secondary amenorrhoea. This can lead to endometrial hyperplasia in the long-term if untreated.
5. C Prolactinoma can cause tunnel vision, headaches and breast discharge.

34.

1. I Transcervical resection of fibroids treats the cause of her menorrhagia without affecting her ability to become pregnant.
2. C Low-dose steroids may be effective in treating lichen sclerosis.
3. B Metronidazole is used to treat bacterial vaginosis.
4. E The oral contraceptive pill allows cycle regulation as well as reducing menstrual blood loss.
5. J Total abdominal hysterectomy and bilateral salpingo-oophorectomy is the definitive treatment for severe and unremitting endometriosis in women who have tried medical treatment.

35.

1. D Given the history, it is important to exclude pregnancy.
2. F The diagnosis is likely to be PCOS, which can be diagnosed by a high LH:FSH ratio.
3. G If the endometrial thickness is 5 mm or more, an endometrial biopsy must be taken.
4. A The diagnosis is likely to be a ruptured ectopic pregnancy. As the patient is haemodynamically unstable, the first step is to resuscitate.
5. I Laparoscopy is the choice of investigation to exclude endometriosis or other causes of chronic pelvic pain such as adhesions or pelvic inflammatory disease.

36.

1. K Hyperemesis gravidarum. This typically presents in the first trimester and is commonly associated with multiple pregnancies. In this example, there is evidence of severe dehydration and gastritis secondary to the excessive vomiting.
2. D Retained products of conception. Although the history and findings are consistent with an incomplete miscarriage, this is not on the list of options. The scan findings give the diagnosis of retained products of conception.
3. B Molar Pregnancy. Molar pregnancy is a known cause of hyperemesis and a uterus which is large for dates. The ultrasound appearance is also characteristic of molar pregnancy.
4. C Ectopic Pregnancy. This lady is in clinical shock — most likely secondary to a ruptured ectopic pregnancy. She needs urgent transfer to theatre for life-saving surgery.
5. H Septic Miscarriage. The most likely causative agent is Group A Streptococcus which may have been transmitted from her son. The importance of hand hygiene BEFORE and after using the toilet can not be over emphasised, especially in pregnant women looking after young children.

37.

1. G Depot Provera. Depot provera is the most appropriate choice. It can be administered promptly by a healthcare professional. Other options H, I require specialist referral and training to be administered. Intrauterine options such as B, E, F are offered only after 6 weeks postpartum, when the uterus has involuted.
2. H Implanon. Implanon is the most appropriate choice of long-acting reversible contraception. This is preferable over the copper IUCD and Mirena as it avoids the risk of ascending uterine infection and subsequent pelvic inflammatory disease (PID).
3. E Copper IUCD. This lady is perimenopausal and so her fertility is reduced, thus increasing the effectiveness of a copper IUCD. This option will also solve the problem of her dislike of needles and hormonal options.
4. I Laparoscopic Sterilisation. This woman needs effective long-term, irreversible contraception. A Mirena IUS is not an option in this case as it may have been tried already and it does have the known issue of irregular unscheduled bleeding when initially inserted which would be difficult for a busy mother of 5 to deal with. A laparoscopic sterilisation would enable inspection of her endometriosis and treatment if needed, which Essure cannot do.
5. C Progesterone-only pill. It would not be safe to put this woman on the COCP, however since she is keen to take an oral hormonal contraceptive a progesterone only pill is a reasonable option.

38.

1. J Vaginal Hysterectomy with posterior repair. This lady has significant uterine descent and symptomatic of a large rectocele. She is otherwise fit and well and so could tolerate a surgical option which is potentially curative.
2. L Pelvic floor exercises (Physiotherapy). The cystocele is very mild and so in a young woman who is motivated, pelvic floor exercises are very effective. If the cystocele was more severe, pessaries may be an option. Surgery is not appropriate until her family is complete.
3. D Anterior Colporrhaphy. This would be the most appropriate option since her symptoms are now affecting her quality of life and her family is complete.
4. K Ring / Shelf Pessary. Ring and shelf pessaries can be inserted in clinic, thereby avoiding a general anaesthetic and an operation. However, patients should be reviewed regularly to make sure this continues to be effective treatment and that the pessary is not eroding through the vaginal wall.
5. I Posterior repair with mesh. A revision of prolapse repair is sometimes reinforced with a mesh. As there is no uterine descent she does not require a hysterectomy.

39.

1. F Endometriosis. These are characteristic signs and symptoms of endometriosis.
2. G Chlamydia. Peri-hepatic adhesions also known as Fitz-Hugh-Curtis syndrome, are a sign of previous Chlamydia infection.
3. A Adenomyosis. This condition typically affects older, parous women. The infiltration of endometrium into the myometrial layer causes the uterus to become enlarged, globular and have a distinct consistency often reported as 'doughy'.
4. C Candida Infection. Typically Candida occurs at times of immunosuppression such as pregnancy, steroid therapy or in women with medical conditions such as diabetes. The normal vaginal flora can also be altered by antibiotic therapy causing over-growth of candida.
5. F Urinary Tract Infection. UTI is a cause of acute pelvic pain, particularly in pregnant women when it can be responsible for uterine tightenings.

40.

1. A Bacterial Vaginosis. Bacterial Vaginosis is not a sexually transmitted infection. There is a change in the natural flora of the vagina. Its clinical significance is that it has been linked to second trimester miscarriage.
2. H Toxic shock syndrome. This girl has been distracted with exams and has forgotten to change her tampon. Her symptoms and clinical signs are in keeping with toxic shock syndrome.
3. F Cervical Carcinoma. There is no cervical screening programme in this lady's country of origin. It would be prudent to check her HIV status which is a known risk factor for cervical cancer.
4. D Chlamydia trachomatis. The COCP does not protect against sexually transmitted infections.
5. I Foreign body. This is the most likely option in this scenario. Foreign body insertion into the vagina is not uncommon in this age group and should be suspected if child abuse has been ruled out.

Index

Note: Page numbers followed by *b* indicate boxes and *f* indicate figures.

A

D

E

F

K

L

M

N

O

P

T

U

V

W

X

Y

Z